Index

Note: Page numbers *in italics* indicate illustrations; those followed by *t* indicate tables.

A

Accommodation—*continued*
spasms
associated with organic disease, 1016
from pharmacologic agents, 1018
unassociated with organic disease, 1016–1018, *1017*
stability of, 911
stimulus to, 910
supranuclear control of, 909
testing techniques for, 949–952, *950, 951*
time characteristics of, 911
tonicity of, 951
weakness of, 5729
Accommodative amplitude, 948
Accommodative convergence, 912, 948
Accommodative fatigue, 951
Accumulation of granulocytes and macrophages, 3726
Acellular pertussis vaccines, 4210–4211
Acephalgic migraine, 3678–3680, *3679, 3680*
Acetanilid and headaches, 1718
Acetinobacter, 4104
in meningitis, 4104
Acetylcholine, 841, 1005
Acetylcholine receptor and neuromuscular junction, 1406, 1408
Acetylsalicylic acid, 3558
Achromatopsia, cerebral, 142
Achromobacter, 4245
Achromobacter xylosoxidans, 4245
Acidophil adenomas, 2152
Acidophilic pituitary adenomas, 2153
Acidosis
lactic, 366, 767
metabolic, 671, 673
Acoustic neuroma, 1655, 2308
Acoustic schwannomas, 1294
Acoustic-amnestic defect, 1831
Acquired accommodation paresis, 1012
Acquired alexia, 424, *425,* 437
with agraphia, 424, 431
without agraphia, 424
anatomy, pathology, and mechanisms of pure, *426, 427,* 427–428, *428, 429, 430, 431*
assessment, 436
associated signs of pure, 425
central dyslexias, 434–435
covert reading in pure, 425–427
disconnection, 428, 451
dyslexia related to abnormal vision, attention, or eye movement, 432–434, *434, 435*
functional imaging, 435–436
pure, 424–428
Acquired amnesia and aneurysmal rupture, 3024
Acquired gustolacrimal reflex, 1024–1025
following facial palsy or section of greater superficial petrosal nerve, 1025
Acquired Horner's syndrome in children, 971
Acquired immune deficiency syndrome (AIDS), 3012, 5375–5376, 5721. (*See also* Human immunodeficiency virus (HIV); Human immunodeficiency virus (HIV) infection.)
epidemiology, *5377,* 5377–5379, *5378*
history, 5376*t,* 5376–5377
and incidence of nonendemic Burkitt's lymphoma, 2375
optic neuritis in, 630
relationship between cytomegalovirus infection and, 5098
and retroviruses, 5361–5362, *5362, 5363*
and risk for developing Hodgkin's lymphoma, 2359
systemic manifestations of, 5374
Acquired myopathic ptosis, 1545–1546
Acquired ocular motor apraxia, 1324
Acquired oculomotor nerve palsy
evaluation and management of patients with, 1225–1227
recovery from, 1220
Acquired oculomotor synkinesis, 1220–1225, *1221, 1222, 1223, 1224*
Acquired pendular nystagmus, 1466–1468, *1467,* 1467*t,* 1496
with demyelinating disease, 1468
Acquired protein S deficiency, 3889
Acquired superior oblique tendon sheath syndrome, 3849
Acquired trochlear nerve palsy
differential diagnosis of, 1236
evaluation and management of, 1236–1237
recovery from, 1236
Acquisition phase, 450
Acrodermatitis chronica atrophicans, 4809
Acrodermatitis enteropathica, 674
Acromegaly, 2156–2160, *2157, 2159,* 2987
Acroparesthesias, 2158
Actinobacillus, 4193
Actinobacillus acetinomycetamicomitans, 4193
Actinobacillus ureae, 4193
Actinomyces, 4177–4180, *4178, 4180, 4181*
in intracranial abscess, 3950
Actinomycetales, 4136
atypical mycobacteria, 4176–4177
Actinomyces, 4177–4180, *4178, 4180, 4181*
Nocardia, 4189, 4189–4192, *4190, 4191*
Tropheryma whippelii, 4180–4189, *4182, 4183, 4184, 4185, 4186, 4187, 4188*
mycobacteria, 4136
Mycobacterium bovis, 4167–4168
Mycobacterium leprae, 4168–4176, *4169, 4170, 4171, 4172, 4174, 4175*
Mycobacterium tuberculosis, 4136, 4136–4167, *4137, 4138, 4139, 4140, 4141, 4142, 4143, 4144, 4145, 4146, 4147, 4148, 4149, 4150, 4151, 4152, 4153, 4154, 4155, 4156, 4157, 4158, 4159, 4160, 4161, 4162, 4163, 4164, 4165, 4166, 4167, 4168*
Actinomycosis, 4177–4180, *4178, 4180, 4181*
Acute acquired toxoplasmosis
diagnosis of, in immunocompetent patient, 4693
treatment of
in immunocompetent patients, 4699–4700
in immunodeficient patients, 4700
in pregnant women, 4700
Acute angle closure glaucoma, *1010,* 1010–1011, 1724–1725
Acute aseptic meningitis and meningoencephalitis, 5387, *5388, 5389*
Acute bacterial meningitis, 3990, 4028–4029, 5018–5019
clinical manifestations, 4001, 4004–4007
clinical settings, 3994–3996
diagnosis, 4007–4010, *4008*
etiology, 3990, 3993–3994
pathology, 3998, *3999, 4000,* 4001, *4001, 4002, 4003, 4004, 4005*
pathophysiology, 3996–3998, *3997, 3998*
prognosis, 4011–4012
prophylaxis, 4012–4013
treatment, 4010–4011
Acute cerebellar ataxia, 5016
Acute choroidal ischemia, 3760
Acute confusional migraine, 3698–3699
Acute disseminated encephalomyelitis (ADEM), 5110–5111, 5174, 5649
clinical manifestations, 5649
laboratory and neuroimaging findings, 5649, *5650*
pathogenesis, 5651
pathology, 5649–5651, *5651, 5652, 5653*
prevention, 5653
prognosis, 5653
treatment, 5651, 5653
Acute disseminated histoplasmosis, 4393
Acute encephalopathy, role of radiation therapy in, 2598
Acute febrile cerebrovasculitis, 4738, *4770, 4771,* 4771–4772, *4772*
Acute febrile mucocutaneous lymph node syndrome, 5733
Acute hemorrhagic conjunctivitis (AHC), 5235, 5243–5245, *5244*
Acute hemorrhagic leukoencephalitis, 5653, *5654, 5655,* 5656
Acute hepatitis B virus infection, 4966–4970, *4968, 4969*
Acute hypervitaminosis, 1718
Acute idiopathic demyelinating optic neuritis, 600
demographics, 600–601
diagnostic, etiologic, and prognostic studies, 605–608, *606, 608*
management recommendations for patients with presumed acute, 616
neurologic prognosis, 615–616
pathogenesis of visual loss in, 617
pathology, 616–617
recurrent, 616
relationship of, to multiple sclerosis, 617–620
residual visual deficits after resolution of, *605,* 612–615, *614*
signs of, 601–602, *603, 604,* 604–605, *605*
symptoms of, 601
treatment of, *609,* 609–610, *610*
visual function in fellow eye, 605
visual prognosis, 610–612, *611*
Acute inflammatory demyelinating polyneuropathy (AIDP), 5539
Acute ischemic cerebrovascular disease, headache associated with, 1706–1707
Acute leukemia, 2337
Acute motor axonal neuropathy, 5705–5707, *5706*
Acute necrotizing chorioretinitis, 4681
Acute necrotizing hemorrhagic encephalomyelitis, 3979
Acute necrotizing myopathy, 2530
Acute nonbacterial meningitis, 4013–4015, *4014*
Acute optic neuritis, 987, 5581–5582, *5583, 5584,* 5584–5588, *5585, 5586*
Acute pandysautonomia, 1028–1029
Acute pericarditis, 3816
Acute phthisis bulbi, 5041
Acute posterior multifocal placoid pigment epitheliopathy (APMPPE), 3727, 3739–3741, *3740, 3741, 3742,* 3743–3744, 3919, 4086, 4957–4958, 4974

Acute posttraumatic headache, 1705
Acute pulmonary blastomycosis, 4333, *4335*
Acute pulmonary histoplasmosis, 4392
Acute rectocolitis, 4619
Acute retinal necrosis (ARN) syndrome, 636, 4984, 4986–4987, 5041, 5426
Acute retrobulbar optic neuropathy, 4298, *4300*
Acute rheumatic fever, 4085
Acute schistosomiasis, 4487, 4489
Acute sensorimotor neuropathy, 2523–2524
Acute subarachnoid hemorrhage, 3348–3349
Acute toxoplasmosis
  in immunocompetent patients, *4671,* 4671–4672, *4672*
  in immunodeficient patients, 4672–4673, *4674,* 4675, *4675, 4676,* 4677–4678, *4678, 4679*
    diagnosis of, 4693–4694, *4694, 4695, 4696*
Acyclovir
  for herpes simplex virus (HSV) encephalitis, 5011–5012
  for herpes zoster ophthalmicus, 5079–5080
Adaptation
  dark, 159, 214–215, *215*
  of vestibulo-ocular reflex (VOR), 1147–1148
Addison's disease, 2163
Adducting eye, 1479
Adduction lag, 1294
Adenocarcinomas, 699
Adenohypophysis, 2141
Adenohypophysitis, lymphocytic, *2207,* 2207–2208, *2208*
Adenoid cystic carcinoma, 2453–2457, *2454, 2455, 2456*
Adenoma sebaceum, *2670,* 2671, *2671*
Adenomas
  acidophil, 2152
  acidophilic pituitary, 2153
  basophil, 2152
  chromophobe, 2152, 2153, 2187
  invasive, 2203–2204
  pituitary. (*See* Pituitary adenomas.)
  PRL-secreting, 2195–2196
Adenopathy, bilateral hilar, 5511, *5511*
  associated with pulmonary infiltration, 5511, *5512,* 5514
Adenoviral infection, 4959
Adenoviridae, 4954
  clinical manifestations, 4956
    miscellaneous, 4959
    neurologic, 4958–4959
    ocular, 4956–4958, *4957, 4958, 4960, 4961*
    respiratory, 4956, *4956*
  diagnosis, 4959–4960, *4962*
  structure, 4954, *4955,* 4956
  treatment, 4960
Adenovirus infection, 5417
Adherence syndromes, 1353–1354
Adie's tonic pupil syndrome, 962, 978–983, *979, 980, 981, 983, 984*
Adiposogenital dystrophy, 1814
Adnexal complications of HIV infection, 5430
Adrenal dysfunction, headaches associated with, 1721
Adrenal hyperplasia, 2197
β-Adrenergic blocking drugs, impact of, on postsynaptic neuromuscular transmission, 1442–1443
Adrenergic drugs, 1003–1004, *1004*
Adrenocorticotropic hormone (ACTH), 2147
Adrenoleukodystrophy, 765
  neonatal, 2843, *2844*
  X-linked, 2845–2847, *2846, 2847, 2848*
Adrenomyeloneuropathy, 2846–2847
  lorenzo oil therapy for, 2847
Adult T-cell leukemia-lymphoma, *5435,* 5435–5436, *5436, 5437*
Aerobes, strict, 4066
Aeromonas, 4245
Aerotolerant anaerobes, 4066
Affect, 1765
Afipia felis, 4197–4198
African Tick Bite Fever, 4751–4752
African trypanosomiasis, 4710, *4710,* 4711, *4713–4714*
Agammaglobulinemia, 5240
Age
  and cerebral blood flow, 2970
  in incidence of saccular aneurysms, 3015
  and papilledema, 504
  and pattern of hypoxia, 3325–3326
  and pupillary light reaction, 888
  and relationship between optic neuritis and multiple sclerosis, 617–618
  and visual loss in dementia, 469–470
Agenesis of extraocular muscles, 1352
Agnogenic myeloid metaplasia, 2335–2336
Agnosia, 1841
  associative visual, 3485
  auditory, 1831
  integrative, 5138
  tactile, 1839
  verbal, 1831
  visual, 413, 1848, 2634
Agraphesthesia, 1839
Agraphia, 1841
  alexia with, 431
  alexia without, 3484
Aicardi syndrome, 783, 788, 798, *799,* 800
AIDS. (*See* Acquired immune deficiency syndrome (AIDS); Human immunodeficiency virus (HIV) infection.)
AIDS dementia complex, 5389
AII cells, 41
Air emboli, 3379
Akinesia of lid function, 1539
Akinetopsia
  anatomy, 438–439, *440*
  associated deficits, 437–438
  functional imaging and other techniques, *443,* 443–445, *444, 445*
  manifestations, 437
  motion perception deficits with unilateral cerebral lesions, 438–439, *440, 441, 442*
  physiology of motion perception in nonhuman primates, 439, 441–443
Alaria, 4493, 4494
Alaria americana, 4492
Albendazole for neurocysticercosis, 4477
Albinism, association between optic nerve hypoplasia and, 783
Alcaligenes species, 4245
Alcohol consumption
  in headaches, 1717
  and incidence of atherosclerosis, 3330
  as risk factor in aneurysms, 3012
Aleutian disease of mink, 4029
Alexander's disease, 766
Alexander's law, 1470, 1472
Alexia. (*See also* Acquired alexia.)
  without agraphia, 1846, 3484
Alice in Wonderland syndrome, 3697
Alien hand syndrome, 1821
Alkylating agents
  altretamine, 2579
  busulfan, 2566
  carboplatin, 2578
  chlorambucil, 2565–2566
  cisplatin, 2573
  cyclophosphamide, 2566
  dacarbazine, 2565
  ifosfamide, 2567
  melphalan, 2564–2565
  nitrogen mustards, 2563–2564, *2564*
  procarbazine, 2565
  spiromustine, 2568
  thiotepa, 2578–2579
Allen Cards, 161
Allergic angiitis and granulomatosis, *3752,* 3752–3754, *3753, 3754*
  demographics, 3752
  diagnosis, 3753–3754
  ocular and neuro-ophthalmologic manifestations, *3752,* 3753, *3753*
  pathology, 3753, *3754*
  systemic manifestations, 3752–3753
  treatment and prognosis, 3754
Allergic aspergillosis, 4287–4290, *4288, 4289, 4290*
Allergic conjunctivitis, 5233
Allergic sinusitis, 4287–4288
Allesthesia, visual, 3673, 5596
Allopurinol, 2593
Alopecia, 3815
Alpha effect, 2595
Alpha-1-antitrypsin
  assessment of, in diagnosing aneurysms, 3015
  spontaneous dissecting aneurysm in patients with deficiency, 3207–3208
Alphaviruses, rubivirus (Rubella), 5286–5293, 5296
Alprenolol in controlling blood pressure, 3145
Altafur, 1263
Alterations in mental status in giant cell arteritis, 3756
Alternating contraction anisocoria, 937, 941
Alternating hemiplegia of childhood, 3699
Alternating Horner's syndrome, 968
Alternating skew deviation, 1288, 4375
Altitudinal hemianopia, 2170
Altretamine
  neurotoxicity, 2579
  systemic toxicity, 2579
Alveolar macrophages, 5475–5476
Alzheimer's disease, 469, 2748, 4605
  biochemical pathology, 2750
  clinical features, 2751–2755, 2752*t*
  diagnosis, 2755
  epidemiology, 2748–2749
  laboratory investigations, 2755
  neurofibrillary tangles in, 5723
  neurologic manifestations, 2751–2753
  ocular motor manifestations, 2754–2755
  pathogenesis, 2751
  pathology, *2749,* 2749–2750, *2750, 2751*
  prognosis, 2756
  pupillary disturbances, 2755
  treatment, 2755–2756
  visual sensory manifestations, 2753–2754, *2754, 2755*
Amacrine cells, *38,* 40–42, *42, 43*

Amastigotes, 4702
Amaurosis, gaze-evoked, *1798,* 1798–1799
Amaurosis fugax, 3420, 3553–3555
Amblyomma americanum, 4739, 4763
Amblyomma cajennense, 4739
Amblyopia, 155, 988–989
  and ethambutol, 674
  and ocular dominance columns, 133–134
  tobacco, 674–675
Amenorrhea, 2160
American Optical Polarizing Test, 1772
American Optical Vectograph Project-O-Chart slide, 163
American trypanosomiasis, 4701–4702, *4702*
Amino acid metabolism disorders
  Lowe syndrome, 2814–2815
  maple syrup urine disease, 2813–2814
  phenylalaninemia
    dihydropteridine reductase defect, 2812
    phenylalanine hydroxylase deficiency, 2811–2812
  tyrosinemia, 2812–2813, *2813*
Aminoglycoside group, 1442
Amnesia
  acquired, 3024
  anterograde, 1833
  retrograde, 1833
Amnestic syndrome, 3024
Amoeba. (*See also* Amoebiasis; Free-living amoebae.)
  leptomyxida, 4638, *4639*
Amoebiasis, 4614, *4614*
  clinical manifestations, 4619
  diagnosis, 4621–4623
  Entamoeba histolytica, 4614, *4614*
  epidemiology, 4615
  extraintestinal disease, 4619–4621
  free-living, 4623
    Acanthamoeba species, 4628–4630, *4630, 4631,* 4632, *4632, 4633, 4634,* 4635, *4635, 4636, 4637,* 4638, *4638*
    Balammuthia mandrillaris (Leptomyxida), 4638, *4639, 4640,* 4640–4641, *4641*
    Naegleria fowleri, 4623–4626, *4624, 4625, 4626, 4627,* 4628, *4628, 4629*
  genitourinary, 4620
  intestinal disease, 4619
  life cycle, *4614,* 4614–4615, *4615, 4616*
  pathogenesis, 4615–4617
  pathology, 4617, *4617, 4618,* 4619
  perianal, 4619
  periaxial, 4619
  pericardial, 4620
  pleuropulmonary, 4620
  prognosis, 4623
  treatment, 4623
Amoebic ascites, 4620
Amoebic encephalitis, granulomatous, 4623, 4629–4630, 4632, *4632, 4633, 4634, 4635*
Amoebic intracranial aneurysm, 3973
Amoebic myositis, 4620
Amoeboma, 4619
Amphetamines, 3363, 3585
Amphotericin B
  for allergic aspergillosis, 4317
  for blastomycosis, 4342
  for candidiasis, 4353
  for coccidioidomycosis, 4365
  for cryptococcosis, 4384–4385
  for fungal infections, *4283,* 4283–4284
  for mucormycosis, 4331
Amplification systems, 3726
Amputation neuromas, 1726
Amsler grid, 156, *157,* 174–175
Amusia, 1831
  expressive, 1821–1822
Amyloid, 4563
Amyloid angiopathy, 3351, *3353,* 3586–3588
Amyloidosis, 590, 2389
  extraocular muscle involvement with, 1397–1398, *1399*
  primary generalized, 2401–2403, *2402*
  secondary systemic, 4173
  transmissible, 4561
Amyotrophic lateral sclerosis, 1331, 1333, 4605
  diagnosis, 2800
  epidemiology, 2796
  etiology, 2796–2797
  laboratory and neuroimaging findings, 2800
  neurologic manifestations, 2797–2799
  neuro-ophthalmologic manifestations, 2799–2800
  pathology, 2797, *2797*
  prognosis, 2800
  treatment, 2800
Amyotrophy, neuralgic, 5147
Anabolic steroids, 3362
Anaerobes
  aerotolerant, 4066
  obligate, 4066
Analgesic-abuse headaches, 1719
Anaplastic astrocytomas, 1924–1925, *1925,* 2559
Ancillary information, 178, *181*
Ancylostoma caninum, 4531
Anemia, 527–528, 3816, 4139
  as complication of malaria, 4653
  hemolytic, 5103
  and ischemic optic neuropathies, 553–555
  normochromic normocytic, 3772–3775, *3774*
  pernicious, 668, 669, 675
  sickle cell, 3012
    homozygous, 3349
Anemic hypoxia, 3324
Anesthesia dolorosa, 1749–1750
Aneurysmal bone cysts, 2444, *2444*
Aneurysms, 4361
  arteriovenous, 2725
  bacterial, 3965–3969, *3966, 3968, 3969, 3970*
  berry, 2977
  clipping, 3149–3150
  de novo formation of, 3142
  definitions, 2977
  dissecting, 2977
    clinical manifestations according to site
      of branches of internal carotid artery, 3216
      of extracranial portion of internal carotid artery, 3210–3215, 3211*t, 3212, 3213*
      of intracranial portion of internal carotid artery, 3215–3216
      of vertebral and basilar arteries and their branches, 3216–3218, *3217, 3218, 3219, 3220,* 3220*t, 3221,* 3221–3223
    general considerations, 3203–3210, *3204, 3205, 3206*
  fungal, 3971–3973, *3972, 3973*
  fusiform
    clinical manifestations, treatment, and prognosis according to site
      of basilar artery and its branches, *3198,* 3198–3199, *3199, 3200, 3201,* 3201–3203, *3202, 3203*
      of internal carotid artery and its branches, 3183–3186, *3184, 3185, 3187,* 3188–3192, *3189, 3190, 3191, 3192, 3193, 3194,* 3195, *3195, 3196*
      of vertical artery and its branches, 3195–3198, *3197*
    general considerations, *3180,* 3180–3183, *3181, 3182*
  giant, 3141–3142
  history, 2975–2977, *2976*
  intracranial, 2611–2612, 2983, *2983,* 2985
  intracranial mycotic, 4088
  mycotic, 3965, 4070–4071, 4073, *4090,* 4090–4091, 4304–4305, *4306, 4307*
    bacterial, 3965–3969, *3966, 3968, 3969, 3970*
    fungal, 3971–3973, *3972, 3973*
    intracranial, 4088
    miscellaneous, 3973
    spirochetal (syphilitic), 3973
  pathogenesis, 2977–2978, *2979, 2980,* 2980–2982, *2981*
    arteritis, 3005
    associated risk factors
      congenital extracranial disease, 3010
      hypertension, 3007–3008
      intracranial arteriovenous malformations, 3008–3010, *3009*
      moyamoya disease, 3012, *3013*
      occlusive disease of internal carotid artery, 3010–3011, *3011*
      other, and miscellaneous disorders, 3012, 3014
      smoking, 3012
    connective tissue diseases, 2982
      Ehlers-Danlos syndrome, *2984, 2985,* 2985–2987
      fibromuscular dysplasia, *2982,* 2982–2983, 2985
      Marfan's syndrome, *2986,* 2987, *2987*
      pseudoxanthoma elasticum, 2987, *2988, 2989*
    mycotic, 2998
      bacterial, 2998–3003, *3000, 3001, 3002*
      fungal, *3003,* 3003–3004, *3004*
      miscellaneous, 3005
      spirochetal (syphilitic), 3004–3005
    neoplastic, 3005–3007, *3006, 3008*
    traumatic, 2989–2990, *2991,* 2991*t,* 2992, *2992, 2993, 2994,* 2994–2998, *2995, 2996, 2997, 2998*
    tumors, 2987, 2989, *2989, 2990*
  saccular, 2977, 2978, *2979*
    clinical manifestations according to site, 3037
      arising from anterior cerebral artery, 3091–3093, *3094, 3095, 3096, 3097*
      arising from anterior choroidal artery, 3084–3085, *3086*
      arising from anterior communicating artery, 3100–3104, *3101, 3102, 3103*
      arising from anterior inferior cerebellar artery, 3122, *3122*
      arising from basilar artery, 3111, 3113, *3114, 3115, 3116,* 3116–3122, *3117, 3118, 3119, 3120, 3121*

arising from bifurcation of internal carotid artery, 3085, *3087*, 3087–3091, *3088, 3089, 3090, 3091, 3092, 3093*
arising from cavernous portion of internal carotid artery, *3040*, 3040–3041, *3041, 3042, 3043, 3044, 3045, 3046*, 3046–3047, *3047, 3048, 3049*, 3050, *3050, 3051, 3052, 3053*, 3054, *3054*
arising from clinoid segment of internal carotid artery, *3055, 3056*, 3056–3059, *3057, 3058*
arising from conjunctival arteries, 3074–3075
arising from extracranial portion of internal carotid artery, 3037–3038, *3038, 3039*
arising from intradural portion of internal carotid artery and its branches, 3054, 3056
arising from junction of internal carotid and anterior choroidal arteries, 3084, *3085, 3086*
arising from junction of internal carotid and ophthalmic arteries, *3059*, 3059–3060, *3060, 3061, 3062*, 3062–3063, *3063, 3064, 3065*, 3065–3066, *3066, 3067*
arising from junction of internal carotid and posterior communicating arteries, *3075*, 3075–3083, *3076, 3077, 3078, 3079, 3081, 3082, 3083*
arising from junction of internal carotid and superior hypophyseal arteries, 3059
arising from middle cerebral artery, 3095, 3097, *3097, 3098, 3099*, 3099–3100, *3100*
arising from ophthalmic artery, 3066–3067, *3067, 3068, 3069, 3070*
arising from petrous portion of internal carotid artery, 3038, *3039*, 3040
arising from posterior cerebral artery, 3123, *3125*, 3125–3127, *3126*
arising from posterior communicating artery, 3083, *3084*
arising from posterior inferior cerebellar artery, 3108–3109, *3112, 3113*
arising from proximal supraclinoid portion of internal carotid artery, 3075
arising from retinal arteries, 3067, 3069, *3071, 3072*, 3072–3074, *3073, 3074*
arising from superior cerebellar artery, *3122*, 3122–3123
arising from vertebral artery, 3104, *3106*, 3106–3108, *3107, 3108, 3109, 3110, 3111*
arising from vertebrobasilar arterial system, 3104, *3104, 3105*
diagnosis, 3130–3133, *3132, 3133, 3134, 3136*, 3136–3139, *3137, 3140, 3141, 3142*
of subarachnoid hemorrhage, 3130
location and laterality, 3015, *3016, 3017*
manifestations of ruptured
general considerations, 3019–3020, *3020*
hydrocephalus after rupture of intracranial, *3035*, 3035–3036
intracerebral hemorrhage associated with, 3033–3034, 3034*t*
intraventricular hemorrhage associated with, 3034
neurologic and neuro-ophthalmologic intracranial, 3021–3024, *3022, 3023*
orbital and intraocular effects of subarachnoid and intracranial hemorrhage, *3024*, 3024–3026, *3025, 3026, 3027, 3028*, 3028–3029, *3029, 3030, 3031, 3032*, 3032–3033, *3033*
subdural hematoma from intracranial, *3036*, 3036–3037
warning signs and symptoms before major rupture of intracranial, 3021
multiple, 3016–3018, *3019*
general clinical manifestations, 3018–3019
natural history, 3139
delayed cerebral ischemia and vasospasm, 3145–3147, *3146, 3147*
medical complications, 3144
recurrent hemorrhage, 3144–3145
ruptured, 3142–3144, *3143*
unruptured, 3139–3142
neuro-ophthalmologic signs of unruptured intracranial, 3127
abducens nerve paresis, 3128
combined ocular motor nerve pareses, 3128
miscellaneous, 3130
oculomotor nerve paresis, 3127–3128
oculomotor nerve synkinesis, 3128, *3129*
trochlear nerve paresis, 3128
visual loss, 3128, 3130
prevalence, 3014–3015
sex and age distribution, 3015
size, 3015–3016, *3018*
surgery for
endovascular, 3178–3180, *3179*
for unruptured, 3154–3155, *3156, 3157*, 3157–3159, *3158, 3159, 3160, 3161, 3162*, 3162–3165, *3164, 3165, 3166, 3167*
ruptured, 3176–3178
timing of, and relationship to neurologic status, 3172–3175
unruptured, 3165–3166, *3168*, 3168–3169, *3169*
treatment and results, 3147
of delayed cerebral ischemia, 3170–3172
direct surgical approach, 3147
medical therapy, 3175–3176
of ruptured intracranial, 3169–3170
Vein of Galen, 2263–2266, *2264, 2265*
Angel's trumpet, 1001
Angiitis, 4738–4739
granulomatous, 5468
Angioblastic meningiomas, 2027–2028, *2028*
Angiocentric T-cell lymphoma, 3727, *3786*, 3786–3788, *3787*
Angioendotheliosis, neoplastic, 3351
Angiogenesis, 3334
Angiography
in diagnosis and management of brain tumors, 1896
fluorescein, 159
Angioid streaks, 2985–2987
with and without pseudoxanthoma elasticum pseudoxanthoma elasticum, 817–818
Angioimmunoblastic lymphadenopathy, 702–703
Angiokeratoma, diffuse, 2831
Angiokeratosis naeviformis, 2275
Angioma
cavernous, *2233*, 2233–2236, *2234*, 2235, *2235, 2236, 2237*, 2238, *2238, 2239, 2241, 2242*, 2242–2244, *2243*
choroidal, 2710–2712
cortical, 2236
diffuse, 2710–2711
extraparenchymal, 2236
extraparenchymal cavernous, 2236
infratentorial, 2235
intracranial cavernous, 2236–2237, *2240*
intraparenchymal, 2235–2236
meningeal, 2712, *2716*, 2716–2718
of optic disc, 2707
orbital, *2243, 2244*, 2244–2245
racemose, 2725
retinal, *2245*, 2245–2246
sclera, 2712, *2714, 2715*
subcortical, 2236
venous, 2246, *2247, 2248, 2249, 2250*, 2250–2252, *2251, 2252*
Angiomatosis
bacillary, 4208
encephalotrigeminal. (*See* Encephalotrigeminal angiomatosis.)
noncalcifying diffuse corticomeningeal, 2275
of retina and cerebellum. (*See* von Hippel-Lindau (VHL) disease.)
systemic, 2275
universal, 2275
Angiomyolipomas, 2688
Angiopathy
amyloid, 3351, *3353*
neoplastic, 3351
radiation, 3350–3351, *3352*
Angioplasty, 3562
Angiostrongyliasis, 4494
intraocular, 4496–4497, *4498*
Angiostrongylus cantonensis, 4494
clinical manifestations, *4496*, 4496–4497, *4497, 4498*
diagnosis, 4500
epidemiology, 4494, 4496
in intracranial brain abscess, 3952
life cycle, 4494, *4496*
pathogenesis and pathology, 4497–4499, *4498, 4499*
treatment and prognosis, 4500
Angiotensin-converting enzyme (ACE), 5516, 5518
Angle closure glaucoma, 3424
Angle kappa, 1180, *1181*
Angular artery, 2940
Angular vestibulo-ocular reflex (VOR), 1139
Anhidrosis, 966
congenital familial sensory neuropathy with, 1027
Anicteric leptospirosis, 4837–4842, *4840, 4841, 4842*
Aniline compounds and headaches, 1718
Animal prion diseases, 4567
bovine spongiform encephalopathy, 4567
scrapie, 4567
Aniridia, 782, 1006, *1007*

Anisocoria, 961, *962,* 5433
  alternating contraction, 937, 941
  benign, 884–885
  causes of, 962*t*
  central, 962
  differentiation of, 986–987, *988*
  in Horner's syndrome, 965
  in lateral gaze, 885, 984–986
  physiologic, 936
  see-saw, 1782–1783
  simple, 962–963, *963*
Anisometropia, 1732
Ankylosing spondylitis, 3852–3854, *3853*
Annulus of Zinn, 1511
Anomalies of extraocular muscle location, *1352,* 1352–1353, *1353*
Anomalous trichromacy, 33
Anomia, tactile, 1839
Anomic sensory aphasia, 3484
Anophthalmic socket syndrome, 2615, 2617
Anosmia, 1794–1795, 1825, 2043, 2044
Anosognosia, 391, 1842
Anoxia, 3323–3324
  of occipital lobes, 363
Ansa lenticularis, 1863
Anterior cavernous sinus, 1668
Anterior cerebral arteries, 2891, *2892, 2893, 2894, 2895, 2896,* 2897, *2897.* (*See also* Cerebral arteries.)
  aneurysms arising from, 3091–3093, *3094, 3095, 3096, 3097*
Anterior chamber hemorrhage, 3426
Anterior chiasmal syndrome, 1807, 1811, *1811,* 2171
Anterior choroidal arteries, 15, 2886, 2889, *2891.* (*See also* Choroidal arteries.)
  aneurysms arising from, 3084–3085, *3086*
  interior carotid artery, aneurysms arising from junction with, 3084, *3085, 3086*
Anterior communicating artery, 2898
  aneurysms arising from, 3100–3104, *3101, 3102, 3103*
Anterior compressive optic neuropathies, 649–653, *650, 651, 652*
Anterior inferior cerebellar artery (AICA), 2914, *2914, 2915, 2916,* 2916–2917, 3005
  aneurysms arising from, 3122, *3122*
  syndrome of, 1287, *1288*
    skew deviation and ocular tilt reaction, 1287–1289
Anterior ischemic optic neuropathy (AION), 58, 259–260, *263, 264,* 2333, 3339, 3760–3761
Anterior optic chiasm syndrome, 294, *297, 298*
Anterior optic neuritis, 4682–4683, 4753, 4872–4873, *4874, 4875,* 5197
Anterior optic neuropathy, 717, *5501,* 5503–5504
  from rhinocerebral mucormycosis, 4321, *4324*
Anterior parietal artery, occlusion of, 3440
Anterior scleritis, 1724
Anterior segment disease, 5429–5430
Anterior spinal artery, 2910–2911, *2911*
Anterior thalamoperforating artery, 2886
Anterior tympanic artery, 2945
Anterior uveitis, 5581
  with hypopyon, 3803–3804
Anterior visual pathways, astrocytomas of, 1941–1947, *1942, 1943, 1944, 1945, 1946, 1948, 1949, 1952, 1954, 1957, 1958, 1959*
Anterior visual sensory pathway, compression of, 3050
Anterior-posterior circulation anastomoses, 2936, 2940
Anterograde amnesia, 1833
Anterograde prosopagnosia, 423–424
Anthracycline antibiotics, 2579–2580
  neuro-ophthalmologic toxicity, 2579–2580
  neurotoxicity, 2579
  ocular toxicity, 2579
  systemic toxicity, 2579
Anthrax, 4105–4106, *4106*
  cutaneous, 4106, *4106*
  gastrointestinal, 4106
  inhalation, 4106
Anti-acetylcholline receptor antibody assay, 1423–1424
Antiadrenergic drugs, 1005
Antiarrhythmic drugs, impact of, on postsynaptic neuromuscular transmission, 1441–1442
Antibiotics
  anthracycline, 2579–2580
    neuro-ophthalmologic toxicity, 2579–2580
    neurotoxicity, 2579
    ocular toxicity, 2579
    systemic toxicity, 2579
  for bacterial meningitis, 4010–4011
  bleomycin, 2580
  for contaminated or infected wounds, 4116–4117
  impact of, on postsynaptic neuromuscular transmission, 1442
  for intracranial abscess, 3962–3963
  mithramycin, 2580
  mitomycins, 2580
  monobasic amino acid, 1442
  suramin, 2580–2581
Antibodies
  anticryptococcal, 4384
  Anti-Ri, 2512
  for bacterial meningitis, 4011
  detection of, 5379–5380
Anticholinergic drugs, *1000, 1001,* 1001–1003, *1002, 1003*
Anticholinesterase agents
  impact of, on postsynaptic neuromuscular transmission, 1440–1441
  for Lambert-Eaton myasthenic syndrome, 1436
Anticoagulant therapy
  in managing cerebrovascular disease, 3557–3558, 3571, 3579
  for septic cavernous sinus thrombosis, 3898
  for septic thrombosis, 4038
Anticonvulsants, impact of, on postsynaptic neuromuscular transmission, 1442
Anticryptococcal antibodies, 4384
Antidiuretic hormone (ADH, Vasopressin), 2146
Antifreeze, 1262
Antigen detection, 5380
Antigenemia, 5417
Anti-Hu antibody, 2502
Anti-Hu syndrome, *2504,* 2504–2505, *2505*
Antihypertensive therapy, 3581
Antimetabolites
  cytosine arabinoside, 2560–2562
  5-fluorouracil, 2558–2560
  hydroxyurea, 2563
  purine analogs, 2562
  pyrimidine analogs (bromodeoxyuridine), 2563
Antimicrobial drug therapy for septic cavernous sinus thrombosis, 3898
Antiphospholipid antibodies, 3362–3363
Antiphospholipid antibody syndrome, 3012, 3391–3392
Antiplatelet therapy in managing cerebrovascular disease, 3558–3561, *3559,* 3571, 3581
Antirabies vaccine, 1261
Anti-Ri antibody, 2512
Antisaccades, *1106,* 1114
Antituberculosis vaccines, 4167
Anton's syndrome, 370, 1830, 3486, 3492
  and cyclosporine, 2634
  inverse, 3486–3487
Anturane, 3560–3561
Aorta, coarctation of
  and development of aneurysms, 3010
  and polycystic kidney disease, 3008
Aortic arch
  occlusion of major branches of, 3522–3524, *3523*
  syndromes involving, *3519,* 3519–3524, *3520, 3521, 3522, 3523*
Aortic bodies, 2462
Aortocranial disease, symptoms and signs of, 3518
Apert's disease, 796
Apert's syndrome, 783
Aphasia
  anomic sensory, 3484
  fluent, 1841
  optic, 3484–3485
  primary progressive. (*See* Primary progressive aphasia.)
  tactile, 1839
  transcortical motor, 3434
  transcortical sensory, 3484
  transient, 3676
Aphthous stomatitis, 3803
Aplasia, optic nerve, *801,* 801–802
Apolipoprotein E (APOE) gene on chromosome 19, 2751
Aponeurosis, 1511
Aponeurotic defects of eyelid, 1545
Apophysomyceae, 4318
Apoplexy
  optic chiasmal, 2258
  optic nerve, 2258
Apoprion, 4565
Apoptosis, 14, 19
Apparent enophthalmos, 964
Apparent erythrocytosis, 2332
Apparent sex-linked optic atrophy, 758
Apperceptive prosopagnosia, 416
Appetite center, 1814
Applanation tonometry, 158
Apraxia, 1841
  acquired ocular motor, 1324
  affecting left arm, 3433
  of eyelid closure, 2775
  of eyelid opening, *1538,* 1539, 2775
  gait, 1820
  ocular, 445
  ocular motor, *1325,* 1325–1326, 2661
  oculomotor, 2722
  unilateral, 1859
Apresoline and headaches, 1718
Aqueductal stenosis, 2660
  and papilledema, 515
Arachnoid cap cells, 2018
Arachnoid cysts, *2020,* 2020–2021, *2021, 2022, 2023,* 2117–2118

external cellular layer of, as barrier to infection, 3941
granulations, 2020, 2956
infratentorial, 2120–2121, *2121, 2122*
in other locations, 2123, *2124*
suprasellar, 2123–2125
supratentorial, 2118–2120, *2119, 2120*
Arachnoid villi, 2956
Arachnoiditis, 589
optochiasmatic, 4153, 4373–4374, 4876, 4878–4880
Arcanobacterium haemolyticum, 4105
Archipallium, 19
Arcuate neuroretinitis, 636
Arden gratings, 622
Arden ratio, 224
Area 17 of Brodmann. (*See* Striate cortex.)
Area V1 (primary visual cortex; striate cortex; area 17 of Brodmann), 126
anatomy and histology, 126, *127,* 128, *128, 129*
layer 1, 128
layer 2, 128
layer 3, 128
layer 4, 128
layer 5, 128–129
layer 6, 129
color vision mechanisms in striate cortex, *138,* 138–139, *139*
physiology, 129–132
binocularity and ocular dominance columns, *132,* 132–133, *133, 134, 135*
ocular dominance columns and amblyopia, 133–134
organization and modularity, 134–135, *135, 136*
representation of brightness in striate cortex, 138
representation of visual field in striate cortex, 135–137, *137*
Area V5, 1126–1127
human homologues of, 1127–1128
Arecoline, 1005
Areflexia, 1029, 5059
Arenaviridae, *5154,* 5154–5158, *5155, 5156, 5157, 5158*
Areolar choroiditis, 4867
Arginine vasotocin, 1867
Argyll Robertson pupils, *991,* 991–993, 4887, 4889–4890, 5510, *5511,* 5614
inverse, 993
Arnold-Chiari malformation, 1291, 1292*t*
Arrhythmias as cause of embolism, 3386–3389
Arsenic, 1261
Arsphenamine, 1261–1262
Artemisinin compounds, 4656–4657, 4664
Arterial dissections, headaches associated with, 1708
Arterial ectasia, 3181
Arterial emboli, 3401–3405, *3403, 3404*
Arterial system of brain
circle of Willis, 2932, 2934, *2938*
external carotid artery, 2940
anterior branches of, 2940–2941
ascending branch of, 2941–2942
posterior branches, 2941
terminal branches of, 2942, *2944,* 2944–2946, *2945*
internal carotid artery and its branches, 2869–2870, *2871*
cavernous segment, *2873,* 2873–2874, *2874, 2875, 2876*
cervical segment of, 2870–2871
clinoid segment, 2877
communicating segment, 2884, 2886, 2889, *2890*
lacerum segment, 2871, *2871,* 2873, *2873,* 2876–2877
ophthalmic segment, 2877, *2878, 2879, 2880,* 2880–2881, *2881, 2882, 2883,* 2884, *2884, 2885, 2886, 2887, 2888*
petrous segment, 2871, *2871, 2872*
terminal branches of, 2889, 2891, *2892, 2893, 2894, 2895, 2896, 2897,* 2897–2899, *2898, 2899, 2900, 2901,* 2902, *2902, 2903,* 2904
internal carotid-basilar anastomoses, 2934
anterior-posterior circulation, 2936, 2940
persistent primitive acoustic (otic) artery, 2936, *2940*
persistent primitive hypoglossal artery, 2936, *2939, 2941, 2942*
persistent primitive trigeminal artery, 2935, *2939*
leptomeningeal arterioles, 2932
origin of cerebral arterila blood supply from aortic arch, 2869, *2870*
vertebrobasilar, and its branches, 2904
basilar artery, *2910,* 2911–2914, *2912, 2913, 2914, 2915, 2916,* 2916–2917, *2918, 2919, 2920,* 2920–2922, *2921, 2922, 2923, 2924, 2925, 2926, 2927, 2928,* 2928–2929, *2929, 2930, 2931,* 2931–2932, *2932, 2933, 2934, 2935, 2936, 2937*
vertebral artery, 2904–2905, *2905, 2906, 2907,* 2907–2911, *2908, 2909, 2910, 2911*
Arterial wall constriction and compression, 3353–3355, *3354, 3355, 3356, 3357*
Arterialization of conjunctiva and episcleral veins, 3275, *3276*
Arteriosclerosis, 3329–3330
Arteriovenous aneurysm, 2725
Arteriovenous malformations (AVMs), 2252, 3671–3672, *3672*
associations, 2274–2275
as cause of spontaneous subarachnoid and intracranial hemorrhage, 3020
clinical manifestations, 2256–2261, *2258, 2259, 2260, 2261, 2262, 2263,* 2263–2274, *2264, 2265, 2266, 2267, 2268, 2269, 2270, 2271, 2272, 2273*
diagnosis of, 2275, *2276*
dural, *2268,* 2268–2274, *2269, 2270, 2271, 2272*
embolization for, 2280, *2280, 2281,* 2282
embryogenesis, 2252–2253
incidence, 2253, 2255
natural history of, 2275–2280, *2280, 2281,* 2282, *2283,* 2284
orbital, 2266
and papilledema, 516
pathology, 2253, *2253, 2254, 2265, 2266*
posterior fossa, 2261, 2263
radiation therapy for, 2282
retinal, *2266,* 2266–2268, *2267*
stereotactic radiosurgery for, 2282, 2284
supratentorial, 2257–2261, *2258, 2259, 2260, 2261*
surgical therapy for, 2279–2280
Arteritic anterior ischemic optic neuropathy, 571–572
Arteritic ischemic optic neuropathy, 5047–5048
Arteritic posterior ischemic optic neuropathy, 583–585, *585*
Arteritis, 3005, 3339–3340, *3340, 3341,* 3342, *3343,* 3344, *3345, 3346, 3347,* 3347–3348, 4028–4031, *4029*
giant cell, 3340, 3342, *3343,* 3424, 3755–3761, *3756, 3757, 3758, 3759, 3760*
demographics, 3755
diagnosis, 3775–3776, *3777, 3778,* 3778–3779, *3779, 3780*
headaches associated with, 1712
laboratory studies, 3772–3775, *3774*
neurologic manifestations, 3757–3758, *3758, 3759*
ocular and neuro-ophthalmologic manifestations, 3758–3761, *3760, 3761, 3762, 3763,* 3763–3769, *3764, 3765, 3766, 3767, 3768, 3769, 3771*
pathogenesis, 3769, 3771
pathology, 3771–3772, *3772, 3773, 3774*
systemic manifestations, *3756,* 3756–3757, *3757*
treatment and prognosis, 3779–3782
vasculitides other than, 578, *579,* 580, *580, 581, 582*
infectious, 3339–3340
Nissl-Alzheimer, 4912
noninfectious, 3340, 3342
Takayasu, 3012, 3342, *3344,* 3727, *3788,* 3788–3792, *3789, 3791,* 3792, *3793*
demographics, 3788
diagnosis, 3791–3792
history, 3788, *3788, 3789*
neurologic manifestations, 3789, *3791*
ocular manifestations, 3789–3790, *3791, 3792*
pathogenesis, 3790–3791
pathology, 3790, *3793*
systemic manifestations, 3789, *3790*
treatment and prognosis, 3792, *3793*
Artery of pterygoid canal, 2946
Artery-to-artery embolism, 3401
Arthralgia, 5288
Arthritides, 3725, 3845
juvenile rheumatoid arthritis, 3850–3852, *3852*
rheumatoid arthritis, 3845, *3846, 3847,* 3847–3850, *3848, 3849, 3850, 3851*
seronegative (HLA-B27-associated spondyloarthropathies), 3852
ankylosing spondylitis, 3852–3854, *3853*
arthritis with inflammatory bowel disease, 3857–3859, *3859, 3860, 3861, 3862, 3863*
Reiter's syndrome, *3854,* 3854–3857, *3855, 3856*
Arthritis, 4335, 5288
cervical, 1727
enteropathic, 3857–3859, *3859, 3860, 3861, 3862, 3863*
with inflammatory bowel disease, 3857–3859, *3859, 3860, 3861, 3862, 3863*
juvenile rheumatoid, 3850–3852, *3852*
psoriatic, 3857, *3857, 3858*
rheumatoid, 1735, 3845, *3846, 3847,* 3847–3850, *3848, 3849, 3850, 3851,* 5145
Arthroconidia, 4355
Arthrokinetic nystagmus, 1462, 1471
Arthropod envenomation, 1437–1438
Ascites, amoebic, 4620

Aseptic cavernous sinus thrombosis
  causes, 3898
  clinical manifestations, 3898
  prognosis, 3898
  treatment, 3898
Aseptic lateral sinus thrombosis, 3901–3902, *3902, 3903, 3904, 3905*
Aseptic meningitis, 2561, 4983, 5053, 5111, 5130–5131, 5146–5147, 5156, 5165, 5237–5238, 5241–5242, 5245, 5261
  OKT3 as cause of, 2628–2629
Aseptic thrombosis
  of internal jugular vein, 3927
  of superior sagittal sinus, *3907,* 3907–3910, *3908, 3909, 3910, 3911, 3912*
Aseptic venous occlusion, 3888–3890
Asperger syndrome, 420
Aspergillomas, 4287, 4290–4294, *4291, 4292, 4293*
  intracranial, 4292–4293, *4293*
Aspergillosis, 4281, 4286–4287, *4287,* 5421
  allergic, 4287–4290, *4288, 4289, 4290*
  clinical manifestations, 4287
    allergic, 4287–4290, *4288, 4289, 4290*
    aspergillomas, 4290–4294, *4291, 4292, 4293*
    invasive, 4294–4299, *4295, 4296, 4297, 4298, 4299, 4300, 4301,* 4301–4306, *4302, 4303, 4304, 4305, 4306, 4307, 4308,* 4308–4310, *4309, 4310, 4311,* 4312, *4312, 4313, 4314, 4315, 4316,* 4316–4317
  intraocular, 4297–4298
  invasive, 4294–4299, *4295, 4296, 4297, 4298, 4299, 4300, 4301,* 4301–4306, *4302,* 4302–4303, *4303, 4304, 4305, 4306, 4307, 4308,* 4308–4310, *4309, 4310, 4311,* 4312, *4312, 4313, 4314, 4315, 4316,* 4316–4317
  orbital, *4296, 4297,* 4298–4299
  treatment, 4317
Aspergillus, 4286–4287, *4287*
  clinical manifestations
    allergic, 4287–4290, *4288, 4289, 4290*
    aspergillomas, 4290–4294, *4291, 4292, 4293*
    invasive aspergillosis, 4294–4299, *4295, 4296, 4297, 4298, 4299, 4300, 4301,* 4301–4306, *4302, 4303, 4304, 4305*
  in endophthalmitis, 4295–4296
  in fungal aneurysms, 3003, 3971
  in intracranial brain abscess, 3952
  intraocular, 4297–4298
  invasive, 4302–4303, *4311,* 4312, *4312, 4313, 4314, 4315, 4316,* 4316–4317
  in meningitis, 4305, 4308–4309, *4313, 4314*
  orbital, *4296, 4297,* 4298–4299
  treatment, 4317
Aspergillus amstelodami, 4287
Aspergillus candidus, 4287
Aspergillus flavus, 4286
Aspergillus fumigatus, 4286, *4287,* 4289, 4290
  in fungal aneurysms, 3971
Aspergillus nidulans, 4287
Aspergillus niger, 4287
Aspergillus oryzae, 4287
Aspergillus restrictus, 4287
Aspergillus sydowi, 4287
Aspergillus terreus, 4287
Aspergillus ustus, 4287
Aspergillus versicolor, 4287
Aspiration of brain abscess, 3963
Aspirin, 1262, 3558
Associated cutaneous eruption, 5053–5055
Associative prosopagnosia, 416
Associative visual agnosia, 3485
Astereognosis, 1878
Asterixis, 1820
Asthenopia, retinal, 1731
Asthma, 4287, 5193
Astroblastomas, 1931, *1932*
Astrocytes, 7, 44
  fibrillary, 1865, 1920
  gemistocytic, 1921, *1921*
  in optic nerve, 65–66
  in optic nerve head, 58–59, *62*
  pilocytic, 1921, *1922*
  protoplasmic, 1920
Astrocytic hamartomas, 690, *691,* 2676, *2678, 2679, 2680*
Astrocytic tumors, 1920, *1921*
Astrocytomas, 1921–1922
  anaplastic, 1924–1925, *1925,* 2559
  of anterior visual pathways, 1941–1947, *1942, 1943, 1944, 1945, 1946, 1948, 1949, 1952, 1954, 1957, 1958, 1959*
  of brainstem, 1937–1939, *1938*
  of cerebellum, 1939–1941, *1940*
  of cerebral hemispheres, 1935–1936
  fibrillary, 1922
  granular cell, 1932–1933
  of hypothalamus, 1936–1937, *1937*
  infantile desmoplastic, 1933–1934
  pilocytic, *1930,* 1930–1931, *1931*
  and pineal gland, 1936–1937, *1937*
  protoplasmic, 1934–1935, *1935*
  of septum pellucidum, 1937
  subependymal giant-cell, 1935, 2687–2688, *2689, 2690*
  of third ventricle, 1936–1937, *1937*
Asymmetric papilledema, *498,* 498–499, *499, 500*
Asymptomatic arteriovenous malformations, natural history of, 2277
Asymptomatic carotid artery disease, prognosis of patients with, 3550–3552
Asymptomatic cervical bruit
  management of patients with, 3569–3570
  prognosis of patients with, 3550
Asymptomatic demyelinating optic neuritis, 620–622, *621, 622*
Asymptomatic neurocysticercosis, 4463
Asymptomatic neurosyphilis, 4882–4883
Asymptomatic optic neuritis, *5589,* 5589–5590, *5590*
Asymptomatic phase of HIV infection, 5369–5370
Ataxia, 1029, 4568, 5699. (*See also* Friedreich's ataxia.)
  acute cerebellar, 5016
  autosomal-dominant cerebellar, 762
  cerebellar, 1869, 1878, 2410
    with associated features, 2790
  congenital cerebellar, 2784–2785, *2785*
  familial paroxysmal, 1479–1480
  gait, 5568
  hereditary, 762–763
  late-onset inherited, 2790*t,* 2790–2795, *2791, 2793*
  Marie, 762
  metabolic, 2785–2786, *2786*
  optic, 445, 448, 451, *451, 452*
  spinocerebellar, 762, 763
  with vitamin E deficiency, 2786
Ataxia telangiectasia, 1292, 2721–2723, *2723, 2724,* 2725, 2786
  cutaneous manifestations, 2787, *2787*
  laboratory findings, 2787
  neurologic manifestations, 2786–2787
  neuro-ophthalmologic manifestations, 2787, *2787*
  pathology, 2786
  prognosis, 2787
  treatment, 2787
Ataxia-oculomotor apraxia syndrome of Aicardi, 1326
Ataxic hemiparesis, 3517
Atherogenesis, prominent feature of, 3334
Atheromatous emboli, 3424
Atherosclerosis
  distribution of, 3330, *3331,* 3332, *3333*
  factors predisposing to, 3329–3330
  of internal and external carotid arteries, 970
  pathology of, 3332, *3334*
  pathophysiology of, 3333–3335
  radiation-induced, 2611, *2611*
  as risk factor in aneurysms, 3012
ATM protein, 2721
Atresia, aural, 1564
Atrial fibrillation and risk of stroke, 3568
Atrophy
  olivopontocerebellar, 762, 1568
  optic, 1835, 1844, 1848, 2044
  postpapilledema, 494, *495, 496,* 496–497, *497, 498*
Atropine, 1001
Attention in Bálint's syndrome, 450
Attentional dyslexia, 433
Atypical facial neuralgia, *1741,* 1741–1743
Atypical mycobacteria, 4176–4177, 5420–5421
  Nocardia, 4189, 4189–4192, *4190, 4191*
  Tropheryma whippelii, 4180–4189, *4182, 4183, 4184, 4185, 4186, 4187, 4188*
Atypical teratomas, 2085
Audiokinetic nystagmus, 1462, 1471
Auditory agnosia, 1831
  verbal, 1831
Auditory evoked reflex blinks, 1530–1531, *1532*
Auditory hallucinations, 1831–1832
Auditory illusions, 1831
Auditory stimuli, nystagmus induced by, 1471
Aura, 3664
  migraine with prolonged, 3678–3681, *3679, 3680*
  neurologic, 3675–3677
  visual, *3665,* 3665–3675, *3666, 3667, 3668, 3669, 3672, 3673, 3674*
Aural atresia, 1564
Auscultation
  of cervical vessels, 3525
  of eyes, 3525
Australia antigen, 4962
Autoimmune diseases, 5373
Autoimmune optic neuritis, 630
Autoimmune polyendocrinopathy-candidiasis-ectodermal dystrophy (APECED), 4345–4346, *4347*
Automated perimetry, 157, 204
Autonomic dysfunction, 5573
Autonomic fibers, regeneration of, *843,* 843–844
Autonomic function, generalized disturbances of, 1026
  acute pandysautonomia, 1028–1029
  autonomic hyperreflexia, 1029
  congenital cholinergic nervous system dysfunction, 1027

congenital familial sensory neuropathy with anhidrosis, 1027
familial dysautonomia (Riley-Day) syndrome, 1026–1027
Fisher's syndrome (ophthalmoplegia, ataxia, and areflexia), 1029
hereditary anhidrotic ectodermal dysplasia, 1027
neural crest syndrome, 1027
primary acquired autonomic dysfunction (Shy-Drager syndrome), 1028
tonic pupils, areflexia, and progressive segmental hypohidrosis (Ross syndrome), 1027–1028
Autonomic hyperreflexia, 1029
Autonomic nervous system, 825
central levels of regulation
brainstem, 837
cerebellum, 828
hypothalamus
anatomy, 828–830, *829, 830, 831,* 832
fiber connections, *832,* 832–835, *834*
function, *835,* 835–837
neuromediators, 832
limbic system, 828, *829*
general considerations, 827–828
peripheral, 837–838
parasympathetic (craniosacral), 839–840, *840*
physiology of, 840
sympathetic (thoracolumbar), 838–839
pharmacology of
chemical transmission of impulses, 841–842
denervation supersensitivity, 842
neuromuscular junctions, *842,* 842–843
regeneration of fibers, *843,* 843–844
Autonomic neuromuscular junctions, *842,* 842–843
Autoregulation of cerebral blood flow, 2968–2969
Autosomal-dominant cerebellar ataxia, 762
Autosomal-dominant cerebellar ataxia type I
etiology, 2790–2791
laboratory and neuroimaging findings, 2792
neurologic manifestations, 2791–2792
neuro-ophthalmologic manifestations, 2792
pathology, 2791, *2791*
prognosis, 2792
treatment, 2792
Autosomal-dominant cerebellar ataxia type II, 2792
genetics, 2792
laboratory and neuroimaging features, 2792
neurologic manifestations, 2792
neuro-ophthalmologic manifestations, 2792, *2793*
prognosis, 2793
Autosomal-dominant cerebellar ataxia type III, 2793–2794
Autosomal-dominant progressive optic atrophy
with congenital deafness, 759
with progressive hearing loss and ataxia, 759
Autosomal-dominant spinocerebellar atrophy, 763
Autosomal-recessive optic atrophy with progressive hearing loss, spastic quadriplegia, mental deterioration, and death (opticocochleodentate degeneration), 760
Auxotyping, 4101
Avocalia, 1821–1822
Axial proptosis, 1799
Axons
anterograde (Wallerian, ascending) degeneration of, 280–281
degeneration, 2750
in optic nerve head, 58, *61, 62*
retrograde (descending) degeneration of, 281, *283,* 283–284
transport, 48–49
Azathioprine
for Lambert-Eaton myasthenic syndrome, 1437
for myasthenia gravis, 1427–1428
Azotemia as side effect of amphotericin B therapy, 4283
AZT, 5365

B

Babesia, 4642
clinical manifestations, 4644–4645
neurologic, 4645
systemic, 4645
diagnosis, 4645–4646
laboratory findings, 4645
life cycle, *4642,* 4642–4644, *4643, 4644*
pathology, 4644
treatment and prognosis, 4646
Babesiosis, 4642
clinical manifestations, 4644–4645
neurologic, 4645
systemic, 4645
diagnosis, 4645–4646
laboratory findings, 4645
life cycle, *4642,* 4642–4644, *4643, 4644*
pathology, 4644
treatment and prognosis, 4646
Bacillary angiomatosis, 4208
Bacillary dysentery, 4224–4225
Bacille Calmette-Guérin (BCG), 4167, *4168*
Bacillettes, 1993
Bacillus, 4065, *4066, 4067,* 4105–4107, *4106,* 4107–4109, *4109*
in bacterial meningitis, 3993–3994
Bacillus alvei, 4108
Bacillus anthracis, 4105–4107, *4106*
in bacterial meningitis, 3994
in meningitis, 4106
in vasogenic cervical edema, 3981
Bacillus cereus, 4108
in bacterial meningitis, 3993, 3994
Bacillus circulans, 4108
Bacillus licheniformis, 4108
Bacillus megaterium, 4108
Bacillus meningitis, 4108–4109
Bacillus pumilus, 4108
Bacillus sphaericus, 4108
Bacillus subtilis, 4108
Bacteremia, *Salmonella,* 4221, *4222*
Bacteria. (*See also* Gram-negative bacilli; Gram-negative cocci; Gram-positive bacilli; Gram-positive cocci.)
classification of, 4065–4066, *4066, 4067*
definition of, 4065
facultative, 4066
gram-negative, 4065–4066, *4066, 4067*
gram-positive, 4065–4066, *4066, 4067*
microaerophilic, 4066
response to oxygen, 4066–4067
Bacterial aneurysms, 2998–3003, *3000, 3001, 3002,* 3965–3969, *3966, 3968, 3969, 3970*
of basilar artery, 3111, 3113
Bacterial disease, 5415
optic neuritis from, 628–629
Bacterial encephalitis, 3986
Bacterial endocarditis, 3000, *3000, 3966,* 3966–3967, 4081
Bacterial meningitis, 3946, 4069–4070, *4070, 4071, 4076,* 4076–4077, *4077,* 5419–5421, *5420*
Bacterial meningoencephalitis, 4029
Bacterium tularense, 4228
Bacteroides, 4193–4195, *4194, 4195*
in empyema, 3983
in intracranial brain abscess, 3952
Bacteroides distasonis, 4194
Bacteroides fragilis, 4193, *4195*
in bacterial meningitis, 3993
in intracranial brain abscess, 3955
Bacteroides intermedius, 4194–4195
Bacteroides melaninogenicus, 4195, 4218
Bailey-Lovie chart, 160
Balamuthia mandrillaris, 4638, *4639, 4640,* 4640–4641, *4641*
Bálint's syndrome, 445–446, 1324–1325, 1519, 2752, 3487, 3489–3490, 3492, 5138, 5413
attention in, 450
critique of classic cases, *448,* 448–450
and cyclosporine, 2634
historical review, 446–448
Balloon angioplasty for delayed cerebral ischemia, 3172, *3173*
Balloon occlusion, 3152–3153
Baló's concentric sclerosis, 5539
Bannwarth's disease, 4783
Bannwarth's syndrome, 4794–4795
Barlow's syndrome, 3390–3391
Bartonella, 4196
Basal cell carcinomas of skin, *2457,* 2457–2458
Basal cell nevus syndrome, 2735
Basal cisterns, 2020, *2021*
Basal epithelial nerve plexus, 1598
Basal ganglia
abscesses of, 3957
blepharospasm associated with lesions in, 1568–1569
ocular motor abnormalities and disease of, 1316
Huntington's disease, 1318–1319
Parkinson's disease, 1316–1318, *1318*
projections, *1519,* 1519–1520
in saccadic eye movements, 1120
tumors involving, *1861,* 1861–1865, *1862, 1864*
Basal tear secretion, 955
Basal vein (of Rosenthal), 2951, *2952*
Basement membrane, 900–901
Basilar arteries
aneurysms arising from, 3111, 3113, *3114, 3115, 3116,* 3116–3122, *3117, 3118, 3119, 3120, 3121*
dissecting aneurysms of, 3216–3218, *3217, 3218, 3219, 3220,* 3220*t, 3221,* 3221–3223
and its branches, *2910,* 2911–2914, *2912, 2913, 2914, 2915, 2916,* 2916–2917, *2918, 2919, 2920,* 2920–2922, *2921, 2922, 2923, 2924, 2925, 2926, 2927, 2928,* 2928–2929, *2929, 2930, 2931,* 2931–2932, *2932, 2933, 2934, 2935, 2936, 2937*
fusiform aneurysm of, *3198,* 3198–3199, *3199, 3200, 3201,* 3201–3203, *3202, 3203*

Basilar artery dolichoectasia, 3202
Basilar artery migraine, 3681
Basilar sinus, 2964
Basophil adenomas, 2152
Basophils, 2329
Bassen-Kornzweig disease, 2785–2786, *2786,* 2851–2852
Baylisascaris procyonis, 4528, *4530,* 4531
BCNU and radiation therapy, 2596
Bean's syndrome, 2235
Behçet's disease, 631, 3346, 3802–3803, 3888
  clinical manifestations, 3803–3808, *3804, 3805, 3806, 3807*
  demographics, 3803
  diagnosis, 3809, 3811
  pathogenesis, 3808–3809
  pathology, 3808, *3810*
  treatment and prognosis, 3811
Behçet's syndrome, 523
Behr's syndrome, 761–762
Bejel, 4844, 4850, *4852,* 4853, *4853, 4854*
Belladonna alkaloids, 1001
Bell's palsy, 1562, 1563, 4982
  diagnosis of, 1563
  treatment of, 1563–1564
Bell's phenomenon, 1176, 5703
  and eye movements associated with blinking, 1535–1536
Bence Jones proteinuria, 2390
Benedikt's syndrome, 1199–1200, 1873
Benign anisocoria, 884–885
Benign childhood epilepsy with occipital spikewaves, 463
Benign cough headache, 1702–1703, *1703*
Benign essential blepharospasm, 1537
Benign exertional headache, 1703–1704, *1704*
Benign paroxysmal torticollis, 3698
Benign paroxysmal vertigo in migraine, 3697–3698
Benign recurrent meningitis, 5721
Benton Facial Recognition Test (BFRT), 413, 416
Benton Visual Retention Test (BVRT), 470
Benton Visual Retention Test—revised (BVRT-revised), 470, *471*
Benzodiazepines for tetanus, 4115
Bergmeister's papilla, 6, *9*
Beriberi, 669
Berry aneurysms, 2977
Beta effect, 2595
Bifurcation of retinal ganglion cell axons, 49–50
Bilateral, simultaneous, light-induced transient visual loss, 3421, *3422*
Bilateral abducens nerve paresis, 4373, 5087, 5248
Bilateral adrenalectomy, 2197
Bilateral anterior optic neuritis, 4116
Bilateral carpal tunnel syndrome, 5147
Bilateral cerebral ptosis, 3466, *3467*
Bilateral ''checkerboard'' altitudinal hemianopia, 300, 302, *302*
Bilateral chorioretinitis, 5235
Bilateral conjugate downbeat nystagmus, 3501
Bilateral cortical ptosis, *1538,* 1539
Bilateral cryptococcosis, 710
Bilateral dolichoectasia, 3188
Bilateral dyschromatopsia, 674–675
Bilateral hilar adenopathy, 5511, *5511*
  associated with pulmonary infiltration, 5511, *5512,* 5514
Bilateral hilar lymphadenopathy, 5480
Bilateral homonymous hemianopia, 357, *359,* 360
Bilateral horizontal gaze paresis, 5603
Bilateral inferior hemianopia, *299,* 300, *300, 301*
Bilateral internal ophthalmoplegia, 5023
Bilateral internuclear ophthalmoplegia, 4375
Bilateral intracavernous aneurysms, 3041
Bilateral lesions of optic nerves, 298, *299,* 300, *300*
  superior or inferior (altitudinal) hemianopia, *299,* 300, *300, 301*
Bilateral nasal hemianopia, 302–304, *303, 304, 305, 306, 307*
Bilateral nonsimultaneous homonymous hemianopia, 360
Bilateral occipital lobe disease, *359,* 361, *362, 363, 364*
Bilateral optic nerve gliomas, 1951
Bilateral optic neuritis, 5248
Bilateral optic neuropathy, 2582, 5184
Bilateral ptosis, 4117
Bilateral punctate keratitis, 5207
Bilateral pupillary dilation, 4373
Bilateral retinal necrosis, 5091
Bilateral retrobulbar optic neuritis, 4552
Bilateral simultaneous visual loss, 3426
Bilateral striate ablation, 1126
Bilateral subacute progressive optic neuropathy, 2561
Bilateral superior hemianopia, *299,* 300, *300, 301*
Bilateral tonic pupils, 5145
Bilateral toxic optic neuropathy, 4142
Bilateral trigeminal neuropathy, 5248
Bilateral vestibular schwannomas, 2667
Bilateral visual field loss, 2171
Binary fission, 4613
Binocular diplopia, 1169, 3673, 3694
Binocular vision, 117–118
  loss of, 3337–3338
Binocularity, 132–133
Binswanger's disease, 3518
Biologic response modifiers, 2589–2592
  neuro-ophthalmologic toxicity, 2591–2592
  neurotoxicity, 2590, *2590*
  ocular toxicity, 2590–2591, *2591*
  systemic toxicity, 2589
Biomicroscopy, slitlamp, in diagnosing traumatic optic neuropathy, 720
Biopsy
  conjunctival, 5523, *5527*
  in diagnosing cylindromas, 2454
  transbronchial, 4140
Biotin-responsive opsoclonus, 1497
Bipolar cells, *38,* 39–40, *40, 41*
Bipolaris species, 4290
Birdshot retinochoroidopathy, 631
Bitemporal hemianopia, 706, 756, 1794, 2171
  from optic chiasmal ischemia, 3692–3693
Bitemporal visual field defects, 2168, 3467, *3469,* 3764–3765
Bjerrum screen, *175,* 175–176, *176*
BK virus, *5132,* 5132–5133
Black eschars and discharge, formation of, 4330, *4331*
Blastomyces dermatitidis, 4282, 4332, *4333*
  acute pulmonary, 4333, *4335*
  clinical manifestations, 4333
    acute pulmonary blastomycosis, 4333, *4335*
    central nervous system blastomycosis, 4336–4338, *4338*
    chronic pulmonary blastomycosis, 4333
    cutaneous blastomycosis, 4333–4334, *4336, 4337*
    extrapulmonary blastomycosis, 4333
    genitourinary tract blastomycosis, 4335–4336
    ocular and orbital blastomycosis, 4338, *4339–4340, 4341,* 4341–4342, *4342*
    paranasal sinus blastomycosis, 4338
    skeletal blastomycosis, 4334–4335
  demographics, 4332
  diagnosis, 4342, *4343*
  in intracranial brain abscess, 3952
  pathophysiology, 4333, *4334*
  treatment, 4342–4343
Blastomycosis, 4282, 4332, *4333,* 5421
  acute pulmonary, 4333, *4335*
  central nervous system, 4336–4338, *4338*
  chronic pulmonary, 4333
  clinical manifestations, 4333
  cutaneous, 4333–4334, *4336, 4337*
  demographics, 4332
  extrapulmonary, 4333
  genitourinary tract, 4335–4336
  ocular, 4338, *4339–4340, 4341,* 4341–4342, *4342*
  orbital, 4338, *4339–4340, 4341,* 4341–4342, *4342*
  paranasal sinus, 4338
  pathophysiology, 4333, *4334*
  skeletal, 4334–4335
  treatment, 4342–4343
Blastomycotic meningitis, 4337–4338, *4338*
Blastoschizomyces capitatus, 4282, 4343, *4344*
Blastoschizomycosis, 4282, 4343, *4344*
Bleeding disorders as cause of intracerebral hemorrhage, 3584–3585, *3585*
Bleomycin, 2580
Blepharoclonus, 1569
Blepharocolysis, 1539
Blepharophimosis, 783
Blepharoplasts, 1963
Blepharoplegia, 5730, *5730*
Blepharoptosis. (*See* Ptosis.)
Blepharospasm, 1565–1568, 1784, 1785, 2560, 2580, 4113, 4887, 5730, *5730*
  associated with drug-induced tardive dyskinesia, 1569–1570
  associated with lesions of brainstem and basal ganglia, 1568–1569
  benign essential, 1537
  cause of, 1566–1567
  essential, 1565, *1566*
  nonorganic, 1570
  ocular, 1569
  reflex, 1569
    stretch, 1569
Blind spot, 256, *258,* 259
Blindness. (*See also* Cortical blindness; Cerebral blindness.)
  caused by retinal emboli, 3383, *3383,* 3385
  monocular, 2257
Blindsight
  in nonhuman primates, 400–402, *402*
  relation to nonstriate visual areas in human, 147–148
  and residual vision
    discrimination of color, 395–396
    discrimination of form, 395, *397*
    effects of training, 398, *398, 399*
    in hemidecorticate patients, 397–398, *398*
    localization of targets, *392,* 392–395, *393, 394, 395, 396, 397*
    in nonhuman primates, 400–402, *402*

Blinking
basic pattern and eyelid movements, 1523–1526, *1524*
Bell's phenomena and eye movements associated with, 1535–1536
movement in, 1509
reflex, *8,* 1523, 1526, 1653–1656
auditory evoked reflex, 1530–1531, *1532*
excitability of trigeminal, and spasms of lid closure, 1529–1530, *1531, 1532*
from stimulation of cornea, 1529, *1530*
trigeminal reflex, *1526,* 1526–1529, *1527,* 1527*t, 1528*
visual evoked, 1531–1532
spontaneous, 1523, 1532–1533
from stimulation of cornea, 1529, *1530*
trigeminal reflex, *1526,* 1526–1529, *1527,* 1527*t, 1528*
voluntary, 1523
Blink-saccade synkinesis, 1534–1535, *1535*
Block design tasks, 471
Blood flow velocity, measurement of, 3923–3924
Blood vessels
in ciliary body, 905
hamartomas of, 2230
arteriovenous malformations, 2252
associations, 2274–2275
clinical manifestations, 2256–2261, *2258, 2259, 2260, 2261, 2262, 2263,* 2263–2274, *2264, 2265, 2266, 2267, 2268, 2269, 2270, 2271, 2272, 2273*
diagnosis of, 2275, *2276*
embryogenesis, 2252–2253
incidence, 2253, 2255
natural history of, 2275–2280, *2280, 2281,* 2282, *2283,* 2284
pathology, 2253, *2253, 2254, 2265, 2266*
capillary telangiectases, 2230–2231, *2231, 2232,* 2233, *2233*
cavernous angiomas
intracranial, *2233,* 2233–2236, *2234, 2235, 2236, 2237,* 2238, *2238, 2239, 2241, 2242,* 2242–2244, *2243*
orbital, *2243, 2244,* 2244–2245
retinal, *2245,* 2245–2246
venous angiomas, 2246, *2247, 2248, 2249, 2250,* 2250–2252, *2251, 2252*
in optic nerve, 59, 61–62, *63, 64*
retinal, 51–54, *52, 53*
tumors of
hemangioblastomas, 2223–2226, *2224, 2225, 2226, 2227,* 2228
hemangiopericytomas, *2228,* 2228–2230, *2229*
Blood viscosity and cerebral blood flow, 2969
Blood-brain barrier (BBB), 2553
to infection, 3942
of optic nerve head, 59
and vasogenic edema, 3942, *3942*
Blood-CSF barrier to infection, 3942
Blood-flow mechanism as cause of arteriovenous malformations, 3009
Blood-retinal barrier, 53, 2554, 2556
Bloody tears, 1785
Bloom's syndrome, 2336
Blue-rubber-bleb-nevus-syndrome, 2235, *2733, 2734,* 2735
Blurred vision, 1170
B-lymphocytes, 2329, 2330
B-mode ultrasonographic scanners, *3534,* 3534–3535
Bobbing
converse ocular, 3512
inverse ocular, 3512
ocular, 3511
reverse, 3511–3512
Bobble-head doll syndrome, 2122
Body dysmorphic disorder, 1766
Bone cartilage, tumors of, 2437
benign, 2442–2444, *2443, 2444, 2445*
chordomas, 2437–2442, *2438, 2439,* 2440, *2441, 2442*
Bone lesions in cryptococcosis, 4381–4382, *4383*
Bone marrow, 2330
Bone marrow transplantation
neuro-ophthalmologic complications, 2634–2635, *2636*
ocular complications, 2632, *2633,* 2634, *2634, 2635, 2636*
systemic complications, 2626
cerebrovascular disease, 2631–2632, *2632*
general, 2626
immunosuppression, 2626–2627
neurologic infections, 2630
neurologic malignancy, 2630–2631
neurotoxicity, 2627–2630, *2628, 2629, 2630*
Bone metastatic tumors, 2477, *2480*
Bonnet, Charles, syndrome, 456
Bonnet-Dechaume-Blanc syndrome, 2725
Bony abnormalities, role of radiation therapy in, 2597
Bordetella, 4208–4211
Bordetella avium, 4208
Bordetella bronchiseptica, 4208–4209
Bordetella parapertussis, 4208, *4209,* 4209–4210
Bordetella pertussis, 4208, *4209,* 4209–4210
in bacterial encephalitis, 3986
Bornholm disease, 5235
Borrelia, 4779, *4780, 4782*
in Lyme disease, 4779–4780, 4783
arthritis, 4809, *4810*
cardiac manifestations, 4789, *4789*
chronic disseminated, 4808–4818, *4810, 4811, 4812, 4813, 4814, 4815, 4816, 4817, 4818*
clinical course, 4787
clinical manifestations, 4786–4787
cutaneous manifestations, 4787, *4788,* 4788–4789, *4789,* 4809–4810, *4810*
diagnosis, 4820, 4822, *4822, 4823, 4824,* 4824–4825, *4825, 4826, 4827,* 4827–4828
early disseminated, 4787–4791, *4789, 4790, 4792, 4793,* 4793–4797, *4794, 4796, 4797, 4798, 4799,* 4799–4803, *4800, 4801, 4802, 4803, 4804,* 4805, *4805, 4806, 4807,* 4807–4808, *4808, 4809*
early localized, 4787
epidemiology, 4783–4786, *4784, 4785*
neurologic manifestations, 4787, 4789–4791, *4790, 4792, 4793,* 4793–4795, *4794, 4796,* 4810–4816, *4811, 4812, 4813, 4814, 4815, 4816*
neuro-ophthalmologic manifestations, 4800–4803, *4802, 4803, 4804,* 4805, *4805, 4806,* 4807–4808, *4808, 4809,* 4816–4818, *4817, 4818*
ocular manifestations, 4787, 4795–4797, *4796, 4798, 4799,* 4799–4800, *4800, 4801, 4816,* 4816–4818, *4817, 4818*
pathogen, 4786
pathogenesis, 4818–4820
pathology, 4820, *4820, 4821*
prevention, *4831,* 4831–4832
seronegative, 4828–4829
systemic manifestations, 4787
treatment, 4829–4831
in lymphocytoma, 4788–4789, *4789*
in relapsing fever, 4832
clinical manifestations, 4833–4834
diagnosing, *4834,* 4834–4835
epidemiology, *4832,* 4832–4833, *4833*
pathogenesis, 4833
prevention, 4836
treatment and prognosis, 4835, *4835, 4836*
Borrelia burgdorferi, 3339, 5721
in chronic basal meningitis, 4030–4031, *4032*
Boston Diagnostic Aphasia Examination (BDAE), 436, 445, 471
Boston Naming Test, 470
Botryomycosis, 4085, *4085*
Botulinum antitoxin, 4120
Botulinum toxin
for eyelid and facial spasms, 1577–1580
for nystagmus, 1498
Botulinum toxin blocks, 1002
Botulinum toxin type A for blepharospasm, 1568
Botulism, 999, 1013, 1438–1440, *1439,* 4109, 4117, *4118, 4119,* 4119–4123, 4120–4121, *4122*
clinical manifestations, 4117, *4118,* 4119, *4119*
diagnosis, 4119–4120
in food poisoning, 4117
clinical manifestations, 4117, *4118,* 4119, *4119*
diagnosis, 4119–4120
treatment, 4120
infant, 4117, *4118, 4119,* 4119–4123, 4120–4121, *4122*
clinical manifestations, 4117, *4118,* 4119, *4119*
diagnosis, 4119–4120
in neuritis, 4026
treatment, 4120
in vasogenic cervical edema, 3981
in neuritis, 4026
treatment, 4120
unclassified, 4122–4123
in vasogenic cervical edema, 3981
wound, 4117, 4121–4122, *4122*
Boutonneuse fever, *4748,* 4748–4751, *4749, 4750, 4751*
Bovine spongiform encephalopathy, 4567
and Creutzfeldt-Jakob disease, 4579–4580
Bowman's membrane, 1598–1599
Brachial plexitis, 5147
Brachial plexopathy, 2607–2609
Brachytherapy, 2595
Bradykinin and optic nerve injury, *727,* 727–728
Bradyzoites, 4667

Brain
agents to increase viability, 3562
arterial system of. (*See* Arterial system of brain.)
extra-axial tumors at base of, 1887–1890, *1888, 1889, 1890, 1891, 1892,* 1893
local infiltration of parenchyma, 1928
microangiopathy of, *3732,* 3732–3734, *3733*
Brain abscesses, 4090, 4108
Brucella species in, 4214
papilledema from, 516
Pasteurella in, 4240
Pseudomonas in, 4242
Serratia marcescens in, 4224
Brain damage, patients with, 391–392
Brainstem, 837
abscesses of, 3957, 3959
afferent, 1624, *1627,* 1627–1628
astrocytomas of, 1937–1939, *1938*
generation of horizontal saccades, 1110–1111, *1111*
generation of smooth pursuit, 1132–1134, *1133*
generation of vertical and torsional saccades, 1111–1113, *1112*
gliomas of, 2659–2660
hematomas, 3611
hemorrhage, 3597–3598
immediate premotor structures of, 1080–1082, *1081*
insufficiency of eyelid closure caused by disorders of, 1560
intrinsic tumors of, 1871–1875, *1872, 1874, 1876, 1877,* 1877–1878
involvement of trigeminal pathways in, 1677–1678
lesions of medulla, *1678,* 1678–1680, *1679*
lesions in, 1018
blepharospasm associated with, 1568–1569
ocular motor dysfunction from damage to, 2619
projections and eyelid control, 1520, 1520*t*
and spinal cord inhibition of pupillary constriction, 879
and spinal cord sympathetic pathways, 879
veins in, 2953
Brainstem auditory evoked potentials (BAEPs), 749, 5626
Brainstem encephalitis, 2498–2500, *2500*
Branch artery occlusion, 3759, *3761*
Branch retinal artery occlusion (BRAO), *3446, 3447,* 3447–3450, *3448,* 5023
Branch retinal vein occlusion (BRVO), 3925–3926, *3926*
Branchiomeric paragangliomas, 2464–2468, *2466, 2467, 2468, 2469, 2470,* 2470–2471
Branhamella catarrhalis, 4103
in meningitis, 4103
Bridging veins, 2953
Brightness, representation of, in striate cortex, 128
Brightness comparison test, 944–945
Brill-Zinsser disease, 4755
Bromocriptine
for pituitary adenomas, 2191–2192, 2194–2195, 2196, 2199
teratogenic effects of, 2203
Bromodeoxyuridine
ocular toxicity, 2563
hydroxyurea, 2563
systemic toxicity, 2563
Bromodeoxyuridine (BUdR) labeling index, 2028
Bronchiolitis obliterans as side effect of amphotericin B therapy, 4283
Bronchopulmonary disease, 4287
Brood capsules, 4445
Brown's syndrome, 3849
Brown-Sequard syndrome, 2605, 3822
Brucella, 4211–4214, *4212, 4214*
in bacterial encephalitis, 3986
in empyema, 3983
Brucella abortus, 4211
in bacterial meningitis, 3994
Brucella canis, 4211
Brucella melitensis, 4211
Brucella ovis, 4211
Brucella suis, 4211
Bruch's membrane, 900–901
Brudzinski sign, 4201
Bruit, 3050, 3277–3278
Bruns' nystagmus, 1294, 1480, 2311
Bruns' syndrome, 1887, 4467
Buboes, 4226, 4227
Bubonic plague, *4226,* 4226–4227, *4227*
Budding, 4282, 4613
Buds, 4282
Buildup neurons, 1115
Bulbar paralysis, 5245
Bulbar paralytic poliomyelitis, 5255–5256
Bunyaviridae, 5158, *5159*
bunyaviruses, 5158–5162
characteristics of, 5159–5160, *5160*
clinical manifestations, 5160–5161
diagnosis, 5161
epidemiology of, 5160, *5161*
pathology, 5161, *5162*
prevention, 5162
treatment, 5161
phlebovirus, *5163,* 5163–5165, *5164*
Bunyaviruses, 5158–5162
characteristics of, 5159–5160, *5160*
clinical manifestations, 5160–5161
diagnosis, 5161
epidemiology of, 5160, *5161*
pathology, 5161, *5162*
prevention, 5162
treatment, 5161
Burian-Allen contact lens electrode, 218
Burkitt's lymphoma, 2375–2378, *2376, 2377*
Burst neurons, 1109–1110, *1110, 1111, 1112, 1113, 1114,* 1115, *1115, 1116, 1117, 1119, 1121, 1122,* 1122–1123
Busulfan
neurotoxicity, 2566
ocular toxicity, 2566
systemic toxicity, 2566
Butterfly rash, 3813, *3813*
B-VAT vision tester, 161
Bystander effect, 5682

C

Cabergoline, 2192
Cachectic myopathy, 2530–2531
Café-au-lait spots, *2648,* 2648–2649, *2670,* 2675–2676
Caffeine and headaches, 1719
Cajal, interstitial nucleus of, 1308, 1310
Calabar swelling, 4503, 4505
Calcarine artery, 2931–2932
Calcinosis, Raynaud's phenomenon, esophageal motility abnormalities, sclerodactyly, and telangiectatic lesions, 3014
Calciosomes, 728
Calcium, 1005–1006
and optic nerve injury, 728–729
Calcium emboli, 3372–3373, *3374, 3375, 3376*
Calcium-channel blockers
for delayed cerebral ischemia, 3171–3172
and headaches, 1718
Calculi, urinary, 5257
California encephalitis, 5158–5162
characteristics of, 5159–5160, *5160*
clinical manifestations, 5160–5161
diagnosis, 5161
epidemiology of, 5160, *5161*
pathology, 5161, *5162*
prevention, 5162
treatment, 5161
Callosal disconnection syndrome, 5574
Callosomarginal artery, 2897
Caloric irrigation, 1175
Caloric stimulation, peripheral vestibular nystagmus induced by, 1471–1472
Caloric testing, 1175–1176
Campylobacter, 4214–4217, *4215, 4216*
Campylobacter fetus, 4215, 4216–4217
Campylobacter fetus intestinalis, 4215
Campylobacter jejuni, 4215–4216, *4216*
in neuritis, 4026
Campylobacter jejuni infection, 5678–5679, 5695–5696, 5704, 5705
Canaliculitis, 4178
Canalolithiasis, 1470–1471
Canavan's disease, 766
Cancer. (*See also* Carcinoma.)
cone dysfunction associated with, 2537
and Epstein-Barr virus infection, 5091
hepatocellular, 4972
retinopathy associated with, 219, 2533, *2534, 2535,* 2535–2537, *2536, 2537*
Candida, 4282, 4343, *4345,* 5421
clinical manifestations, 4345
deep organ involvement, 4346–4349, *4348, 4349, 4350,* 4351–4352, *4352*
disseminated candidiasis, 4352–4353
mucocutaneous candidiasis, 4345–4346, *4347*
in cystitis, 4348
in endocarditis, 4347
in fungal aneurysms, 3003
in intracranial aneurysms, 3971
in intracranial brain abscess, 3952
in meningitis, 4349, 4351
in myocarditis, 4347
pathology, 4344, *4346*
pathophysiology, 4343–4344
in pneumonia, 4346–4347
treatment, 4353
in vaginitis, 4347
Candida albicans, 4343
Candida albicans infections, 2627
Candida parapsilosis endophthalmitis, 4353
Candidiasis, 4281, 4282, 4343, *4345*
cardiac, 4347
central nervous system, 4348–4349, *4350,* 4351–4352, *4352*
clinical manifestations, 4345
deep organ involvement, 4346–4349, *4348, 4349, 4350,* 4351–4352, *4352*
disseminated candidiasis, 4352–4353

mucocutaneous candidiasis, 4345–4346, *4347*
in endocarditis, 4347
in intracranial aneurysms, 3971
in intracranial brain abscess, 3952
in meningitis, 4349, 4351
mucocutaneous, 4345–4346, *4347*
ocular, 4348, *4348, 4349*
pathology, 4344, *4346*
pathophysiology, 4343–4344
respiratory tract, 4346–4347
treatment, 4353
urinary tract, 4347–4348
in vaginitis, 4347
vascular, 4348
Candle wax drippings, 5491
Capillary hemangiomas, 691–694, *692, 693, 694*
Capillary telangiectases, 2230–2231, *2231, 2232,* 2233, *2233*
Capnocytophaga, 4245
Capsaicin cream in herpes zoster, 5080–5081
Capsid, 4946, *4951*
Capsomeres, 4946
Capsular arteries, 2876–2877
Capsulopalpebral fascia, 1512–1513
Carbachol, 1005
Carbamazepine
for neuromyotonia, 2532
for trigeminal neuralgia, 1737–1738
Carbohydrate and lipid metabolism, myopathies resulting from errors in, 1405
Carbon monoxide and headaches, 1719
Carbon tetrachloride, 1262
Carboplatin, 2578
Carcinoma. (*See also* Cancer.)
adenoid cystic, 2453–2457, *2454, 2455, 2456*
basal cell skin, *2457,* 2457–2458
embryonal, 2091–2092, *2092*
nasopharyngeal, 2444–2450, *2446, 2447, 2449, 2450*
ophthalmoplegia with acute necrotizing myopathy and, 1397
pituitary, *2205,* 2205–2206
renal cell, 2690
squamous cell skin, *2457,* 2457–2458
Carcinomatosis, meningeal, 700–701, 701, 2485–2488, *2486, 2487,* 3351
Carcinomatous meningitis, 701, 2485–2488, *2486, 2487*
Carcinomatous neuromyopathy, 2524
Cardiac candidiasis, 4347
Cardiac disease
as cause of decreased cerebral perfusion, 3407
as cause of embolism, 3386–3396, *3389, 3390, 3391, 3392, 3393, 3394, 3395, 3396, 3397,* 3398, *3398, 3399, 3400,* 3400–3406, *3401, 3402, 3403, 3404, 3405, 3406*
Cardiac function, tests of, 3546, 3548–3549, *3549*
Cardiac migraine, 3699
Cardiac tumors, 3396, 3398, 3400, *3401*
Cardiac valvular disease, 3816
Cardiobacterium, 4245
Cardiobacterium hominis in bacterial aneurysms, 2999
Cardiomegaly, 2158
Cardiomyopathies, 3396, *3400*
Cardiovascular syphilis, *4881,* 4881–4884
Caroticotympanic artery, 2871
Carotid arterial system transient ischemic attacks, 3427
symptoms of, 3419–3426, *3421, 3422, 3425, 3426*
Carotid arteries. (*See also* External carotid arteries; Interior carotid arteries; Internal carotid arteries.)
atherosclerosis of internal and external, 970
collateral circulation with occlusion of
common, 3417
internal, 3414–3415, *3416*
disease in, 585–586
extracranial pseudoaneurysms of, 3038
generalized disease of, 3518–3519
right common, 2869
right internal and external, 2869
theory of distention and pulsation of external, as cause of migraine headaches, 3703–3704
Carotid bifurcation aneurysms, 3085
Carotid body paragangliomas, 2465–2468, *2468*
Carotid endarterectomy, 3575
headache after, 1713–1714
Carotid siphon, 2877
collateral channels to, 3415–3416
Carotid-cavernous sinus fistulas, *3263, 3264, 3265, 3266*
direct, 3263
anatomy, 3263–3264, *3267*
diagnosis, 3284–3285, *3286*
natural history, 3285–3287
nonocular manifestations, 3268–3269
ocular manifestations, 3269, *3269, 3270, 3271, 3272, 3273, 3274,* 3275, *3275, 3276, 3277,* 3277–3284, *3278, 3279, 3280, 3281, 3282, 3283*
pathogenesis, 3264, 3266–3268, *3268*
prognosis after treatment, 3292–3293, *3293, 3294, 3295, 3296*
treatment, *3287,* 3287–3292, *3288, 3289, 3290, 3291*
dural
anatomy, 3297–3298
clinical manifestations, 3298–3306, *3303, 3304, 3305, 3306, 3307, 3308*
diagnosis, 3306–3307, *3308,* 3309
natural history, 3309, *3310, 3311*
pathogenesis, 3298, *3299*
prognosis after treatment, 3315–3316, *3316, 3317,* 3318
treatment, 3309–3312, *3313, 3314,* 3315
Carotid-choroidal aneurysms, 3084, *3085, 3086*
Carotid-opthalmic aneurysms, *3059,* 3059–3060, *3060, 3061, 3062,* 3062–3063, *3063, 3064, 3065,* 3065–3066, *3066, 3067*
Carotidynia, 1708
Carpal-tunnel syndrome, 2158
Cataracts, 989, 1366, 3837, 5292, *5295, 5296*
post bone marrow transplantation, 2632
central posterior, 2667
formation of, 1997
peripheral wedge-shaped, 2667
posterior subcapsular, 2667
Catecholamine, excessive output, 4112
Cat-like (elliptic) pupils, 1006
Cat-scratch disease, *4196,* 4196–4208, *4197, 4198,* 4199, *4200, 4201, 4202, 4203,* 4204, *4205, 4206,* 5721
clinical manifestations, 4199–4200
diagnosis, 4207
epidemiology, 4199
etiology, 4196–4199, *4201*
neurologic manifestations, *4201,* 4201–4202
neuro-ophthalmologic manifestations, 4202–4207, *4204, 4205, 4206*
ocular manifestations, 4202, *4202, 4203*
systemic manifestations, 4200–4201
treatment, 4207–4208
Cat-scratch encephalopathy, *4201,* 4201–4202
Cat-scratch fever, 637
Caudate hemorrhage, 3594, *3594*
Caudate nucleus, 1862
Cavernous angiomas, 2235
extraparenchymal, 2236
intracranial, *2233,* 2233–2236, *2234, 2235, 2236,* 2236–2237, *2237,* 2238, *2238, 2239, 2240, 2241, 2242,* 2242–2244, *2243*
orbital, *2243, 2244,* 2244–2245
retinal, *2245,* 2245–2246
Cavernous hemangiomas, 691–694, *692, 693, 694*
Cavernous segment of internal carotid artery, *2873,* 2873–2874, *2874, 2875, 2876*
Cavernous sinus, 2962–2964, *2963, 2964*
aneurysms of, 3018
dural arteriovenous malformations (AVMs) of, *2270,* 2270–2273, *2271, 2272, 2273,* 2278
headaches in, 1709
meningiomas in, 2031, *2032, 2033, 2034,* 2034–2036, *2035*
oculomotor nerve involvement in, 1215, *1216, 1217*
septic thrombosis of, 4034–4039, *4035, 4036, 4037, 4038,* 4305
and superior orbital fissure syndromes, 1212–1215, *1214*
thrombosis of, 1709, 3894–3898, *3896, 3897*
tumors in, 1804–1805, *1805, 1806,* 1807, *1807, 1808, 1809*
Cavum septi pellucidi, 2125
CCNU and radiation therapy, 2596
CD4 + T-cell quantitation, 5380–5381
Cecocentral scotomas, 602
Celiac disease, ocular myopathy associated with, 1405
Cell-mediated immunity, 4137, 5371–5372
Cell-mediated inflammation and optic nerve injury, 729
Cells
aII, 41
amacrine, *38,* 40–42, *42, 43*
bipolar, *38,* 39–40, *40, 41*
cone, 39–40
rod, 39
clump, 855
complex, 130–131
dural border, 2017
end-stopped, *130,* 130–131, *131*
foam, 3332
gaze velocity Purkinje, 1132
glial, 43–44
horizontal, 36, *38,* 39
hypercomplex, *130,* 130–131, *131*
interdigitating, 2404
intermediate dendritic, 2404
interplexiform, 42–43
Kupffer, 2329, 2403

Cells—*continued*
Langerhans, 2404
lining, 2404
lymphoid stem, 2329
magnocellular, 46, 47
mast, 855
mesangial, 2403–2404
microglial, 2404
motion-sensitive, 130–131
Müller, *38*, 43–44, *44*
myeloid stem, 2329
neuroglial, 1919, 1920
parasol, 46, 47
parvocellular, 46
plasma, 2329, 2330
pluripotential stem, 2329
Reed-Sternberg, 2352, 2356
number and appearance of, 2351
origin of, 2351
retinal ganglion, 107–108
anatomy and physiology of, *45*, 45–48, *46*, 47*t*, *48*, *49*
sézary, 2386
simple, 130
true pursuit, 1129
W-, 48
Cellulitis, 4035
orbital, 1725, 3945–3946, *3947*, 4035
as cause of brain abscess, 3945–3946, *3947*
as cause of septic cavernous sinus thrombosis, 3894–3895
peritonsillar, 4085
Central achromatopsia. (*See* Cerebral achromatopsia.)
Central anisocoria, 962
Central core myopathy, 1354
Central dazzle, 2177, 3484
Central disorders of visual function, 387–388
acquired alexia, 424, *425*, 437
with agraphia, 431
anatomy, pathology, and mechanisms of pure, *426*, *427*, 427–428, *428*, *429*, *430*, *431*
assessment, 436
associated signs of pure, 425
central dyslexias, 434–435
covert reading in pure, 425–427
disconnection, 428, 451
dyslexia related to abnormal vision, attention, or eye movement, 432–434, *434*, *435*
functional imaging, 435–436
pure, 424–428
akinetopsia
anatomy, 438–439, *440*
associated deficits, 437–438
functional imaging and other techniques, *443*, 443–445, *444*, *445*
manifestations, 437
motion perception deficits with unilateral cerebral lesions, 438–439, *440*, *441*, *442*
physiology of motion perception in nonhuman primates, 439, 441–443
approach to patients with brain damage, 391–392
Bálint's syndrome, 445–446
attention in, 450
critique of classic cases, *448*, 448–450
historical review, 446–448
blindsight and residual, 392, 403–404
discrimination of color, 395–396
discrimination of form, 395, *397*
effects of training, 398, *398*, *399*
explanations of, 398–400, *400*, *401*
in hemidecorticate patients, 397–398, *398*
localization of targets, *392*, 392–395, *393*, *394*, *395*, *396*, *397*
in nonhuman primates, 400–402, *402*
other, 396–397
cerebral achromatopsia
anatomy, 404–406, *405*
associated deficits, 406
color and shape, 410, *410*, *411*
color anomia, 412–413
and color constancy, 409–410
color perception, language, and memory, 410–412, *412*
color perception and color testing in, 406–408, *407*, *408*, *409*
hemiachromatopsia, 408–409
historical perspective, 404
disorders of visually guided reaching and grasping, *450*, 450–451
anatomic correlates, 451, *452*, *453*, 453–454
optic ataxia, 451, *451*, *452*
historical perspective, 388, *389*
loss in aging and dementia, 469–470
positive phenomena, 454
perseveration, 454–457
visual distortions, 467–469
visual hallucinations, 457–464, *458*, *459*, *460*, *461*, *464*, *465*, *466*, 466–467
prosopagnosia
anatomy, 417–419, *418*, *419*, *420*
anterograde, 423–424
associated deficits, 414–415
covert facial recognition, 414, *415*
face perception in nonhuman primates, 421–423
forms of, 416
functional imaging, 423, *423*
neuropsychology of face perception, 415–416
other disorders of face perception, 424
pathology, 419–420
perceptual deficit in, 416–417
recognition deficit in, 417, *417*
specificity of impairment for faces in, 413–414
symptoms, 413
segregation of inputs, 388–391, *390*, *391*
tests of higher, *470*, 470–471, *471*, *472*
Central dyslexias, 434–435
Central European and Russian spring-summer tick-borne encephalitis viruses, *5186*, 5186–5188, *5188*
clinical manifestations, 5187
diagnosis, 5187
epidemiology, *5186*, 5186–5187
pathology, 5187, *5188*
prevention, 5188
prognosis, 5187–5188
treatment, 5187
Central facial nerve paresis, 1845–1846
Central mesencephalic reticular formation (cMRF), 1120
Central midbrain reticular formation in saccadic eye movements, 1120
Central nervous system (CNS), 3727, 5471
angiostrongyliasis, 4496
barriers to infection, 3941–3942
blastomycosis, 4336–4338, *4338*
candidiasis, 4348–4349, *4350*, 4351–4352, *4352*, 4353
coccidioidomycosis, 4360–4361, *4361*, *4362*, *4363*
cryptococcosis, 4370–4375, *4374*, *4375*, *4376*, *4377*, 4378
DNA viruses that infect, 4954–5154
adenoviridae, 4954, 4955, *4956*, 4956–4960, *4957*, *4958*, *4959*, *4960*
clinical manifestations, 4956
miscellaneous, 4959
neurologic, 4958–4959
ocular, 4956–4958, *4957*, *4958*, *4960*, *4961*
respiratory, 4956, *4956*
diagnosis, 4959–4960, *4962*
treatment, 4960
hepadnaviridae, 4961–4962, 4961–4975, *4962*, *4963*, *4966*, *4967*, *4969*, 4970, *4971*, *4974*, 4975
structure of, 4962–4963, *4963*
clinical syndromes caused by infection, 4965–4972, *4966*, *4968*, *4969*, *4970*, *4971*
epidemiology of infection, 4964
extrahepatic disease caused by, 4972
prevention of infection, 4973–4975, *4974*, *4975*
replication of, *4963*, 4963–4964
routes of transmission, 4964–4965
tropism of, 4964
herpesviridae, 4975–4979, *4976*, *4977*, 4979, *4980*
cellular transformation, 4978–4979
classification and structure, *4976*, 4976–4977
epidemiology and transmission, 4979
herpes simplex virus, 4979–4980, *4980*
congenital and neonatal infection, 4990–4991, *4991*, *4992*, *4993*
diagnosis, *5009*, 5009–5011
encephalitis, 4991–4992, 4994–4997, *4995*, *4996*, *4997*, *4998*, *4999*, 4999–5002, *5000*, *5001*, *5002*, *5003*, *5004*, 5004–5005, *5005*, *5006*, *5007*, 5007–5008, *5008*
epidemiology, 4980
idiopathic neurologic syndromes, 5008–5009
pathogenesis, 4980–4981, *4981*
primary infections, 4981–4984, *4982*, *4983*, *4984*, *4985*, 4985–4987, 4986
prophylaxis, 5012
treatment and prognosis, *5011*, 5011–5012
latency, 4978, *4978*, *4979*
pathogenesis, 4979
replication, 4977, *4977*
tropism, 4977–4978
varicella-zoster virus, 5012–5013, *5013*
epidemiology, 5025–5026
neurologic manifestations, 5029, 5031–5033, *5033*, *5034*, 5035, *5035*, *5036*, *5037*, 5037–5039, *5038*, *5040*, *5041*, *5042*, *5043*, 5043–5047, *5044*, *5045*, 5051–5054, 5056–5059, 5070, *5071*
systemic manifestations, 5028–5029, *5031*

varicella, 5013
clinical manifestations, 5014, *5015, 5016,* 5016–5025, *5018, 5020, 5021, 5022,* 5024
congenital and perinatal infection, 5025
epidemiology, 5013–5014, *5014, 5015, 5016,* 5016–5025, *5018, 5020, 5022, 5024*
pathogenesis, 5013
pathology, 5013, *5014*
papovaviridae, 5131, *5131*
BK virus, *5132,* 5132–5133
JC virus, *5133,* 5133–5139, *5134, 5135, 5136, 5137, 5138, 5139, 5140, 5141,* 5141–5142, *5142*
papillomaviruses, 5132
polyomaviruses, 5132
parvoviridae, 5142–5143, *5143, 5144, 5145,* 5145–5147, *5146*
vaccinia virus, 5149–5154, *5151, 5152, 5153*
variola, 5148–5149, *5150*
poxviridae, 5147–5148, *5148, 5149*
echinococcosis, 4447, *4450*
eosinophilic meningoencephalitis, 4503, *4505*
gnathostomiasis, 4496
infections in, 4145, 4245
Fusarium in, 4387
invasive aspergillosis of, 4316–4317
lesions produced by infection
acute bacterial meningitis
clinical manifestations, 4001, 4004–4007
clinical settings, 3994–3996
diagnosis, 4007–4010, *4008*
etiology, 3990, 3993–3994
pathology, 3998, *3999, 4000,* 4001, *4001, 4002, 4003, 4004, 4005*
pathophysiology, 3996–3998, *3997, 3998*
prognosis, 4011–4012
prophylaxis, 4012–4013
treatment, 4010–4011
acute nonbacterial meningitis, 4013–4015, *4014*
chronic meningitis, *4015,* 4015–4017, *4016*
demyelination, 3974
etiology, 3975, 3978–3979
normal myelin and, 3974–3975, *3975, 3976, 3977, 3978*
pathology, 3979, *3979, 3980*
remyelination after central, 3981, *3981*
edema, 3981–3982
empyema, 3982, *3982*
causes, *3982,* 3982–3983
clinical manifestations, 3983
diagnosis, 3983–3984, *3984, 3985*
pathology, 3983
prognosis, 3985
treatment, 3984–3985
encephalitis (meningoencephalitis), 3985–3989, *3986, 3987, 3988*
encephalomyelitis, 3989
granuloma, 3989–3990, *3990, 3991, 3992*
intracranial abscesses, 3943–3945, *3944*
diagnosis, 3960–3962, *3961, 3962, 3963*
etiology, 3950–3952, *3953,* 3954, *3954*
general and neurologic manifestations, 3955–3958
neuro-ophthalmologic manifestations, *3958,* 3958–3960, 3959
pathogenesis, 3945–3950, *3946, 3947, 3948, 3949, 3950, 3951, 3952*
pathology, *3954,* 3954–3955, *3955, 3956, 3957*
prognosis, 3963–3965
treatment, 3962–3963, *3964, 3965*
meningitis (leptomeningitis), 3990
mucoceles, 4017
clinical manifestations, 4017, *4019,* 4019–4023, *4020, 4021, 4022, 4023, 4024*
diagnosis, 4024–4025
general features, 4017, *4018*
prognosis, 4025
treatment, 4025
mycotic aneurysms, 3965
bacterial, 3965–3969, *3966, 3968, 3969, 3970*
fungal, 3971–3973, *3972, 3973*
miscellaneous, 3973
spirochetal (syphilitic), 3973
neuritis, 4026, *4027,* 4028, *4028*
pyoceles, 4017
clinical manifestations, 4017, *4019,* 4019–4023, *4020, 4021, 4022, 4023, 4024*
diagnosis, 4024–4025
general features, 4017, *4018*
prognosis, 4025
treatment, 4025
sinusitis, 4025–4026
subacute, *4015,* 4015–4017, *4016*
vasculitis, 4028
arteritis, 4028–4031, *4029*
septic occlusion of deep cerebral veins, 4034
septic occlusion of superficial cerebral veins, 4032–4034
septic thrombophlebitis, 4032
diagnosis of, 4042–4043, *4043*
treatment, 4043
septic thrombosis
of cavernous sinus, 4034–4039, *4035, 4036, 4037, 4038*
of dural sinuses, 4034
of lateral sinus, *4039,* 4039–4041, *4040*
of superior sagittal sinus, 4042
loiasis, 4505–4506
mucormycosis, *4320,* 4327–4329, *4328, 4329, 4330*
natural immunity of, 3941
pseudoallescheriasis, 4414–4415
RNA viruses that infect, 5154–5296
arenaviridae, *5154,* 5154–5158, *5155, 5156, 5157, 5158*
bunyaviridae, 5158, *5159*
bunyaviruses, 5158–5162
characteristics, 5159–5160, *5160*
clinical manifestations, 5160–5161
diagnosis, 5161
epidemiology of, 5160, *5161*
pathology, 5161, *5162*
prevention, 5162
treatment, 5161
phlebovirus, *5163,* 5163–5165, *5164*
coronaviridae, *5165,* 5165–5166, *5166*
filoviridae, 5166–5167
flaviviridae, 5167, 5179–5184, *5181, 5183*
Central European and Russian spring-summer tick-borne encephalitis, *5186,* 5186–5188, *5188*
clinical manifestations, 5187
diagnosis, 5187
epidemiology, *5186,* 5186–5187
pathology, 5187, *5188*
prevention, 5188
prognosis, 5187–5188
dengue virus, 5167–5170, *5168, 5169*
Hepatitis C virus (HCV), 5190
Japanese encephalitis, 5170
clinical manifestations, *5171,* 5171–5172, 5187
diagnosis, 5173–5174, 5187
epidemiology, 5170–5171
pathology, *5172,* 5172–5173, *5173,* 5187, *5188*
prevention, 5174, *5175*
prognosis, 5174, 5187–5188
treatment, 5174
Kunjin virus, 5174–5175
Kyasanur Forest disease virus, 5188–5189
Louping III virus, 5189
Murray Valley encephalitis virus, 5175–5176, *5177, 5178,* 5178–5179, 5179, *5179*
clinical manifestations, 5175–5176
diagnosis, 5178–5179
epidemiology, 5175
pathology, 5176, 5178, *5178, 5179, 5180*
prevention, 5179
prognosis, 5179
treatment, 5179
Negishi virus, 5189
Powassan virus, 5189–5190
St. Louis encephalitis virus, 5179–5184, *5181, 5183*
clinical manifestations, 5182
diagnosis, 5182–5183
epidemiology, 5179, *5181,* 5181–5182
pathogenesis, 5182
pathology, 5182, *5183*
prevention, 5183–5184
prognosis, 5183
treatment, 5183
West Nile virus, 5184
yellow fever virus, 5184–5186, *5185*
clinical manifestations, 5184
diagnosis, 5185
epidemiology, 5184, *5185*
pathogenesis and pathology, 5184–5185
prevention, 5185–5186
prognosis, 5185
treatment, 5185
orthomyxoviridae
characteristics of, 5190, *5191*
influenza viruses, 5190–5198, *5191, 5194, 5195, 5197*
clinical manifestations of infections, 5192
diagnosis, 5196
epidemiology, 5190–5192
nonpulmonary complications of, 5193–5196, *5195*
prevention, 5196–5198
prognosis, 5196
pulmonary complications of, 5192–5193

Central nervous system—*continued*
treatment, 5196
uncomplicated, 5192
paramyxoviridae, 5198, *5199,* 5200
measles, 5200
clinical manifestations, 5201, *5201*
complications, 5201, *5202,* 5203–5208, *5204, 5205, 5206, 5208, 5209, 5210*
diagnosis, 5209–5210
epidemiology, 5200
pathogenesis, 5208–5209
prevention and complications of vaccination, 5210–5213, *5211, 5212, 5213*
treatment, 5210
morbilliviruses, 5200–5201, *5201, 5202,* 5203–5217, *5204, 5205, 5206, 5208, 5209, 5210, 5211, 5212, 5213, 5214, 5215, 5216, 5217, 5218, 5219,* 5220, *5220*
characteristics of, 5200
measles, 5200
parainfluenza viruses, 5231
characteristics of, 5231, *5231*
clinical manifestations, 5232
paramyxoviruses, 5220
mumps virus, 5223
characteristics of, 5223, *5225*
clinical manifestations of, 5225, *5226*
complications of, 5225–5229, *5227*
diagnosis of, 5229–5230
epidemiology of, 5223, 5225
pathogenesis of, 5225
prevention, 5231
prognosis of, 5230–5231
treatment of, 5230
pneumoviruses, *5232,* 5232–5233, *5233*
subacute sclerosing panencephalitis, 5213
clinical manifestations, *5214,* 5214–5216, *5215, 5216, 5217*
diagnosis, 5217, 5220, *5223, 5224*
epidemiology, 5213–5214
pathogenesis, 5217
pathology, 5216–5217, *5218, 5219*
treatment and prognosis, 5220, *5224*
picornaviridae, 5233–5234, *5234*
coxsackieviruses, 5235–5241
echoviruses, 5241–5243
enteroviruses, 5234–5235, 5243–5250, *5244, 5246*
polioviruses, 5250–5258, *5251, 5252, 5253, 5254*
clinical manifestations, 5253–5257
diagnosis, 5257
epidemiology, 5250–5251
pathogenesis, 5251–5252, *5252*
pathology, 5252–5253, *5253, 5254*
prevention, 5258
rhinovirus, 5258
prognosis, 5257–5258
treatment, 5257
rabdoviridae
rabies virus
pathology, *5269,* 5269–5271, *5270, 5271,* 5273
prevention, 5274–5276
prognosis, 5274
treatment, 5274
vesiculoviruses, 5263
reoviridae, 5258
Colorado tick fever virus
clinical manifestations, 5259–5260
diagnosis, 5260
epidemiology, 5259
prevention, 5261
prognosis, 5261
treatment, 5260–5261
orbiviruses, *5259,* 5259–5261, *5260*
orthoreoviruses, 5261
rotaviruses, 5261, *5261,* 5263
retroviridae, 5263
rhabdoviridae, 5263
lyssaviruses, 5263–5271, *5264, 5265, 5266, 5267, 5268, 5269, 5270, 5271, 5272, 5273,* 5274–5276
rabies virus, 5263
clinical manifestations, *5266,* 5266–5268, *5267*
diagnosis, 5274
differential diagnosis, 5273–5274
epidemiology, 5264, *5264*
pathogenesis, 5264–5266, *5265, 5266*
pathology, *5269,* 5269–5271, *5270, 5271,* 5273
prevention, 5274–5276
prognosis, 5274
treatment, 5274
vesiculoviruses, 5263
togaviridae, 5277
alphaviruses, 5277–5281, *5278, 5279, 5280, 5281, 5282,* 5283, *5283, 5284, 5285,* 5285–5286
clinical manifestations, 5279–5281, *5280, 5281, 5282, 5283, 5284, 5285,* 5285–5286
pathology of, 5278–5279, *5279, 5280, 5281, 5282*
rubivirus (Rubella), 5286–5293, 5296
clinical manifestations, 5287–5293, *5288, 5289, 5294, 5295,* 5296, *5296*
diagnosis, 5293
epidemiology, 5286–5287
pathogenesis, 5287
prevention, 5293, 5296
treatment, 5293
sporotrichosis, 4415
toxoplasmosis, 4673
pathology of, 4685
acquired, *4686,* 4686–4687, *4687, 4688*
trichinosis, 4525, *4526,* 4527–4528
tuberculosis, 4145, 4167
tumors in, 2667–2668
and viruses, 4954
Central nervous system hemangiopericytomas, 2229
Central nervous system leukemia, 2337
Central nervous system sarcoidosis, 5471–5472
Central neurocytoma, 1977–1978, *1978*
Central neurogenic hyperventilation, 1878
Central pontine myelinolysis, 4662
Central posterior cataracts, 2667
Central retinal artery, 2884
occlusion, 3339, 3758–3759
occlusion of, 2333, 4321, *4323,* 5023
Central retinal vein, 2966, *2967*
occlusion of, 3464–3465, 3918–3925, *3920, 3921, 3922, 3923, 3924*
Central retinal vein occlusion (CRVO), 988, 1957, 2333
Central scotomas, 602, 674
Central syndrome of Rostral-Caudal deterioration, 996–997
Central vestibular nystagmus, pathogenesis of, 1473–1475, *1474, 1475*
Central vision, loss of, 514
Central visual acuity, loss of, in optic neuritis, 601
Centronuclear (myotubular) myopathy, 1355, *1356, 1357*
Cephalic tetanus, 4111, 4113, *4113*
Cercariae, 4479
Cercopithecine herpesvirus, 5129
Cercopithecine herpesvirus 1, 5129
Cerebellar and spinocerebellar disorders
ataxia telangiectasia, 2786
cutaneous manifestations, 2787, *2787*
laboratory findings, 2787
neurologic manifestations, 2786–2787
neuro-ophthalmologic manifestations, 2787, *2787*
pathology, 2786
treatment and prognosis, 2787
autosomal-dominant ataxia type I
etiology, 2790–2791
laboratory and neuroimaging findings, 2792
neurologic manifestations, 2791–2792
neuro-ophthalmologic manifestations, 2792
pathology, 2791, *2791*
prognosis, 2792
treatment, 2792
autosomal-dominant ataxia type II, 2792
genetics, 2792
laboratory and neuroimaging features, 2792
neurologic manifestations, 2792
neuro-ophthalmologic manifestations, 2792, *2793*
prognosis, 2793
autosomal-dominant ataxia type III, 2793–2794
congenital ataxias, 2784–2785, *2785*
Friedreich's ataxia, 2787–2787*t*
etiology and genetics, 2789
laboratory and neuroimaging findings, 2789
neurologic manifestations, 2789
neuro-ophthalmologic manifestations, 2789
pathology, 2787, *2788,* 2789
prognosis, 2789–2790
treatment, 2789
hereditary spastic paraplegia, 2794, 2795*t*
complicated forms of, 2795
pure, 2794–2795
idiopathic late-onset ataxias, 2794
clinical manifestations, 2794
diagnosis and investigations, 2794
pathology, 2794
metabolic ataxias, 2785–2786, *2786*
Cerebellar ataxia, 1869, 1878, 2410
with associated features, 2790
Cerebellar control
of saccades, 1120, *1121,* 1122–1123
of vergence eye movements, 1136
Cerebellar cortical degenerations, 1292
Cerebellar dysfunction as sign of tumor, 1797
Cerebellar encephalitis, 2500–2501
Cerebellar hemangioblastomas, 2707
Cerebellar hemorrhage, 3024, 3604–3607, *3606*

Cerebellar syndrome, 2560–2561
Cerebello-olivary degeneration of Holmes, 762
Cerebellopontine angle (CPA) chordoma, 2442
Cerebellopontine angle (CPA) meningiomas, 2052–2053
Cerebellosubarcuate artery, 2917
Cerebellum, 828
  abscesses of, 3957, 3959
  astrocytomas of, 1939–1941, *1940*
  in eye movement control, 1092, *1093,* 1094, *1094*
  in eyelid control, 1520
  and ocular motor control, 1153
    regulation of saccadic amplitude and dysmetria, 1153
    regulation of vestibulo-ocular reflex (VOR), 1153
    stabilization of images on retina, 1153
  ocular motor syndromes caused by disease of, 1290, 1290*t*
    degenerative, 1292–1293
    developmental anomalies of hindbrain, 1291–1292, 1292*t*
    location of lesions and their manifestations, 1290–1291
    mass lesions, 1293–1294
    vascular, *1292,* 1293, *1293*
  and smooth pursuit, 1131–1132
  tumors of, *1878,* 1878–1884, *1879, 1881*
Cerebral achromatopsia, 142
  anatomy, 404–406, *405*
  associated deficits, 406
  color and shape, 410, *410, 411*
  color anomia, 412–413
  and color constancy, 409–410
  color perception, language, and memory, 410–412, *412*
  color perception and color testing in, 406–408, *407, 408, 409*
    hemiachromatopsia, 408–409
  historical perspective, 404
  prosopagnosia, 413
    specificity of impairment for faces in, 413–414
    symptoms, 413
Cerebral angiitis, 3973
Cerebral angiography in diagnosing migraines, 3707–3708, *3708*
Cerebral arteries. (*See also* Anterior cerebral arteries; Posterior cerebral arteries.)
  infarction in territory of posterior, *3476,* 3477, *3477, 3478,* 3478–3479, *3479,* 3480, *3480, 3481,* 3482–3487, *3486, 3487, 3488*
  occlusion of, 3432–3434, *3433*
    middle, 3436–3438, *3439*
Cerebral autosomal-dominant arteriopathy with subcortical infarcts and leukoencephalopathy (CADASIL), 3363
Cerebral blindness, 361, 363, 366, 368–369, *369,* 2634–2635, *2636,* 2637
  with denial of blindness, 370
  optokinetic nystagmus in, 370
  visual-evoked responses in, 369–370
Cerebral blood flow
  and age, 2970
  autoregulation of, 2968–2969
  and blood viscosity, 2969
  and metabolism, 2969–2970
  sympathetic nervous system and, 2970
Cerebral control
  of saccadic eye movements, 1114
    basal ganglia, 1120
    central midbrain reticular formation, 1120
    frontal eye fields, 1114–1115, *1115, 1116, 1117*
    parietal cortex, 1118–1120
    prefrontal cortex, 1118, *1119*
    superior colliculus, 1115–1118
    supplementary eye field, 1118
    thalamus, 1120
  of vergence eye movements, 1135–1136
Cerebral cortex in controlling eye movements, 1082–1087, *1084, 1085, 1086*
Cerebral diplopia, 454
Cerebral diplopia-polyopia, 1170
Cerebral edema, *3942,* 3942–3943, *3943*
  interstitial, 3943, 3982
Cerebral embolism via vertebral venous system, 3929–3930
Cerebral encephalitis, 2498, *2499*
Cerebral hemispheres
  astrocytomas of, 1935–1936
  ocular motor syndromes caused by lesions in, 1319
    abnormal eye movements and dementia, 1326–1327
    acute, 1319–1320, *1320*
    apraxia, *1325,* 1325–1326
    eye movements in stupor and coma, 1327–1330
    focal lesions, 1322
    frontal lobe, 1324–1325
    manifestations of seizures, 1327
    occipital lobe, 1322
    parietal lobe, 1322–1323
    persistent deficits caused by large unilateral, 1320–1322, 1321*t, 1322*
    temporal lobe, 1323–1324
  visual disturbances originating from, *3673,* 3673–3674, *3674*
Cerebral hemorrhage, 2611–2612
Cerebral infarcts, 4302
Cerebral ischemia
  in Lyme disease, 4795, *4796*
  treatment of delayed, 3170–3172
Cerebral malaria, 4657–4658
Cerebral metamorphopsia, 469
Cerebral micropsia, 468, *468*
Cerebral phaeohyphomycosis, 4353
Cerebral polyopia, 456–457, 1170
Cerebral ptosis, 2990, 3037, 3465, *3465,* 3466, *3466, 3467,* 3767, 3797
  postganglionic, 3043
Cerebral toxoplasmosis, 5409–5411, *5410*
Cerebral vasculitis, delayed, 5061, *5062, 5063,* 5063–5064, *5064, 5065, 5066, 5067, 5068*
Cerebral veins, 2946–2947, *2948, 2949,* 2949–2952, *2950, 2951, 2952*
Cerebral venous and dural sinus thrombosis
  causes, 3887–3890
  of cavernous sinus, 3894–3898, *3896, 3897*
  of deep cerebral veins, 3893, *3894*
  diagnosis, *3905,* 3912–3914, *3913*
  of dural sinuses, 3893
  evaluation, 3914–3915
  of lateral (transverse) sinus, *3899,* 3899–3903, *3900, 3901, 3902, 3903, 3904, 3905*
  pathophysiology, 3890–3891
  of sigmoid sinus, 3912
  of straight sinus, 3910, 3912
  of superior sagittal sinus, 3905–3910, *3906, 3907, 3908, 3909, 3910, 3911, 3912*
  thrombosis of superficial veins, *3891,* 3891–3893, *3892, 3893*
  treatment, 3915
Cerebral vessels, collateral circulation between, 3414
Cerebriform cells, 2386
Cerebritis, 4125
  hemorrhagic, 4303, *4303*
Cerebrohepatorenal syndrome, 765–766
Cerebrospinafluid in patients with intracranial abscess, 3960–3961
Cerebrospinal fluid
  analysis of, 1896, 5614–5616, *5615*
  changes in, and relationship between optic neuritis and multiple sclerosis, 619
Cerebrovascular accident, 3947
Cerebrovascular disease, 3323, 5413–5415, *5414.* (*See also* Hemorrhagic cerebrovascular disease; Ischemic cerebrovascular disease.)
  and bone marrow transplantation, 2631–2632, *2632*
  radiation therapy in, 2609, *2609, 2610, 2611,* 2611–2612
Cerebrovascular infarcts, related to neurofibromatous, 2660–2661
Cerebrovascular thromboembolic disorders, 2515
  disseminated intravascular coagulation, 2515–2518, *2516, 2517, 2518*
  venous and dural sinus thrombosis, 2518–2520, *2520*
    nonbacterial thrombotic endocarditis, 2520–2521
Cerebrovasculitis, acute febrile, 4738, *4770, 4771,* 4771–4772, *4772*
Ceruloplasmin, 2801
Cervical arthritis, 1727
Cervical segment, 2870–2871
  of internal carotid artery, 2870–2871
Cervical spondylosis, 1722, 3353
Cervicofacial infections, 4177
Cervico-ocular reflex, 1138
Cervicothoracic sympathectomy, 1696
Cestodes (tapeworms), 4439–4440, *4440*
  Coenurus cerebralis, 4440–4441, *4441, 4442, 4443*
  Diphyllobothrium latum, 4441, 4443, *4444*
  Diphyllobothrium nihonkaiense, 4441, 4443, *4444*
  Echinococcus, 4443, *4445,* 4445–4447, *4446, 4447, 4448, 4449,* 4449–4453, *4450, 4451, 4453, 4454*
  Spirometra species, 4453–4455, *4455, 4456, 4457, 4458, 4459,* 4460, *4460*
  Taenia crassiceps, 4479
  Taenia solium, 4460
    clinical manifestations, 4462–4469, *4463, 4464, 4465, 4466, 4467, 4468, 4469, 4470,* 4471, *4471, 4472*
    diagnosis, 4474–4477, *4475, 4476, 4477*
    epidemiology, 4460
    neuropathology, 4471–4474, *4473, 4474*
    ocular pathology, 4474
    pathogenesis, 4460–4461, *4461, 4462*
    treatment, 4477–4479, *4478*
Chagas' disease, 4701–4702, *4702,* 5416
  acute, 4705, *4705, 4706*
  chronic, 4705–4706, *4707, 4708*
  indeterminate phase, 4705

Chagoma, 4706, 5416
Changuinola virus, 5261
Chapman-Cook Speed of Reading Test, 436, 470
Charcot-Leyden crystals, 4287, 4288
Charcot-Marie-Tooth disease (CMT), 763–764
Charcot's sign, 1539
CHARGE association, 788
Charles Bonnet syndrome, 456
Cheiro-oral-pedal syndrome, 1682
Chemical meningitis, 2339
Chemodectomas, paragangliomas of head and neck, 2462–2464, *2463, 2464, 2465*
 branchiomeric, 2464–2468, *2466, 2467, 2468, 2469, 2470,* 2470–2471
 intravagal, 2471–2472, *2472*
Chemoprophylaxis, 5198
 and bacterial meningitis, 4012
Chemosis of conjunctiva, *3268,* 3271, *3274, 3275*
Chemotherapy, 1902–1903, 2553–2554
 alkylating agents
  altretamine, 2579
  busulfan, 2566
  carboplatin, 2578
  chlorambucil, 2565–2566
  cisplatin, 2573
  cyclophosphamide, 2566
  dacarbazine, 2565
  ifosfamide, 2567
  melphalan, 2564–2565
  nitrogen mustards, 2563–2564, *2564*
  procarbazine, 2565
  spiromustine, 2568
  thiotepa, 2578–2579
 allopurinol, 2593
 antibiotics
  anthracycline, 2579–2580
  bleomycin, 2580
  mithramycin, 2580
  mitomycins, 2580
  suramin, 2580–2581
 antimetabolites, 2554
  cytosine arabinoside, 2560–2562
  5-fluorouracil, 2558–2560
  hydroxyurea, 2563
  methotrexate, 2554–2558, *2556, 2557, 2558*
  purine analogs, 2562
  pyrimidine analogs (bromodeoxyuridine), 2563
 biologic response modifiers, 2589–2592
 hormones
  corticosteroids, 2586–2589
  tamoxifen, 2584
 implication of agents in increased radiation toxicity, 2596
 laetrile, 2592–2593
 L-asparaginase, 2593
 misonidazole, 2593
 mitotane, 2583–2584
 retinoids, 2593
 vinca alkaloids, 2581
  taxoids, 2583
 VP-16, 2593
Chest roentgenogram, diagnosis, 4139–4140
Cheyne-Stokes respiration, 998
 comatose patients with, 1550
Chiari malformation, 1703, 2660
Chiasmal compression, 2176
Chiasmal gliomas, 2652–2654, *2653, 2654, 2655*
Chiasmal infarction, 5433
Chiasmal syndromes, 321–323, 3130
Chickenpox, 5013
 clinical manifestations, 5014, *5015, 5016,* 5016–5025, *5018, 5020, 5021, 5022,* 5024
 congenital and perinatal infection, 5025
 and development of viral encephalitis, 3986
 epidemiology, 5013–5014, *5014, 5015, 5016,* 5016–5025, *5018, 5020, 5022, 5024*
 pathogenesis, 5013
 pathology, 5013, *5014*
Children
 acquired Horner's syndrome in, 971
 alternating hemiplegia in, 3699
 aneurysms in, 3015
 electroretinogram (ERG) in, 219–220
 glaucoma in, 1012–1013
 HIV-associated progressive encephalopathy in, 5403–5407, *5405, 5406, 5407*
 migraines in, 3696–3697
  acute confusional in, 3698–3699
  Alice in Wonderland syndrome in, 3697
  alternating hemiplegia of, 3699
  benign paroxysmal torticollis in, 3698
  benign paroxysmal vertigo in, 3697–3698
  cyclic vomiting in, 3698
  motion sickness in, 3697
  somnambulism in, 3698
 optic neuritis in, *36,* 632–634
 traumatic aneurysms in, 2989
Chinese restaurant syndrome, 1718
Chlamydia botulinum, 5681
Chlamydia trachomatis in encephalitis, 3987
Chlorambucil, 2565–2566
 neuro-ophthalmologic toxicity, 2566
 neurotoxicity, 2566
 ocular toxicity, 2566
 systemic toxicity, 2565–2566
Chloromas, 2338–2339, 2341
Chloroquine, 1262
 impact of, on postsynaptic neuromuscular transmission, 1443
Chlorpheniramine maleate, 1004
Cholecystitis, 5105
Cholera, 4244–4245
Cholesteatomas, 2108–2110, *2109*
Cholesterol emboli, 3365–3367, *3366, 3367, 3368, 3369*
Cholinergic drugs, 1005, *1006*
Cholinesterase inhibitors for myasthenia gravis, 1424–1425
Chondrodysplasia punctata, 783
Chondrodysplasia-hemangioma syndrome, 2275
Chondrodystrophic myotonia, 1377
Chondroid chordomas, 2439
Chondromas, 2437–2442, *2438, 2439,* 2440, *2441, 2442,* 2443, *2443*
 cerebellopontine angle, 2442
 chondroid, 2439
 clivus, 2440–2441
 intracranial, 2438–2439
Chondrosarcoma, 2068–2069
 mesenchymal, 2068
Chorea, 2783
 in tuberous sclerosis, 2684
Choriocarcinoma, 2094–2095, *2095*
Chorioretinal inflammation, 4183, *4186*
Chorioretinal scarring, 4902
Chorioretinitis, 4671, 4687, 4866, 4905–4906, 5289, 5491, *5493, 5494,* 5495
 acute necrotizing, 4681
 bilateral, 5235
 circumscribed, 4906
 diffuse, *4866,* 4866–4867, *4867*
 localized central, 4867–4868, *4868, 4869, 4870, 4871,* 4871–4872
 multifocal, *4866,* 4866–4867, *4867*
Chorioretinopathy, 5040
Choristomas, 2083
 intracranial epidermoids and dermoids, 2110
  dermoids, 2113–2115, *2114, 2115*
  epidermoids, 2110–2113, *2111, 2112*
  relationship of, to other lesions of maldevelopmental origin, 2115
 of neurohypophysis (pituicytoma; granular cell myoblastoma), 2116–2117, *2117, 2118*
 of optic disc, nerve, and chiasm, 2115–2116, *2116*
Choroid, photocoagulation of, 1725
Choroid plexus tumors, *1968,* 1968–1970, *1969*
Choroidal angiomas, 2710–2712
Choroidal arteries, 2917. (*See also* Anterior choroidal arteries.)
 occlusion of anterior, 3434–3436, *3435, 3436, 3437, 3438*
Choroidal effusion or detachment, 3283
Choroidal folds, *1803,* 1803–1804, *1804*
Choroidal hypoxia, 3458, 3460
Choroidal ischemia, 3463, *3465*
 permanent visual defects from, 3694
Choroidal metastases, 1013
Choroiditis, 4128, 4671
 areolar, 4867
 disseminated, 4867
 multifocal, 4380–4381
Choroidopathy, 3823, *3825*
 peripapillary central serous, 814
Chromagraph, 212
Chromoblastomycosis and cerebral phaeohyphomycosis, 4353–4355, *4354, 4355, 4356*
Chromomycosis and cerebral phaeohyphomycosis, 4353–4355, *4354, 4355, 4356*
Chromophobe adenomas, 2152, 2153, 2187
Chromosomal-deletion retinoblastoma, 1992
Chromosome, 783
Chromosome 3, 2696
Chromosome 9, 2669
Chromosome 11, 2721
Chromosome 16, 2669
Chromosome 17, 2648
Chromosome 22, 2666
Chronic active plaques, 5552, 5555
Chronic basal meningitis, 3339, 4030–4031, *4031, 4032*
Chronic daily headache, 1752
Chronic demyelinating optic neuritis, 620, *620*
Chronic disseminated histoplasmosis, 4397–4401, *4399, 4400, 4401*
Chronic encephalitis, 5104
Chronic fatigue syndrome, 5091
Chronic granulomatous disease of childhood, 3950
Chronic hepatitis B, 4970–4972, *4971*
Chronic hypervitaminosis, 1718–1719
Chronic inactive plaques, 5552, *5553, 5554, 5555*

Chronic inflammatory demyelinating polyneuropathy (CIDP), 5539, 5707
clinical manifestations, 5709–5710, *5710, 5712, 5713*
diagnosis, 5711–5712
epidemiology, 5707
laboratory findings, 5710–5711
natural history, 5712
papilledema in, 518–519, *519*
pathogenesis, 5708–5709
pathology, 5707–5708, *5708*
prognosis, 5712
treatment, 5712
Chronic leukemia, 2337
Chronic meningitis, *4015*, 4015–4017, *4016*
Chronic meningoencephalitis, 5240, 5243
Chronic mononucleosis syndrome, 5091
Chronic mucocutaneous candidiasis (CMC), 4345–4346, *4347*
Chronic nondysenteric syndrome, 4619
Chronic obstructive pulmonary disease, 5193
Chronic ocular ischemia, 3457–3458, *3458, 3459, 3460*, 3460–3462, *3461, 3462, 3463*
Chronic open angle glaucoma, 253, *255*, 255–256, *256, 257*
Chronic optic neuritis, *5588*, 5588–5589
Chronic papilledema, 494, *494*
Chronic posttraumatic headache, 1705–1706
Chronic progressive external ophthalmoplegia (CPEO), 1545
Chronic progressive sensorimotor neuropathy, 2522–2523
Chronic pulmonary blastomycosis, 4333
Chronic pulmonary histoplasmosis, 4392
Chronic pulmonary hypertension and sarcoidosis, 5483
Chronic relapsing herpes zoster keratouveitis, 5080
Chronic respiratory insufficiency, 528
Chronic schistosomiasis, 4487–4488, 4489
Chryseomonas luteola, 4245
Churg-Strauss disease, 3727
Churg-Strauss syndrome, 3342, *3344*
Churg-Strauss vasculitis, *3752*, 3752–3754, *3753, 3754*
demographics, 3752
diagnosis, 3753–3754
ocular and neuro-ophthalmologic manifestations, *3752*, 3753, *3753*
pathology, 3753, *3754*
systemic manifestations, 3752–3753
treatment and prognosis, 3754
Ciliary body
blood vessels of, 905
nerves of, 907
Ciliary epithelium
pigmented, 900
unpigmented, 900
Ciliary ganglion, *864*, 864–868, *865, 866*
damage to, and its roots in orbit, *977*, 977–978
Ciliary muscle, 905
motor control of, 907–909
optic function of, 909–910
parasympathetic outflow to, 908–909
Ciliary nerves, short, 867
Ciliary processes, photocoagulation of, 1725
Ciliary zone, 850
Cilioretinal arteries, 2881
Circle of Willis, 85, 3414, *3414, 3415*
incidence of asymmetry in, 3018
Circle of Zinn-Haller, 61–62
Circumscribed chorioretinitis, 4906
Cisplatin
impact of, on postsynaptic neuromuscular transmission, 1443
neuro-ophthalmologic toxicity, 2576–2578, *2577, 2578*
neurotoxicity, 2573–2574
ocular toxicity, *2574*, 2574–2576
systemic toxicity, 2573
Citrobacter, 4218
in bacterial meningitis, 3993
in intracranial abscess, 3950
Citrobacter amalonaticus, 4218
Citrobacter diversus, 4218
in brain abscess, 3946
Citrobacter freundii, 4218
Citrullinemia, late-onset, and papilledema, 521
Cladosporium carrionii, 4353
Cladosporium trichoides, 4353, 4354
in intracranial brain abscess, 3952
Classic dengue fever, 5167–5170, *5168, 5169*
Classic migraine, 3658, 3664, 3664*t*
aura, 3664
neurologic, 3675–3677
pupillary signs, 3675, *3676*
visual, *3665*, 3665–3675, *3666, 3667, 3668, 3669, 3672, 3673, 3674*
headache, 3677–3678
Clathrin, 4948
Claude Bernard-Horner syndrome, 963
Claude-Bernard syndrome, 1555
Claustrum, 1863
Clindamycin, 4699
Clinically definite multiple sclerosis, 600, 5627
Clinically probable multiple sclerosis, 5627
Clinoid segment of internal carotid artery, 2877
Clivus, meningiomas of, *2053*, 2053–2054
Clivus blumenbachii, 2053, *2053*
Clivus chordomas, 2440–2441
Clonal erythrocytosis, 2332
Clopidogrel, 3561
Clostridia cadaveris, 4123
Clostridia paraputrificum, 4123
Clostridia perfringens, 4123
Clostridia septicum, 4123–4125
Clostridia welchii, 4123
Clostridium, 4109, *4123*, 4123–4125, *4124, 4125*
Clostridium botulinum, 4117, *4118, 4119*, 4119–4123, 4120–4121, *4122*
clinical manifestations, 4117, *4118*, 4119, *4119*
diagnosis, 4119–4120
in neuritis, 4026
treatment, 4120
in vasogenic cervical edema, 3981
Clostridium paraputrificum in intracranial abscess, 3947
Clostridium perfringens
in bacterial meningitis, 3993, 3995
in intracranial abscess, 3947
Clostridium septicum, 4125
Clostridium tetani, *4109*, 4109–4117
diagnosis, 4115
epidemiology, 4111
general manifestations, 4111–4113, *4112, 4113*
in neuritis, 4026
neurologic manifestations, 4114–4115
neurological manifestations, 4114–4115
ocular and neuro-ophthalmologic manifestations, 4113–4114, *4114*
pathogenesis, 4109–4111, *4110, 4111*
prevention, 4116–4117
prognosis, 4116
treatment, 4115–4116
in vasogenic cervical edema, 3981
Clostridium welchii in bacterial meningitis, 3993
Clump cells, 855
Clumsy hand syndrome, 3517
Cluster headaches, 970
relationship between episodic paroxysmal hemicrania, migraine and, 3699–3701
Cluster-tic headache, 1752
Coagglutination (CoA) tests, 4100
in diagnosing bacterial meningitis, 4009
Coagulase, 4068
Coarctation of aorta
and development of aneurysms, 3010
and polycystic kidney disease, 3008
Coated vesicle, 4948
Cocaine, 1003–1004, 3363–3364, 3585–3586
in blocking re-uptake of norepinephrine, 966
Coccidioidal meningitis, 4360, *4361*
Coccidioides immitis
in chronic basal meningitis, 4030
in fungal aneurysms, 3004, 3971
in intracranial brain abscess, 3952
in meningitis, 4282, 4355, 4356, 4364
clinical manifestations, 4357–4362, *4358, 4359, 4360, 4361, 4362, 4363, 4364, 4365, 4366*
demographics, 4355–4356
diagnosis, 4364–4365, *4367*
pathology, 4357, *4357*
pathophysiology, 4356–4357, *4357*
prognosis, 4367
treatment, 4365, 4367
Coccidioidin, 4361
Coccidioidomycosis, 4281, 5422
in chronic basal meningitis, 4030
cutaneous, 4359–4360, *4360*
in fungal aneurysms, 3971
genitourinary tract, 4360
in intracranial brain abscess, 3952
in meningitis, 4282, 4355, 4356, 4364
clinical manifestations, 4357–4362, *4358, 4359, 4360, 4361, 4362, 4363, 4364, 4365, 4366*
demographics, 4355–4356
diagnosis, 4364–4365, *4367*
pathology, 4357, *4357*
pathophysiology, 4356–4357, *4357*
prognosis, 4367
treatment, 4365, 4367
musculoskeletal, 4359, *4359*
ocular orbital, 4361–4362, *4364, 4365, 4366*
pulmonary, 4357–4358, *4358*
Coccygeal ganglion, 838
Cockayne syndrome, 766, 1326
Coenurosis, 4440–4441, *4441, 4442, 4443*
Coenurus cerebralis, 4440–4441, *4441, 4442, 4443*
Cogan's lid twitch, 1411, 1541
Cogan's syndrome, 3727, 3733, *3734*, 3734–3736, *3735*
Cogwheel rigidity, 2769
Cohen syndrome, 3889
Coital headache, 1704
Colchicine, 1262, 3811
Cold, sensations of, 1650

Cold stimulus headache, 1702
Colitis, fulminant, 4619
Collagen, 2978
Collarette, 850
Collateral nerve sprouting, 843–844
Collier's sign, 1549, *1551*
Collins' law, 1989
Colloid cysts of 3rd ventricle, 1970–1972, *1971*
Coloboma of iris, 1006
Coloboma syndromes, 777
Color
  discrimination of, 395–396
  and shape, 410, *410, 411*
Color anomia, 412–413
Color arrangement tests, 407
Color blindness, congenital, 33
Color constancy and cerebral achromatopsia, 409–410
Color discrimination and area V4, 142–143
Color Doppler flow imaging, 3535
Color dysphasia, 412
Color perception
  and color testing
    in cerebral achromatopsia, 406–408, *407, 408, 409*
    in hemiachromatopsia, 408–409
  language, and memory in, 410–412, *412*
Color testing, general principles of, 212, 213*t*
Color vision, 209–212, *210, 211, 212, 213,* 213*t,* 214, 214*t*
  in assessing traumatic optic neuropathy, 719
  and brightness comparison, 156, 156*t*
  clinical tests of, 210–211
  mechanisms in striate cortex, *138,* 138–139, *139*
  normal mechanisms, 210, *210, 211*
  in optic neuritis, 601, 602, 612
  in retinal disease, 238, 240
Colorado tick fever, 5259
  clinical manifestations, 5259–5260
  diagnosis, 5260
  epidemiology, 5259
  prevention, 5261
  prognosis, 5261
  treatment, 5260–5261
Coma
  disturbances in, 995–998
  eye movements in, 1327–1330
  from metabolic disease, 998
Coma somnonole, 5722
Combined head and eye saccades, 1138–1139
Combined ocular motor nerve pareses, 3128
Common carotid artery, signs of occlusive disease of, *3427,* 3427–3428
Common migraine, 3658, 3662–3664, *3663,* 3663*t*
Communicating hydrocephalus, 1568
Communicating segment of internal carotid artery, 2884, 2886, 2889, *2890*
Complete hemianopia, 5640
Complete ophthalmoplegia, 2722
Complete spontaneous necrosis with regression, 1994
Completed stroke, 3324
Complex cell, 130–131
Complex partial seizures, 1834
Complicated hereditary infantile optic atrophy, 761–762
Complicated migraine
  basilar artery, 3681
  familial hemiplegic, 3678
  without headache, 3678–3680, *3679, 3680*
Compression ophthalmodynamometry (ODM), 3537, 3538, *3538*
Compressive optic neuropathy, 264
  with optic disc swelling, 649–653, *650, 651, 652*
  without optic disc swelling, *653, 654, 656,* 657
Compulsive eye opening, 1560
Computed tomography (CT) scanning
  in diagnosing aneurysms, 3137–3139, *3138*
  in diagnosing cerebrovascular disease, 3525–3527, *3526*
  in diagnosing migraines, 3708–3709, *3709*
  in imaging multiple sclerosis, *5616,* 5616–5617, *5617*
Concentric sclerosis of Baló, 628
Conduction, 841
Cone bipolar cells, 39–40
Cone pedicles, 35
Confluence of sinuses, 2961–2962
Confrontation visual fields, 172–174, *173, 174*
Confusion in intracranial abscess, 3955
Congenital abnormalities of iris color, 1009
Congenital acetylcholinesterase deficiency, 1432, *1433*
Congenital adduction palsy with synergistic divergence, 1191–1192, *1192, 1193*
Congenital adherence and fibrosis syndromes, 1353–1354
Congenital and hereditary accommodation insufficiency and paralysis, 1011–1012
Congenital anomalies of optic disc, 777–778
Congenital bulbar paralysis, 1238–1240, *1239*
Congenital cerebellar ataxias, 2784–2785, *2785*
Congenital cholinergic nervous system dysfunction, 1027
Congenital color blindness, 33
Congenital comitant strabismus, 1176
Congenital diffuse hemangiomatosis, 2234–2235, *2236, 2237*
Congenital extracranial disease, 3010
Congenital familial sensory neuropathy with anhidrosis, 1027
Congenital fiber type disproportion, 1357–1358, *1359, 1360*
Congenital glaucoma, 2652
Congenital gustolacrimal reflex, 1024
Congenital Horner's syndrome, 971–973, *972, 973*
Congenital hypothesis of aneurysm formation, 2977
Congenital malformations, 3947
Congenital miosis, 1008–1009
Congenital muscular dystrophies, 1361
  Fukuyama, 1361
  muscle-eye-brain disease, 1361–1362
  nosologic relations of, 1362
  Walker-Warburg syndrome, 1362
Congenital myasthenic syndromes, 1431–1432
Congenital mydriasis, 1009
Congenital myopathies, 1359
  background and classification, 1354
    central core, 1354
    centronuclear (myotubular), 1355, *1356, 1357*
    fiber type disproportion, 1357–1358, *1359, 1360*
    with intracytoplasmic inclusion bodies, 1358–1359
    miscellaneous, 1359
    multicore disease, 1357, *1358*
    nemaline, 1354–1355, *1355*
  with cytoplasmic bodies, 1358
  with intracytoplasmic inclusion bodies, 1358–1359
  relationship among different, 1359–1360
Congenital neoplasms
  cholesteatomas, 2108–2110, *2109*
  craniopharyngiomas, *2098,* 2098–2106, *2099, 2100, 2101, 2104, 2105*
  germ cell tumors, 2083–2085, *2084*
    choriocarcinoma, 2094–2095, *2095*
    embryonal carcinoma, 2091–2092, *2092*
    endodermal sinus tumors, 2092, *2093,* 2094, *2094*
    germinoma, 2085–2089
    teratoma, 2089–2091, *2090, 2091*
  lipomas, 2095–2098, *2096, 2097, 2098*
  pearly tumors, 2108–2110, *2109*
  Rathke's cleft cysts, 2106–2108, *2107, 2108*
  suprasellar epidermoid cysts, 2108–2110, *2109*
Congenital nystagmus
  clinical features, *1482,* 1482–1483
  pathogenesis of, 1483–1484
Congenital ocular motor apraxia (COMA), *1325,* 1325–1326
Congenital ocular oscillations, nature of, 1482
Congenital optic disc pigmentation, 798, *798*
Congenital paradoxic gustolacrimal reflex, 1018
Congenital ptosis, 1545, *1545, 1546*
Congenital recessive optic atrophy, 758
Congenital rubella, 5289–5293, *5290, 5291*
Congenital strabismus, 1170
Congenital syphilis, 4902–4908
  tests for, 4928
Congenital tilted disc syndrome, 794, *794, 795,* 796
Congenital toxoplasmosis, 4678, *4680,* 4681
  diagnosis of, 4698
  neuropathology of, 4687, *4690*
  treatment of, 4700
Congenital unilateral lower lip paralysis, 1564
Congenital universal absence of pain, 1686–1687
Conidia, 4287
Conjugate deviation of eyes and head, 4151
Conjugate eye movements, 1102
Conjugate gaze palsies, 1848
Conjunctiva, 2712, *2714, 2715*
  chemosis of, *3268,* 3271, *3274, 3275*
  leukemic involvement of, 2350
  sensory nerve endings in, 1601, *1602*
Conjunctival arteries, aneurysms arising from, 3074–3075
Conjunctival biopsy, 5523, *5527*
Conjunctival granulomatosis, 5487, *5488, 5489*
Conjunctival hamartomas, 2658
Conjunctivitis, 3855, 4128, 5226
  acute hemorrhagic, 5235, 5243–5245, *5244*
  allergic, 5233
  radiation therapy as cause of, 2613–2614
Connective tissue diseases, 2982, 3346, 3725
  associations, 3829–3830
  cardiovascular manifestations, 3815–3816, *3816*
  constitutional symptoms, 3812
  demographics, 3812
  diagnosis, 3830–3831, 3831*t*
  drug-induced lupus, 3830
  Ehlers-Danlos syndrome, *2984, 2985,* 2985–2987

fibromuscular dysplasia, *2982,* 2982–2983, 2985
gastrointestinal manifestations, 3817–3818
hematologic manifestations, 3816–3817
Marfan's syndrome, *2986,* 2987, *2987*
mucocutaneous lesions, *3813,* 3813–3815, *3814, 3815*
musculoskeletal symptoms and signs, *3812,* 3812–3813
neurologic and psychiatric manifestations, 3819–3822, *3820, 3821, 3822*
neuro-ophthalmologic manifestations, 3826–3829, *3827, 3828, 3829*
ocular manifestations, 3822–3823, *3823, 3824, 3825, 3826*
orbital manifestations, 3825–3826, *3826*
pathogenesis, *3818,* 3830, *3830*
prognosis, 3831
pseudoxanthoma elasticum, 2987, *2988, 2989*
pulmonary manifestations, 3815, *3816*
renal manifestations, *3817,* 3817–3818, *3818, 3819*
systemic lupus erythematosus, 3811
history, 3811–3812
treatment, 3831–3833, *3832*
Consensual testing light response, 937
Constant speed rotations, 1142
Constructional disorders, 1840
Continuous tears, 926
Continuous-wave Doppler, 3533
Contralateral trochlear nerve palsy, 968
Contrapulsion, 1123
of saccades, 1286, 3512
Contrast sensitivity, 164–169, *165, 166, 167, 168, 169,* 612–613
in optic neuritis, 601
Contusion of globe, 1013
Convergence, 947, 948
absent, 5729
accommodative, 948
excess, 947
fusional, 948
insufficiency, 947, 1780, *1780*
paralysis, 1780, *1780*
reduced, 5729
relation between accommodation and, 912
relative, 948
testing, 952
tonic, 948
voluntary, 948
Convergence nystagmus, 1781–1782
Convergence spasm, 1304, 1869
Convergence zone, 415–416
Convergence-accomodative micropsia, 467–468
Convergence-retraction nystagmus, 1304–1305, 1480–1481, *1481,* 1794, 3501–3502
Convergent accommodation, 912
Convergent-divergent components, 1328
Convergent-divergent pendular oscillations, 1469
Converse bobbing, 1328, 1493
ocular, 3512
Conversion disorder, 666, 1766
Convexity meningiomas, *2036,* 2036–2037, *2038, 2039*
Cookie Theft Picture, 470, 471
Coprion, 4565
Cor pulmonale and sarcoidosis, 5483
Coracidia, 4443, 4453
Corectopia, midbrain, 996
Cornea
anatomy of trigeminal nerve fiber endings, 1595–1596, *1596, 1597,* 1598, *1598, 1599,* 1600, *1600*
calcification of, 5487–5488
changes in, 1997
clouding of, 2820–2821
complications from radiation therapy, 2614
damage to, 5038–5039, *5039*
examination of, 934
involvement in neurofibromatosis, 2658, *2660*
leukemic involvement of, 2349–2350
reflex blinks from stimulation of, 1529, *1530*
superficial disease of, 1723–1724
thermal sensation, 1604–1605
touch and pressure sensation, 1604
transplants of, 5264
ulceration of, 4090, 4128
Corneal anesthesia, 4172
Corneal arcus, 3465–3466
Corneal erosion, pain of, 1724
Corneal hypesthesia, 1844
congenital, 1666
due to acquired disease, 1664–1666, *1665*
inherited, 1666
Corneal reflex, absence of, 1893
Corneal sensation
alterations in, 1663–1666, *1665*
tests of, *1651,* 1651–1652
Corneal sensibilometer, *1651,* 1652
Corneomandibular reflex, 1571, 1657–1658
Cornification of vaginal epithelium, 4102
Corollary discharge, 1106–1107
Coronary artery disease, 3816
Coronaviridae, *5165,* 5165–5166, *5166*
Corpus callosum, tumors involving, 1855, *1857,* 1857–1859, *1858*
Corrected Loss Variance (CLV), 180
Corrected Pattern Standard Deviation (CPSD), 180
Corrective saccade, 1106
Corrugator superciliaris, 1513, *1513*
Cortical anesthesia, 3433
Cortical angiomas, 2236
Cortical blindness, 361, 363, 366, 368–369, *369,* 2339, 3485–3487, 3765, 4160, 4351, 5433, 5640
and cyclosporine, 2634
with denial of blindness, 370
optokinetic nystagmus in, 370
visual-evoked responses in, 369–370
Cortical branches, occlusion of, 3440, *3441*
Cortical connections, between visual areas, *146,* 147
Cortical deafness, 1830
Cortical inhibition of pupillary constriction, 878–879
Cortical projections to upper facial motoneurons, *1518,* 1519
Cortical tubers in tuberous sclerosis, *2684,* 2684–2686, *2685, 2686*
Corticobasal ganglionic degeneration (CBGD)
laboratory studies, 2780, *2781*
neurologic manifestations, 2779–2780
neuro-ophthalmologic manifestations, 2780
pathology, 2779, *2779*
pathophysiology, 2780
treatment, 2780
Corticogeniculate pathway, 108
Corticosteroids, 2586–2589
for bacterial meningitis, 4011
for endocrine myopathies, 1405
impact of, on postsynaptic neuromuscular transmission, 1441
for Lambert-Eaton myasthenic syndrome, 1437
for myasthenia gravis, 1425–1427
neuro-ophthalmologic toxicity, 2588–2589, *2589*
neurotoxicity, 2587–2588
ocular toxicity, 2588
for septic cavernous sinus thrombosis, 3898
for septic thrombosis, 4038
systemic, 4699, 5692
systemic toxicity, 2587
for traumatic optic neuropathy, 733
Corticothalamic projections, 1637
Corticotropin deficiency, 780
Corynebacteria, 4125
Corynebacterium diphtheriae, 4125–4128, *4126, 4127*
other, 4128–4130, *4129*
Corynebacterium, in intracranial brain abscess, 3952
Corynebacterium afermentans, 4129
Corynebacterium bovis, 4128
Corynebacterium diphtheriae, 4125–4128, *4126, 4127*
in neuritis, 4026
in vasogenic cervical edema, 3981
Corynebacterium equi, 4128–4129
Corynebacterium haemolyticum, 4128
Cotransmission, 841
Cotton thread test, 955
Counter rolling, 1172
Counterimmunoelectrophoresis, 4100
in diagnosing bacterial meningitis, 4009
Countertorsion, static, 1172
Countertorsion rolling, 1172
Cover tests, 1180–1181
Covert familiarity, 414
Covert semantic knowledge, 414
Cover-uncover test, 952, 1181
Cowdry inclusion bodies, 5216, *5219*
Cowdry type A inclusions, 5005, *5006*
Coxiella burnetii, 4737, 4766–4767
Coxsackieviruses, 5235–5241
Cranial bone, headaches associated with disorders of, 1722
Cranial fossa, dural arteriovenous malformations (AVMs) of anterior, 2269
Cranial hypertrophic pachymeningitis, 4136
Cranial nerves
dysfunction and aneurysmal rupture, 3022
pareses, 5087, 5245
schwannomas of lower, 2316
testing of, 158
tumors of, 2321–2322
Cranial neuropathies, 1835, 2269, 2362–2363, *2363,* 2391, 3214, 3837, 4127, 4878, 4889, 4907–4908, *5032,* 5032–5033, *5033, 5034,* 5035, *5035, 5036, 5037,* 5037–5041, *5038, 5040, 5041,* 5042, *5043,* 5043–5047, *5044, 5045, 5046, 5047, 5048, 5049,* 5049–5051, *5050, 5051,* 5238–5239, 5242, 5492, 5699–5700
caused by venous compression, 3930, *3930*
and Lyme disease, 4791, 4793–4794
radiation therapy in, 2612
as sign of tumors, 1794–1797

Cranial traction or stabilization procedures, 3947
Craniocervical junction, organic disease at, 1747–1748
Craniopharyngiomas, 1814, *2098*, 2098–2106, *2099, 2100, 2101, 2104, 2105*
Craniosynostosis, papilledema and, 520
Craniotomy, 2189–2190
  and development of intracerebral abscess, 3947–3948
Craniotopic defects, 1130
C-reactive protein (CRP), 3774–3775, 3961–3962
  in diagnosing bacterial meningitis, 4010
CREST syndrome, 3014, 3835, 3838
Creutzfeldt-Jakob disease, 366, 631, 1560, 2030, 4568–4569
  diagnosis, 4584, *4587*, 4587–4591, *4588, 4589, 4590, 4591*
  epidemiology, 4569, 4571
  familial, 4576–4577
  iatrogenic, *4578*, 4578–4579
  panencephalic, 4584, *4586*
  pathology, 4580–4581, *4581, 4582, 4583,* 4584, *4584, 4585, 4586*
  prevention of Iatrogenic, 4592
  relationship of, and Bovine Spongiform Encephalopathy, 4579–4580
  sporadic, 4571–4574, *4572, 4574, 4575,* 4576, *4576*
  treatment, 4592
Critical flicker frequency (CFF), 206
Crocodile tears, 1022–1025, *1023*
Crohn's disease, 3857, 3888
Crossed quadrant hemianopia, 361, *364, 365–366, 367*
Crouzon's disease, 796
Crow-Fukase syndrome, 2399
  papilledema in, 520
Cryoglobulin, 3783–3784
Cryoglobulinemia, 3727
  mixed, 3783–3786, *3785*
Cryptococcal granulomas, 4370, 4378
Cryptococcal meningitis, 4371, 4374, 4387
Cryptococcal optic neuropathy, 710
Cryptococcomas, 4370, 4378, *4379, 4380, 4381*
Cryptococcosis, 4281, 5421–5422
  bilateral, 710
  intraocular, 4378–4381, *4379, 4380, 4381*
  ocular, 4378–4381, *4379, 4380, 4381*
  orbital, 4378–4381, *4379, 4380, 4381*
  pulmonary, 4370, *4373*
Cryptococcus neoformans, 4281, 4282, 4367–4368, *4368*
  in chronic basal meningitis, 4030
  clinical manifestations
    central nervous system cryptococcosis, 4370–4375, *4374, 4375, 4376, 4377,* 4378
    ocular and orbital cryptococcosis, 4378–4381, *4379, 4380, 4381*
    other sites of cryptococcosis, 4381–4382, *4382*
    pulmonary cryptococcosis, 4370, *4373*
  diagnosis, 4382–4384, *4384, 4385*
  in intracranial brain abscess, 3952
  intraocular, 4378–4381, *4379, 4380, 4381*
  in neuritis, 4026
  ocular, 4378–4381, *4379, 4380, 4381*
  orbital, 4378–4381, *4379, 4380, 4381*
  pathology, *4369*, 4369–4370, *4370*
  pathophysiology, 4368–4369
  prognosis, 4387
  pulmonary, 4370, *4373*
  treatment, 4384–4387, *4386*
CSF IgG index, 5614
CSF lactic dehydrogenase (LDH) in diagnosing bacterial meningitis, 4010
CSF pleocytosis, 4072
CSF rhinorrhea, 510
Cunninghamellacaeae, 4318
Cupping, appearance of atrophic optic disc with respect to, *286*, 286–287, *287*
Curvularia lunata, 4290
Curvularia species in intracranial brain abscess, 3952
Cushing's disease, *2160*, 2160–2162, *2161*
  radiation for, 2198
Cushing's syndrome, 321–323, 1404–1405, 2160–2162
  of chiasm, 2062
  evaluating patients with, 2186–2187
Cutaneous anergy, 5518
Cutaneous anthrax, 4106, *4106*
Cutaneous blastomycosis, 4333–4334, *4336, 4337*
Cutaneous coccidioidomycosis, 4359–4360, *4360*
Cutaneous granulomas, 5480, *5481*
Cutaneous lymphedema, 4509
Cutaneous mucormycosis, 4325–4326
Cutaneous neurofibromatosis, 2664
Cutaneous schwannomatosis, 2668
Cutaneous sensation, tests of, 1649–1650
Cutaneous sporotrichosis, 4415
Cutaneous T-cell lymphoma, *2386*, 2386–2389, *2387, 2388*
Cyanide optic neuropathy, 675
Cyclic esotropia and its relationship to abducens nerve palsy, 1258
Cyclic oculomotor paresis, 1192–1194, *1196*
Cyclic vomiting in migraine, 3698
Cyclooxygenase, 3558
Cyclopentolate, 1001–1002
Cyclophosphamide, 2566
  neuro-ophthalmologic toxicity, 2567
  ocular toxicity, 2567
  systemic toxicity, 2566–2567
Cycloplegic refraction, 154
Cyclosporine
  for aneurysms, 3175
  for headaches, 1718
  for immunosuppression, 2627–2628
  for myasthenia gravis, 1428–1429
  in preventing graft-versus-host disease (GVHD), 2626–2627, 2632
Cyclovergence nystagmus, 1469
Cylindromas, 2453–2457, *2454, 2455, 2456*
  treatment of, 2454–2456
Cyproheptadine for pituitary adenomas, 2192
Cysticercosis, 631, 4460
  intraocular, *4471, 4472*
  ocular, 4468–4469, *4469, 4470,* 4471, *4471, 4472, 4473*
  orbital, 4468–4469, *4470*
  spinal, 4472
Cysticercus
  in intracranial brain abscess, 3952
  intraventricular, 4476
Cystitis, hemorrhagic, 4959
Cysts, 4614
  ependymal, *43*, 2123–2124, *2125*, 2126, *2127, 2128*
  hydatid, 4445
  involving 3rd ventricle, 1849, *1851, 1852,* 1852–1855, *1853*
  leptomeningeal, 4452
  lung, in patients with tuberous sclerosis, 2692
  pancreatic, 2705
  Racemose, 4473
  Rathke's cleft, 2098, *2107*, 2107–2108, *2108*
  renal, 2705
  of septum pellucidum, 1855, *1855, 1856,* 2124–2126, *2128*
  suprasellar arachnoid, 2123–2125
  suprasellar epidermoid, 2108–2110, *2109*
  supratentorial arachnoid, 2118–2120, *2119, 2120*
Cytokines in diagnosing bacterial meningitis, 4010
Cytomegalic inclusion disease (CID), 5098
Cytomegalovirus (CMV), 5096–5097, 5417
  acquired infection in immunocompetent children and adults, 5102–5104, *5103*
  acquired infection in immunosuppressed persons, 5104–5113
  characteristics of, 5097
  clinical manifestations, 5098
  congenital infection, 5098–5100, *5099, 5101*
  diagnosis, 5115, 5118–5119
  in encephalitis, 5108–5110
  epidemiology, 5097–5098
  in intrauterine infection, 5097
  in multifocal neuropathy, 5112–5113
  pathology, *5113*, 5113–5115, *5114, 5115, 5116, 5117, 5118, 5119*
  perinatal infection, 5100–5102, *5102*
  prophylaxis, 5122
  retinitis caused by, 5426–5427
  treatment, 5119–5122, *5120, 5121*
Cytoplasmic body myopathy, 1359
Cytosine arabinoside, 1262, 2560–2562
  neuro-ophthalmologic toxicity, 2561–2562
   purine analogs, 2562
  neurotoxicity, 2560–2561, *2561*
  ocular toxicity, 2561
  systemic toxicity, 2560
Cytotoxic brain edema, 3943, *3943*
Cytotoxic cerebral edema, 3982

D

D-15 panel, 436, 749
Dacarbazine
  neurotoxicity, 2565
  systemic toxicity, 2565
Dacryoadenitis, 5226
Dacryocystitis, 2350, 4178, 5289
Dacryocystography, 956
Dandy-Walker syndrome, 782
Dapiprazole hydrochloride, 1005
Dark adaptation, 159, 214–215, *215*
Darkness
  paradoxical reaction of pupils to, 990
  poorly reacting from midbrain disease, 990
  pupillary response to, 892
Dawson's encephalitis, 5213
Dawson-Trick-Litzkow electrodes, 218, 219
Dazzle, 1795
De Morsier syndrome, 779, 780, 783
De novo formation of aneurysms, 3142
Decompensation, 1176
Decompression

monitoring optic nerve function during, 657
visual recovery following, 657–658
Decompression sickness, 1015
Decreased cerebral perfusion
causes of, 3407, *3408*, 3409–3413
general considerations, 3407
Decreased intracranial pressure, headache associated with, 1714–1716
Deep auricular artery, 2945
Deep cerebral veins
septic occlusion of, 4034
thrombosis of, 3893, *3894*
Deep dyslexia, 435
Deep organ involvement, 4346–4349, *4348, 4349, 4350*, 4351–4352, *4352*
Defecation, disturbances of, 5573
Deferoxamine in development of mucormycosis, 4319
Deficiency, thiamine, 669–670
Degeneration, 5703
of white matter
Krabbe disease, 2857–2859, *2858, 2859*
Pelizaeus-Merzbacher, 2856–2857
Degenerative hypothesis of aneurysm formation, 2977–2978
Degos disease, 3346, 3725, 3859, 3861, 3863–3864, 3888
Delayed cerebral ischemia, 3353
Delayed cerebral vasculitis, *5020*, 5020–5022, *5021*
Delayed hypersensitivity reactions, 3726–3727
Delleman syndrome, 782
Delta hepatitis virus, 4971
Dementia
and abnormal eye movements, 1326–1327
age as factor in, 469–470
causes of, 2747–2748, 2748*t*
frontotemporal. (*See* Frontotemporal dementia.)
human immunodeficiency virus (HIV)-induced, 5373, 5389–5390
with Lewy bodies
diagnosis, 2758, 2758*t*
epidemiology, 2756
laboratory and neuroimaging findings, 2758
neurologic and psychiatric manifestations, 2757–2758
neuro-ophthalmologic manifestations, 2758
pathology, 2756–2757, *2757*
pathophysiology, 2757
prognosis, 2759
treatment, 2758–2759
primary degenerative. (*See* Primary degenerative dementia.)
as sign of tumors, 1794
subcortical, 2748
thalamic, 3483
Demyelinated optic nerves, 5547
Demyelinating disease, 5539
acquired pendular nystagmus with, 1468
Demyelinating plaque, 5549–5550
Demyelinating polyneuropathy, 2561
Demyelination, 3974, 5539
etiology, 3975, 3978–3979
neuronolytic, 3974, 5539
normal myelin and, 3974–3975, *3975, 3976, 3977, 3978*
pathology, 3979, *3979, 3980*
periaxial, 3974, 5539
remyelination after central, 3981, *3981*
Dendritic keratitis, 5023
Denervation supersensitivity, 842, 1021
Dengue hemorrhagic fever, 5167–5170, *5168, 5169*
Dengue virus, 5167–5170, *5168, 5169*
Dental infections, 3946, 4035
as cause of septic cavernous sinus thrombosis, 3894
Dentatorubropallidoluysian atrophy, 2794
Dentato-rubro-pallidoluysian atrophy, 763
Deoxyribonucleic acid (DNA) hybridization probes in diagnosis of *E. histolytica*, 4622
Deoxyribonucleic acid (DNA) viruses. (*See* DNA viruses.)
Depression, 3819, 5575
theory of spreading, 3703–3706
Depth of field, 949
Dermacentor andersoni, 4739, 4766
Dermacentor variabilis, 4739, 4763
Dermatomyositis, 2527–2530, *2528*, 3838–3841, 3839, *3839, 3840, 3841, 3842*
Dermoids, 2113–2115, *2114, 2115*
Descending palatine artery, 2946
Detection acuity, 160
Developmental anomalies of hindbrain, 1291–1292, 1292*t*
Developmental myopathic ptosis, 1545, *1545, 1546*
Developmental prosopagnosia, 420
Devic's disease, 600, 622, 4164, 4166, 5275, 5539, 5632, *5632, 5635*
clinical manifestations, 5633
loss of vision, 5634–5635, *5637*
miscellaneous, 5637
paraplegia, 5635, 5637
prodrome, 5633–5634
diagnosis, 5637–5638
epidemiology, 5632
laboratory studies and neuroimaging, 5637, *5638*
pathology, *5632*, 5632–5633, *5633, 5634*
prognosis, 5638–5639
treatment, 5638
Devic's syndrome, 5019
Dextrocardia, familial, 796
DI Guglielmo syndrome, 2334, *2334*
Diabetes insipidus, syndrome of, 1812
Diabetes mellitus
and facial dysesthesias, 1751–1752
and incidence of atherosclerosis, 3330
maternal insulin-dependent, 782
as risk factor for stroke, 3567–3568
transient loss of accommodation in patients with, 1015
Diabetic ophthalmoparesis, 3685
Diabetic papillopathy, *564*, 564–565
Diagnostic fiberoptic bronchoscopy with transbronchial biopsy and bronchial washings, 4140
Dialysis, headaches associated with, 1721
3,4-Diaminopyridine for Lambert-Eaton syndrome, 1436
Diaphragma sellae, 90, 2018, 2062, 2142, 2144
Diaphragmatic meningiomas, 2062
Dichloroacetylene, 1262
Dichromacy, 33
Didanosine (DDI), 5365
Diechslera in intracranial brain abscess, 3952
Diencephalic autonomous epilepsy, 1854
Diencephalic syndrome, 1814–1815, *1815*
Diencephalon, 16
Dietary management and phenylketonuria, 2811–2812
Diffuse angiokeratoma, 2831
Diffuse angiomas, 2710–2711
Diffuse brain injury, role of radiation therapy, 2604, *2605*
Diffuse chorioretinitis, *4866*, 4866–4867, *4867*
Diffuse congenital hemangiomatosis, *2731, 2732*, 2735
Diffuse disseminated atheroembolism (DDA), 3404–3405
Diffuse encephalitis, 4394
Diffuse infiltrating retinoblastomas, 1994, *1995*
Diffuse necrosis of subcortical white matter, 4016
Diffuse proliferative nephritis, 3817–3818
Diffuse systemic sclerosis, 3835
Diffuse unilateral subacute neuroretinitis (DUSN), 4531, *4531*
association with neuroretinitis, 636–637
Diffuse uveal melanocytic proliferation (DUMP), 2538–2541, *2540*
differential diagnosis of, 2540
pathogenesis of, 2540
treatment of, 2540–2541
Digital subtraction angiography (DSA), 3545–3546, *3548*
Dihydropteridine reductase defect, 2812
Dilation lag, 938, 965–966
Dilation of pupils, *1000, 1001*, 1001–1003, *1002, 1003*
constriction of, *1004*, 1005
Diltiazem for delayed cerebral ischemia, 3171
Diopters, 948
Diphenylhydantoin (DPH, Dilantin), 1262
Diphtheria, 1015, 4125
Diphtheritic polyneuritis, 4127–4128, 4128
Diphtheroids, 4128
Diphyllobothriasis, 668, 4443
Diphyllobothrium, 4441, 4443, *4444*
Diphyllobothrium latum, 4441–4443, *4444*, 4453
Diphyllobothrium nihonkaiense, 4441, 4443, *4444*
Diplococcus pneumoniae, 4075
Diploic veins, 2954, *2955*
Diplopia, 514, 1169–1170, 2031, 2333, 3278–3281, *3280, 3281*, 3473, 3765–3766, *3767, 3768*
binocular, 1169, 3673, 3694
cerebral, 454
in chordomas, 2439
horizontal, 2439
monocular, 1169–1170, 1777, 3673, 3694
permanent, 3694
and tumors of bone or cartilage, 2437
Diplopia-polyopia, cerebral, 1170
Dipyridamole, 3560
Direct injury to arterial wall, 2990
Direct optic nerve injuries, 715
Direct optokinetic pathway, 1151
Direct parasympathetic pathway to eye, 867
Direct pupillary light reaction, 936
Direct vestibulo-ocular reflex (VOR), 1143
Direction selectivity, 141
Directional Doppler imaging, 3533
Directional pursuit defects, 1126
Dirofilaria, 4528–4529, *4529*
Dirofilaria immitis, 4529, *4530*
Discoid skin lesions, 3813–3814, *3814*
Disconjugate eye movements, 1102

Disconnection alexias, 428, 451
Disembryoplastic infantile gangliogliomas (DIGs), 1977
Disequilibrium syndrome, 1721
Dissecting aneurysms, 2977
  clinical manifestations according to site
    of branches of internal carotid artery, 3216
    of extracranial portion of internal carotid artery, 3210–3215, 3211*t*, *3212, 3213*
    of intracranial portion of internal carotid artery, 3215–3216
    of vertebral and basilar arteries and their branches, 3216–3218, *3217, 3218, 3219, 3220,* 3220*t*, *3221,* 3221–3223
  general considerations, 3203–3210, *3204, 3205, 3206*
Disseminated adenoviral infection, 4959
Disseminated candidiasis, 4352–4353
Disseminated choroiditis, 4867
Disseminated histoplasmosis, 4393–4401, *4394, 4395, 4396, 4397, 4398, 4399, 4400, 4401*
Disseminated intravascular coagulation (DIC), 2515–2518, *2516, 2517, 2518*
Dissociated nystagmus, 1479, *1480*
Dissociated vertical nystagmus, 1296
Distal anterior cerebral artery aneurysms, 3093, 3095, *3097*
Distal embolization, 3209
Distal optic nerve, syndrome of, 1807, 1811, *1811,* 2171
Distal optic nerve syndrome, 294, *297, 298*
Distal optic neuropathy, 294, *297, 298*
Disulfiram, 674
Divergence insufficiency, 1257–1258
Divergence paralysis, 1257–1258
Diving reflex, 1657
DNA probe test, 4402
DNA viruses, 4948
  that infect central nervous system
    adenoviridae, 4954, 4955, *4956,* 4956–4960, *4957, 4958, 4959, 4960*
      clinical manifestations, 4956
        miscellaneous, 4959
        neurologic, 4958–4959
        ocular, 4956–4958, *4957, 4958, 4960, 4961*
        respiratory, 4956, *4956*
      diagnosis, 4959–4960, *4962*
      treatment, 4960
    hepadnaviridae, 4961–4962, 4961–4975, *4962, 4963, 4966, 4967, 4969,* 4970, *4971, 4974,* 4975
      structure of, 4962–4963, *4963*
        clinical syndromes caused by infection, 4965–4972, *4966, 4968, 4969, 4970, 4971*
        epidemiology of infection, 4964
        extrahepatic disease caused by, 4972
        prevention of infection, 4973–4975, *4974, 4975*
        replication of, *4963,* 4963–4964
        routes of transmission, 4964–4965
        tropism of, 4964
    herpesviridae, 4975–4979, *4976, 4977,* 4979, *4980*
      cellular transformation, 4978–4979
      classification and structure, *4976,* 4976–4977
      cytomegalovirus, 5096–5097
        acquired infection in immunocompetent children and adults, 5102–5104, *5103*
        acquired infection in immunosuppressed persons, 5104–5113, *5105, 5106, 5107, 5108, 5109, 5110, 5111, 5112*
        characteristics of, 5097
        congenital infection, 5098–5100, *5099, 5101*
        diagnosis, 5115, *5118–5119*
        epidemiology, 5097–5098
        pathology, *5113,* 5113–5115, *5114, 5115, 5116, 5117, 5118, 5119*
        perinatal infection, 5100–5102, *5102*
        prophylaxis, 5122
        treatment, 5119–5122, *5120, 5121*
      epidemiology and transmission, 4979
      Epstein-Barr virus, 5081–5091, *5082, 5083, 5084, 5086, 5088, 5089, 5090, 5091, 5092,* 5094
        characteristics of, 5081–5082
        clinical manifestations, *5083,* 5083–5091, *5085, 5086, 5088, 5089, 5090, 5091, 5092, 5093,* 5093–5094, *5094*
        diagnosis of, 5095–5096
        epidemiology of, 5082
        pathology of, *5094,* 5094–5095, *5095*
        prevention, 5096
      Herpes B virus, 5128–5129
        characteristics of, 5129
        clinical manifestations, 5129–5131
        diagnosis, 5131
        epidemiology, 5129
        pathogenesis and pathology, 5129
        prevention, 5131
        prognosis, 5131
        treatment, 5131
      herpes simplex virus, 4979–4980, *4980*
        congenital and neonatal infection, 4990–4991, *4991, 4992, 4993*
        diagnosis, *5009,* 5009–5011
        encephalitis, 4991–4992, 4994–4997, *4995, 4996, 4997, 4998, 4999,* 4999–5002, *5000, 5001, 5002, 5003, 5004,* 5004–5005, *5005, 5006, 5007,* 5007–5008, *5008*
        epidemiology, 4980
        idiopathic neurologic syndromes, 5008–5009
        pathogenesis, 4980–4981, *4981*
        primary infections, 4981–4984, *4982, 4983, 4984, 4985,* 4985–4987, 4986
        prophylaxis, 5012
        treatment and prognosis, *5011,* 5011–5012
      human herpesvirus type 6, *5122,* 5122–5127, *5123, 5124, 5125, 5126, 5127*
      human herpesvirus type 7, 5127–5128, *5128*
      human herpesvirus type 8, 5127–5128, *5128*
      latency, 4978, *4978, 4979*
      pathogenesis, 4979
      replication, 4977, *4977*
      tropism, 4977–4978
      varicella-zoster virus, 5012–5013, *5013*
        diagnosis of infections, 5075–5076
        epidemiology, 5025–5026
        neurologic manifestations, 5029, 5031–5033, *5033, 5034,* 5035, *5035, 5036, 5037,* 5037–5039, *5038, 5040, 5041, 5042, 5043,* 5043–5047, *5044, 5045, 5046,* 5051–5054, 5056–5059, 5070, *5071*
        ocular manifestations, 5072, *5073, 5074, 5075, 5076*
        prevention of, 5081
        systemic manifestations, 5028–5029, *5031*
        treatment and prognosis of, 5076–5081, *5078, 5079*
        varicella, 5013
          clinical manifestations, 5014, *5015, 5016,* 5016–5025, *5018, 5020, 5021, 5022,* 5024
          congenital and perinatal infection, 5025
          epidemiology, 5013–5014, *5014, 5015, 5016,* 5016–5025, *5018, 5020, 5022, 5024*
          pathogenesis, 5013
          pathology, 5013, *5014*
    papovaviridae, 5131, *5131*
      BK virus, *5132,* 5132–5133
      JC virus, *5133,* 5133–5139, *5134, 5135, 5136, 5137, 5138, 5139, 5140, 5141,* 5141–5142, *5142*
      papillomaviruses, 5132
      polyomaviruses, 5132
    parvoviridae, 5142–5143, *5143, 5144, 5145,* 5145–5147, *5146*
      vaccinia virus, 5149–5154, *5151, 5152, 5153*
      variola, 5148–5149, *5150*
    poxviridae, 5147–5148, *5148, 5149*
Dolichoectasia, 3180, 3186–3190
  of basilar artery, 1285
  bilateral, 3188
Dolichoectatic aneurysms, 2977, 3182
Dolichoectatic dilation of vertebral artery, 3196–3198
Doll's eyes response, 1782
Dominant optic atrophy, 755–758, *757*
  clinical features, 756–757, *757*
  deafness, 759–760
  etiology, 758
  myopathy, 759–760
  ophthalmoplegia, 759–760
  pathology, 758
  prognosis, 758
Dominantly-inherited neuropathies, 666
Dopaminergic amacrine cell, 42
Dopaminergic pars compacta of substantia nigra, 1317–1318
Dorsal meningeal artery perforates, 2874
Dorsal mesencephalon, 1014
Dorsal midbrain syndrome, 1793, 1794, 1868, 3497, 5433
Dorsal nucleus, 105, 106
Dorsomedial mesencephalic syndrome, 3502, 3506
Dorsum sellae, 2142
Dotumor cerebri, 5023
Double elevator palsy, 1311
Double hemianopia, 357
Double optic neuritis, 2976
Double simultaneous stimulation, 1841
Double-ring sign, 778
Doubling of optic disc, *800,* 800–801

Downbeat nystagmus, 1472, 1472*t*, 1495–1496, 2702
Downgaze paralysis and pseudoptosis, 1547
Down's syndrome, 2336
D-Penicillamine, impact of, on postsynaptic neuromuscular transmission, 1441
DPT immunization, 4116
Dreamy states, 1834
Drop attack, 3472
Droplet nuclei, 4136–4137
Drowsiness in intracranial abscess, 3955
Drug abuse, 3363–3364
  vasculitis associated with, 3754–3755, *3755*
Drug effects in bone marrow transplantation, 2626–2627
Drug-induced lupus, 3830
Drug-induced Parkinsonism, 2771
Drugs. (*See also specific.*)
  and eye movements, 1332*t*, 1333
  iris pigment and pupillary responses to, 1006
  and lacrimation, 1025
  that affect pupils, 1005–1006
  that constrict pupils, *1004*, 1005
  that dilate pupils, *1000, 1001*, 1001–1003, *1002, 1003*
Duane's retraction syndrome, *1240*, 1240–1242, *1241, 1242, 1243*, 1244, *1244, 1245*
Duane's syndrome, 782, 1554
Ductions, 1172
  forced, 1173
Duncan's syndrome, 5091
Dura border cells, 2017
Dura mater, 73, *2017*, 2017–2018, *2019*
  as barrier to infection, 3941
Dural arteriovenous malformations (AVMs), *2268*, 2268–2274, *2269, 2270, 2271, 2272*
  natural history of, 2278
Dural border cells, 2017
Dural sinus thrombosis, 2518–2520, *2520*
Dural sinuses, 2954, *2955*, 2956, *2956, 2957, 2958*, 2959, *2959, 2960, 2961*, 2961–2964, *2962, 2963, 2964, 2965*
  septic thrombosis of, 4034
  thrombosis of, 3893
Dürck's granuloma, 4661, *4665*
Dyad, 45
Dynamic counter-roll, 1141
Dynamic retinoscopy, 951
Dynamic skiametry, 951
Dynamic visual acuity, 1175
Dysarthria, 3472, 3517
Dysautonomia, familial, 764, 1026–1027
Dyscalculia, 1841
Dyschromatopsia, 156, 664, 673–674
  bilateral, 674–675
  unilateral, 653
Dysembryogenesis, 2083
Dysembryoplastic neuroepithelial tumors (DNTs), 1978–1979, *1979*
Dysentery, bacillary, 4224–4225
Dysesthesias, 1750
Dyslexia
  attentional, 433
  central, 434–435
  deep, 435
  hemianopic, 432
  neglect, 433
  phonologic, 435
  related to abnormal vision, attention, or eye movement, 432–434, *434, 435*
  surface, 435
Dysmetria, 1106, 1122–1123
  limb, 5568
  saccadic, 1184, 1326, 1848
Dysmetropsia, 467–469
Dysplasia
  color, 412
  fibromuscular, 3348, *3349*
  hereditary anhidrotic ectodermal, 1027
  optic disc, 1821, 796, *796*
  septo-optic, 779, 780, 783
Dysplastic cerebellar gangliocytomas, 1977, *1978*
Dysthyroid lid retraction, factors in genesis of, 1556–1558
Dysthyroidism, 2163
Dystonia
  focal, 1567, 1840–1841
  focal eyelid, 1539
Dystrophies. (*See also* Muscular dystrophies.)
  adiposogenital, 1814
  infantile neuroaxonal, 766
  oculopharyngeal, 1372–1374, *1373, 1374, 1375*, 1376
Dysuria, postmicturition, 4488

E

E200K mutation, 4577
Eagle's syndrome, 1722
Eales' disease, 3727, 3736–3737, *3737, 3738*, 3739, *3739*
Early delayed encephalopathy, role of radiation therapy in, 2598–2599
Early delayed radiation myelopathy, 2604–2605, *2606*
Early Treatment for Diabetic Retinopathy Study (ETDRS) Chart, 160
Early-onset cerebellar ataxia with retained reflexes, 2790
Early-onset degenerative cerebellar disorders, 2787, 2787*t*, *2788*, 2789–2790
East African trypanosomiasis, 4713–4714, 4715
Eastern equine encephalitis, *5279*, 5279–5281
Eaton-Lambert syndrome
  clinical features, 2524–2525
  diagnostic evaluation, *2525*, 2525–2526
  differential diagnosis, 2526
  pathogenesis, 2526
  treatment and prognosis, 2526–2527
Ebola virus infection, 5166
Eccentric gaze, nystagmus due to abnormality of mechanism for holding, *1478*, 1478–1482, *1480, 1481*
Echinococcal cysts, 4445
  intracranial, 4452
  of orbit, 4452
Echinococcosis, 4439, 4445
  intraocular, 4446–4447, *4448*
  of liver, 4452
  orbital, 4447, *4449*
Echinococcus, 4443, *4445*, 4445–4447, *4446, 4447, 4448, 4449*, 4449–4453, *4450, 4451, 4453, 4454*
Echinococcus cyst, intraventricular, 4447, *4450*
Echinococcus granulosus, 4445
Echinococcus multilocularis, 4445
  cyst of, 4452
Echinococcus oligarthrus, 4445
Echinococcus vogeli, 4445
Echinococcoccosis, 4443, *4445*, 4445–4447, *4446, 4447, 4448, 4449*, 4449–4453, *4450, 4451, 4453, 4454*
Echoviruses, 5241–5243
Ectasia, 3180
Ectopia
  of neural tissue, 2130, *2130*
  posterior pituitary, 782
Ectopic orbital meningiomas, 2051
Ectopic pinealomas, 2085
Ectopic pupils, 1008
Eczema vaccinatum, 5152
Edema, 3981–3982
  cerebral, *3942*, 3942–3943, *3943*
    interstitial, 3943, 3982
  cytotoxic brain, 3943, *3943*
  cytotoxic cerebral, 3982
  eyelid, 4036
  macular, 3462–3463
  vasogenic, 3942, *3942*
  vasogenic cerebral, 3981–3982
  vasogenic cervical, 3981
Edge-light pupil, cycle time, testing, *945*, 945–946
Edinger-Westphal nucleus, 860, 861, 878
  damage to, 974–975
Edwardsiella, 4218
Edwardsiella tarda, 4218
Effector cell, 841
Efference copy, 1106–1107
Effort migraine, 1704
Egocentric localization, past-pointing and disturbances of, 1177
Ehlers-Danlos syndrome, 796, *2984, 2985*, 2985–2987, 3352
Ehrlichia, 4762
Ehrlichia canis, 4762, 4764
Ehrlichia chaffeensis, 4764–4765
Ehrlichia equi, 4763
Ehrlichia phagocytophila, 4763
Ehrlichiosis, 4737–4738, *4762*, 4762–4765, *4765*
Eikenella, 4245
Eikenella corrodens, 4245
Elastase, assessment of, in diagnosing aneurysms, 3015
Electrocardiogram, 3548
Electroencephalograph (EEG) in diagnosing migraines, 3709
Electromyography, single-fiber, 1423
Electro-oculogram (EOG), 223–225, *224*
Electrophysiologic tests, 1422–1424, *1423*
Electroretinogram (ERG), 159, 215–223, *216, 217, 218, 219, 220, 221, 222, 223*
  in children, 219–220
  focal, 159, 220–222
  historical overview, 215–217, *216*
  use of, 219
ELISA in diagnosing bacterial meningitis, 4009
Ellipsoid, 31
Elliptical nystagmus, 1326
Elongation factor 2, 4125–4126, *4126*
Emboli
  air, 3379, 3381
  appearance of, 3365
  arterial, 3401–3405, *3403, 3404*
  atheromatous (and nonatheromatous), 3424
  calcium, 3372–3373, *3374, 3375, 3376*
  causes of, 3386–3396, *3389, 3390, 3391, 3392, 3393, 3394, 3395, 3396, 3397*, 3398, *3398, 3400*, 3400–3406, *3401, 3402, 3403, 3404, 3405, 3406*
  cholesterol, 3365–3367, *3366, 3367, 3368, 3369*

Emboli—*continued*
fat, 3377, 3379, *3379, 3380*
foreign body, 3381–3383, *3383, 3384, 3385,* 3385–3386, *3386, 3387*
general considerations, 3364–3365, 3365*t*
organism, 3379, *3382*
platelet-fibrin, 3367, *3370,* 3370–3371, *3371, 3372*
tumor, 3376–3377, *3378, 3379, 3380*
venous (paradoxical), *3405,* 3405–3407, *3406*
Embolization for arteriovenous malformations (AVMs), 2280, *2280, 2281,* 2282
Embryogenesis, 2252–2253
Embryoid bodies, 2091
Embryonal carcinoma, 2091–2092, *2092*
Embryonal tumors, 1979
ependymoblastoma, 1979
medulloblastoma, 1979–1984, *1981, 1982, 1983*
medulloepithelioma, 1984–1985, *1985, 1986*
neuroblastoma, 1985–1990, *1987, 1988, 1989, 1991*
primitive neuroectodermal, *1999,* 1999–2000, *2000*
retinoblastoma, 1990–1999, *1992, 1993, 1994, 1995, 1996*
Emphysema, orbital, 716–717
Empty delta sign, 3913
Empty space myopia, 910
Empyema, 3943, 3982, *3982,* 4090
causes, *3982,* 3982–3983
clinical manifestations, 3983
diagnosis, 3983–3984, *3984, 3985*
Haemophilus influenzae as cause of, 4234–4236
intracranial subdural or epidural, 4069
pathology, 3983
prognosis, 3985
spinal epidural, 4069
treatment, 3984–3985
En plaque meningiomas, 2057–2058
Encephalitis, 3985–3989, *3986, 3987, 3988,* 4149, 4151, 4309, 4361, 4549–4550
bacterial, 3986
brainstem, 2498–2500, *2500*
California, 5158–5162
characteristics of, 5159–5160, *5160*
clinical manifestations, 5160–5161
diagnosis, 5161
epidemiology of, 5160, *5161*
pathology, 5161, *5162*
prevention, 5162
treatment, 5161
caused by *Haemophilus influenzae,* 4234
cerebellar, 2500–2501
cerebral, 2498, *2499*
chronic, 5104
as complication
of CNS infection with coxsackieviruses, 5238
of CNS infection with echoviruses, 5242
following influenza vaccine, 5197
of herpes zoster, 5053
of HSV infection, 4991–4992, 4994–4997, *4995, 4996, 4997, 4998, 4999,* 4999–5002, *5000, 5001, 5002, 5003, 5004,* 5004–5005, *5005, 5006, 5007,* 5007–5008, *5008*
of influenza, 5193
of postnatally acquired rubella, 5288
cytomegalovirus-induced, 5108–5110
Dawson's, 5213
Eastern equine, *5279,* 5279–5281
enterovirus 71 as cause of, 5245
Epstein-Barr virus (EBV)-associated, 5084–5085
granulomatous amoebic, 4623, 4629–4630, 4632, *4632, 4633, 4634, 4635,* 5415–5416
herpes simplex virus in, 5011–5012
neurotetinitis associated with, 636
Histoplasma, 4394, *4395, 4396, 4397*
human immunodeficiency virus in, 5389
Japanese, 5170
clinical manifestations, *5171,* 5171–5172
epidemiology, 5170–5171
Japanese type A, 5722
Japanese type B, 3985–3986, 5722
LaCrosse, 5158–5162
characteristics of, 5159–5160, *5160*
clinical manifestations, 5160–5161
diagnosis, 5161
epidemiology of, 5160, *5161*
pathology, 5161, *5162*
prevention, 5162
treatment, 5161
lethargic, 5213
Listeria brainstem, 4132
and Lyme disease, 4791, *4792*
measles and development of viral, 3986
measles inclusion body, 5213, 5418
mumps, 5228–5229
and development of viral, 3986
Murray Valley, 5175–5176, *5177, 5178,* 5178–5179, *5179*
clinical manifestations, 5175–5176
diagnosis, 5178–5179
epidemiology, 5175
pathology, 5176, 5178, *5178, 5179, 5180*
prevention, 5179
prognosis, 5179
treatment, 5179
necrotizing, 4686
Negishi, 5189
papilledema in, 517–518
Powassan, 5189–5190
rabies virus in endemic, 3985
St. Louis, 5179–5184, *5181, 5183*
clinical manifestations, 5182
diagnosis, 5182–5183
epidemiology, 5179, *5181,* 5181–5182
pathogenesis, 5182
pathology, 5182, *5183*
prevention, 5183–5184
prognosis, 5183
treatment, 5183
St. Louis type A, 5722
St. Louis type B, 5722
Salmonella, 4222
subacute measles, 5213, 5418–5419
tick-borne, *5186,* 5186–5188, *5188*
clinical manifestations, 5187
diagnosis, 5187
epidemiology, *5186,* 5186–5187
pathology, 5187, *5188*
prevention, 5188
prognosis, 5187–5188
treatment, 5187
Toxocara, 4522
tuberculous, 4149, 4151
Venezuelan equine, *5282,* 5285–5286
viral, 3985–3986, *3986*
Von Economo's, 5722
clinical manifestations, 5723, 5725
acute and subacute, 5725
amyostatic-akinetic type, 5729
hyperkinetic type, 5729
somnolent-ophthalmoplegic type, 5725–5729, *5727*
chronic, 5729
Parkinsonian syndrome, 5729–5732
miscellaneous deficits, 5732
diagnosis, 5732
epidemiology, 5722
etiology, 5733
laboratory studies, 5732
pathology, 5722–5723, *5723, 5724, 5725, 5726, 5727*
prognosis, 5733
treatment, 5733
West Nile, 5184
Western equine, 5280, 5281, 5283, *5283, 5284, 5285*
zoster-related, 5053–5055
Encephalitis lethargica, 1568, 5722
clinical manifestations, 5723, 5725
acute and subacute, 5725
amyostatic-akinetic type, 5729
hyperkinetic type, 5729
somnolent-ophthalmoplegic type, 5725–5729, *5727*
chronic, 5729
Parkinsonian syndrome, 5729–5732
miscellaneous deficits, 5732
diagnosis, 5732
epidemiology, 5722
etiology, 5733
laboratory studies, 5732
pathology, 5722–5723, *5723, 5724, 5725, 5726, 5727*
prognosis, 5733
treatment, 5733
Encephalitis periaxialis concentrica, 628, 5539, 5643–5645, *5646, 5647, 5648*
Encephalocele, 3947
transsphenoidal, 786
Encephalomyelitis, 3989, 4239, 4550, 5088, 5238, 5243
acute disseminated, 5110–5111, 5174, 5649
clinical manifestations, 5649
epidemiology, 5649
laboratory and neuroimaging findings, 5649, *5650*
pathogenesis, 5651
pathology, 5649–5651, *5651, 5652, 5653*
prevention, 5653
prognosis, 5653
acute necrotizing hemorrhagic, 3979
and Lyme disease, 4810–4814, *4811, 4812, 4813, 4814, 4815*
multifocal, 5246
paraneoplastic. (*See* Paraneoplastic encephalomyelitis.)
postinfectious, 3989
Viliuisk, 5741–5744, *5742*
cause, 5744
clinical manifestations, 5743
epidemiology, 5741
laboratory findings, 5743
pathology, 5742–5743
treatment and prognosis, 5743
Encephalomyocarditis syndrome, 5241
Encephalomyopathy with ophthalmoplegia from vitamin E deficiency, 1391
Encephalopathy, 2567, 2588, 3336, 5147

acute, 2598
bovine spongiform, 4567
relationship of, and Creutzfeldt-Jakob disease, 4579–4580
cat-scratch, *4201,* 4201–4202
of childhood, HIV-associated progressive, 5403–5407, *5405, 5406, 5407*
early delayed, 2598–2599
focal, 2599
of fulminant hepatitis B, 4969
hepatic, 4969
human immunodeficiency virus, 5389
human immunodeficiency virus-associated progressive, of childhood, 5403–5407, *5405, 5406, 5407*
hypertensive, headaches associated with, 1713
late delayed, 2599–2602, *2600, 2601, 2603,* 2604, *2605*
metabolic, 2631
in Lyme disease, 4814–4816
mitochondrial, 366, 767
pertussis, 4210
post-treatment reactive, 4719
radiation therapy in, 2598–2599
reactive arsenical, 4719
and *Shigella,* 4225
subacute, 2554–2555
toxic, in Lyme disease, 4814–4816
transmissible spongiform, 4561
Wernicke's, 670, 1331, 5415
Encephalotrigeminal angiomatosis, 2275
cutaneous findings, *2708,* 2708–2709, *2709, 2710*
diagnosis, 2718–2719
management, 2719–2721, *2720, 2721*
neuroimaging, 2718, *2718, 2719, 2720*
neurologic findings, 2712, *2716,* 2716–2718
occurrence, 2707–2708
ocular findings, 2709–2712, *2710, 2711, 2712, 2713, 2714, 2715*
pathogenesis, 2708
Endarterectomy, 3562–3566, *3564, 3565*
carotid, 3575
headache after, 1713–1714
intracranial vertebral artery, 3575
Endemic (Murine) typhus, *4755,* 4755–4758, *4756, 4757, 4758, 4759*
Endocarditis
bacterial, *3966,* 3966–3967, 4081
Candida, 4347
infective, *3393,* 3393–3395, *3394, 3395, 3396, 3397,* 3590, *3592,* 3593
as manifestation of Q fever, 4767–4768
nonbacterial thrombotic, 2520–2521
systemic disease and marantic, 3391
Endocrine abnormalities, 1871, 2597–2598, 3050–3051
in patients, with neurofibromatosis type 1, 2662–2663
Endocrine myopathies, 2531
corticosteroids and, 1405
Cushing's syndrome, 1404–1405
Graves' disease, 1399, *1402, 1403,* 1403–1404
Endodermal sinus tumors, 2092, *2093,* 2094, *2094*
diagnosis of, 2094
treatment of, 2094
Endodyogeny, 4667
Endolymphatic sac tumors, 2703–2704
Endonuclease, 5363
Endophthalmitis, 4090, 4178, 4296, 4298–4299
of meningococcal meningitis, 4096–4097
Endophytic retinoblastomas, 1993–1994, *1994*
Endosome, 4948
Endospores, 4355
Endothelin, 3146–3147
Endotoxin, 4065, 4739
Endovascular surgery
results of, 3178–3180, *3179*
for unruptured aneurysms, 3154–3155, *3156, 3157,* 3157–3159, *3158, 3159, 3160, 3161, 3162,* 3162–3165, *3164, 3165, 3166, 3167*
End-stopped cells, *130,* 130–131, *131*
Enhancers, 4952
Enophthalmos, 1800–1801, *1801*
Entamoeba histolytica, 4614
in intracranial brain abscess, 3952
life cycle, *4614,* 4614–4615, *4615, 4616*
Enteric fever, 4221
Enterobacter, 4218–4219
Enterobacter aerogenes, 4220
Enterobacter cloacae, 4218, 4219
Enterobacter sakazakii, 4218
Enterobacteriaceae, 4217–4218
Citrobacter, 4218
Edwardsiella, 4218
Enterobacter, 4218–4219
Escherichia coli, 4219
Klebsiella, 4219–4220
Proteus, 4220–4221
Salmonella, 4221–4224, *4222, 4223*
carrier state, 4223
clinical manifestations, 4221–4223, *4222, 4223*
prevention, 4223–4224
Serratia, 4224
Shigella, 4224–4225
Yersinia, 4225, 4225–4228
Enterococcal meningitis, 4091
Enterococci, 4090–4091
Enterococcus faecalis, 4090
in bacterial aneurysms, 2999
in bacterial meningitis, 3994
Enterococcus faecium, 4090
Enteropathic arthritis, 3857–3859, *3859, 3860, 3861, 3862, 3863*
Enteroviral infection, pathogenesis of, 5234–5235
Enterovirus 70, 5243–5245, *5244*
Enterovirus 71, 5245–5246
Enterovirus 72, *5246,* 5246–5250
Enteroviruses, 5234–5235, 5243–5250, *5244, 5246*
Entomophthorales, 4318
Entomophthoramycosis, 4318
Env gene, 5364, 5365, 5434
Environmental dependency syndrome, 1822
Enzyme immunoassay test, 5379
in diagnosing bacterial meningitis, 4009
Eosinophilia, peripheral, 4287
Eosinophilic granuloma, 2405
Eosinophilic meningitis, 4496, *4498,* 4498–4499, *4499,* 4503, *4505,* 4681
Eosinophilic meningoencephalitis, 4496, 4503, *4505*
Eosinophils, 2329
Ependyma, neoplastic infiltration of, 1929, *1929*
Ependymal cysts, *43,* 2123–2124, *2125,* 2126, *2127, 2128*
Ependymal tumors, *1963,* 1963–1966, *1964, 1965*
ependymomas, *1963,* 1963–1966, *1964, 1965*
subependymomas, 1966–1967, *1967*
Ependymoblastoma, 1966, 1979
Ependymomas, *1963,* 1963–1966, *1964, 1965*
Ephaptic cross activation, 5566–5567, *5567*
Ephedrine, 1003
Epidemic keratoconjunctivitis (EKC), 4956
Epidemic nutritional optic neuropathy, 667–668
Epidemic pleurodynia, 5235
Epidemic Reiter's syndrome, 3854
Epidemic typhus, *4752,* 4752–4755, *4753, 4754*
Epidermal growth factor (EFG), 3334
Epidermal nevus syndrome, 2735
Epidermoids, 2110–2113, *2111, 2112*
Epididymitis with orchitis, 5225–5226
Epidural abscesses, 3943, *3944,* 4179
by *Aspergillus,* 4308
Epidural empyema, 4105
Epidural hematoma
headaches associated with, 1709
papilledema from, 516
Epidural lipomatosis, 2588
Epidural parasellar echinococcus cyst, 4447, *4450*
Epidural tuberculous granulomas, 4162–4163
Epilepsia partialis continua, 4375
Epilepsy. (*See also* Seizures.)
benign childhood, with occipital spikewaves, 463
diencephalic autonomous, 1854
eye movements during seizures in, 1485–1486
myoclonic, with ragged red fibers (MERRF), 767
psychomotor, 1834
Epileptic nystagmus, 1485–1486
Epimastigotes, 4702, 4711
Epiphora, 953
Episcleritis, 3822
Episodic ataxia type 1, 2794
Episodic ataxia type 2, 2794
Episodic paroxysmal hemicrania, relationship between migraine, cluster headache and, 3699–3701
Epithelial keratitis, 5289
Epithelioid cell, 3989
Epitheliopathy, acute posterior multifocal placoid pigment, 4086, 4957–4958, 4974
Epsilon-aminicaproic acid (Amicar) for aneurysms, 3175
Epstein-Barr virus (EBV)
characteristics of, 5081–5082
clinical manifestations of, *5083,* 5083–5091, *5085, 5086, 5088, 5089, 5090, 5091, 5092, 5093,* 5093–5094, *5094*
epidemiology of, 5082
Epstein-Barr virus (EBV) infection
and cancer, 5091
diagnosis of, 5095–5096
pathology of, *5094,* 5094–5095, *5095*
prevention, 5096
treatment, 5096
Equine morbillivirus, 5200
Equine viral arteritis, 4029
Ergonovine for cough-induced headache, 1703
Eruptive histiocytoma, 2421

Erysipelas, 4130
Erysipeloid, 4130
Erysipelothrix insidiosa, 4130, *4130*
Erysipelothrix rhusiopathiae, 4130, *4130*
Erythema migrans, 4779–4780
Erythema nodosum, 4170–4171, 5480, *5480*
  skin manifestations of, 4170–4171
Erythematous urticarial rashes, 5153
Erythrocyte sedimentation rate, 3772–3773
Erythrocytosis, 2332
  absolute, 2332, 3357
  apparent, 2332
  clonal, 2332
  nonclonal, 2332
  secondary, 2332
Erythroleukemia, 2334, *2334*
Erythropoiesis, 2329
Escherichia coli, 4219
  in bacterial meningitis, 3993
  in empyema, 3983
  in intracranial abscess, 3950
  in vasogenic cervical edema, 3981
Esophageal motility abnormalities in CREST syndrome, 3014
Esotropia, 1316, 3483–3484
  cyclic, and its relationship to abducens nerve palsy, 1258
Essential blepharospasm, 1565, *1566*
Essential thrombocythemia, 2335, 3357
Esthesioneuroblastoma, 1989–1990, *1991*
Estrogen therapy, 3362, 3890
  for pituitary adenomas, 2196
Ethambutol amblyopia, 674
Ethambutol for tuberculosis, 4142–4143
Ethambutol intoxication, 673–674
Ethambutol optic neuropathy, 674
Ethmoid sinus mucoceles, 4019, *4021, 4022*
Ethylene glycol, 1262
  intoxication, 673
Euphoria, 5575
European blastomycosis, 4367
Evaginations, 2981, *2981*
Evoked potentials
  brainstem auditory, 5626
  somatosensory, 5626–5627
  visual, *5625,* 5625–5626
Exanthem subitum, 5123
Excavated optic disc anomalies, 785
  coloboma, *12,* 788–789, 789*t*, 790*t*
  morning glory, *785,* 785–788, *786, 787*
  peripapillary staphyloma, *780,* 789–790
Excessive eyelid closure
  of myopathic origin, 1576–1577, *1577*
  of neuromuscular origin, 1576, *1576*
Excitotoxic hypothesis, 2796–2797
Exertion migraine, 1704
Exflagellation, 4651
Exoantigen test, 4402–4403
Exoerythrocytic forms, 4650
Exogenous agents, 3585–3586, *3586*
Exophiala dermatitidis, 4353, 4354
Exophthalmometers, 1799, *1799*
Exophthalmometry, 158
Exophthalmos, 1799, 2589, 2654–2655, *2656*
  positional, 2655
  pulsating, 3275, 3277, *3279*
Exophytic retinoblastomas, 1994, *1995*
Exotoxin, 4125–4126, *4126*
Exotoxin A, 4241
Exotropia, 324
  paralytic pontine, 1302
Experimental allergic encephalomyelitis (EAE), 3979
Experimental allergic neuritis (EAN), 5682
Exposure keratopathy, 3277, *3280,* 4171
Express saccades, 1105, *1106*
Express smooth pursuit, 1123
Expressive amusia, 1821–1822
External carotid arteries, 2869, 2940. (*See also* Carotid arteries.)
  anterior branches of, 2940–2941
  ascending branch of, 2941–2942
  meningeal branches of, 3298
  posterior branches of, 2941
  terminal branches of, 2942, *2944,* 2944–2946, *2945*
External compression headache, 1702
External maxillary artery, 2940
External ophthalmoplegia, 3837
Extorsion, 1172
Extra-axial tumors at base of brain, 1887–1890, *1888, 1889, 1890, 1891, 1892,* 1893
Extracellular gram-negative bacilli, 4067
Extracellular space of optic nerve, 62–64
Extracranial cerebral veins, *2957, 2962,* 2966–2967, *2968*
Extracranial metastases, 1929
Extracranial pseudoaneurysms of carotid, 3038
Extracranial to intracranial (EC-IC) bypass, 3562, 3566
Extracranial vascular transposition, 3566–3567
Extracranial vertebral artery aneurysms, 3014
Extracutaneous sporotrichosis, 4415
Extradural pachymeningitis, 4337, *4338*
Extrahepatic disease, caused by hepatitis B virus (HBV), 4972
Extramedullary disease, intradural, 4467
Extraocular muscle afferents
  anatomy of, 1641–1642, *1642*
  central trigeminal pathways of, 1643–1644
  peripheral trigeminal pathways of, 1642, *1643*
  trigeminal cells of origin of, 1642–1643
Extraocular muscles, 1072–1075, *1074, 1075, 1076, 1077*
  developmental disorders of
    agenesis of, 1352
    anomalies of location, *1352,* 1352–1353, *1353*
    congenital adherence and fibrosis syndromes, 1353–1354
  dysfunction of, 3077
  evidence for importance of proprioception, 1641
  involvement with amyloidosis, 1397–1398, *1399*
  ischemic myopathy of, 1405
Extraorbital lymphoma, 2378–2379
Extraparenchymal angiomas, 2236
  cavernous, 2236
Extrapulmonary blastomycosis, 4333
Extrapulmonary tuberculosis, 4144
Extrapyramidal signs as sign of tumor, 1797
Extrastriate cortex, lesions of, with defects in visual field, *371,* 371–372
Extra-trigeminal (sympathetic) corneal innervation, 1600–1601
Eye closure, hallucinations during, 467
Eye movements
  abnormal, 1364, 1366, 1462
    dyslexia related to, 432–434, *434, 435*
  effects of drugs on, 1332*t*, 1333
  during epileptic seizures, 1485–1486
  generalized limitations of, 1797–1798
  lid movements that accompany vertical, 1533–1536, *1534, 1535*
  ptosis associated with, *1540,* 1540–1541, *1541*
  quantitative analysis of, 1185
  range of, *1171,* 1171–1176
  types of, 1101
Eye popping reflex, 1550
Eye position command, 1113
Eye velocity command, 1113
Eyebrow, control of, 1513, *1513*
Eye-head movements, 1317
Eyelashes, trichomegaly of, 5374
Eyelid closure, 937
  abnormalities, 1559
    excessive or anomalous, 1565–1580, *1566, 1567, 1572, 1573, 1574, 1575, 1576, 1577, 1578*
    insufficiency, 1560–1565, *1561, 1562, 1565*
  reflexes after, 893
Eyelid control and brainstem projections, 1520, 1520*t*
Eyelid edema, 4036
Eyelid freezing, 1539
Eyelid function, disturbances of, 5730
Eyelid myoclonia, 1570
Eyelid nystagmus, 1486, 1550–1551
Eyelid opening, abnormalities of
  ptosis, 1537–1543, *1538, 1539, 1540, 1541, 1542, 1543, 1544, 1545,* 1545–1547, *1546, 1547, 1548, 1549, 1550, 1551*
  retraction, 47–53, 1547–1551, *1551, 1552, 1553, 1554, 1555, 1556, 1557, 1558, 1559*
    associated oculomotor nerve palsy, 1554
    associated with contralateral ptosis, 1555, *1556*
    evoked by jaw movement, 1553–1554, *1554*
    neuromuscular, and lid-lag, 1555–1556, *1556*
    from paradoxic levator excitation, 1551, *1553,* 1553–1555, *1554, 1555*
    from supranuclear lesions, 1548–1550, *1551, 1552*
    from sympathetic hyperfunction, 1555
Eyelid ptosis from combined paradoxic levator excitation and inhibition, 1554, *1555*
Eyelid retraction, 3466–3467
  from combined paradoxic levator excitation and inhibition, 1554, *1555*
  mechanical, 1559, *1559*
Eyelid retractors, 1511–1513, *1512*
  lower, 1512–1513
Eyelid spasms, botulinum toxin for, 1577–1580
Eyelid system, anatomy of
  basis of passive lid-closing forces, 1513
  innervation of levator palpebrae superioris muscle, 1520–1522, *1521*
  innervation of orbicularis oculi muscle and motoneurons, 1513–1514, *1514, 1515, 1516, 1517,* 1517–1520, *1518, 1519,* 1520*t*
  orbicularis oculi muscle, 1510–1511, *1511*
  other muscles interacting with, 1513, *1513*
  retractors, 1511–1513, *1512*
  surface, 1510, *1510*

Eyelids
aponeurotic defects of, 1545
apraxia of closure, 2775
apraxia of opening, 2775
effects of radiation therapy on, 2613
evaluation of, 1509
leukemic involvement of, *2340,* 2340–2341, *2341, 2342*
motor control and physiology of
adaptation and motility, *1536,* 1536–1537
blinking, 1523–1533, *1524, 1525, 1526, 1527, 1528, 1530, 1531, 1532*
eyelid movements and eye movements, 1533–1536, *1534, 1535*
lid position, 1522–1523, *1523*
nonorganic disturbances of, 1784
sensory nerve endings in, 1601–1602
upward jerking of, 1551
Eyelid-triggered synkinesias, 1570–1571
Eyestrain headaches, 1731–1732

F

Fabry disease, 2831–2832, *2832, 2833,* 3352–3353
Face perception
neuropsychology of, 415–416
in nonhuman primates, 421–423
other disorders of, 424
Facial ganglion neuralgia from herpes zoster, *1742,* 1743–1745, *1745*
Facial impairment, specificity of, in prosopagnosia, 413–414
Facial infections, *4034,* 4034–4035
Facial myokymia, 1571, *1572,* 5685
with peripheral neuropathy, 1571–1572
Facial nerve, 1517, *1517*
dysfunction, 1796–1797
labyrinthine segment, 1517
mastoid segment, 1517
misdirection, 1564, *1565*
paresis of, and Lyme disease, 4793–4794
schwannomas of, 2306–2308, *2307*
tympanic segment, 1517
Facial nerve palsy, insufficiency of eyelid closure from, *1558,* 1560–1564, *1562*
Facial neuropathy, 4373
Facial neuropathy, role of radiation therapy in, 2612
Facial nucleus and nerve, *1513,* 1513–1514, *1514, 1515, 1516, 1517, 1518*
Facial pain with sixth nerve palsy, *1730,* 1730–1731
Facial paresthesia, 1750–1752
Facial Recognition Test, 470, 471
Facial sensation, nonorganic disturbances of, 1784
Facial spasms, botulinum toxin for, 1577–1580
Facial swelling in giant cell arteritis, 3756–3757
Factor V Leiden, 3889
Facultative bacteria, 4066
Faget's sign, 5184
Falcotentorial junction, 2041
False orientation, 1177, *1178*
False-positive serologic tests of syphilis, 4927–4928
Falx cerebelli, 2018
Falx cerebri, 2018
Falx meningiomas, 2037, *2039,* 2039–2041, *2040, 2042,* 2043
Familial aneurysms, 3014–3015
Familial Creutzfeldt-Jakob disease, 4576–4577
Familial dextrocardia, 796
Familial dysautonomia, 764, 1026–1027
Familial episodic ataxia with nystagmus, 1496
Familial hemiplegic migraine, 3678
Familial Mediterranean fever, 529, 631
Familial motor neuron disease, 2799
Familial multiple myeloma, 2390
Familial panencephalopathic Creutzfeldt-Jakob disease, 4584, *4585*
Familial paroxysmal ataxia, gaze-evoked nystagmus in, 1479–1480
Family album tomography, 933
Fanconi's syndrome, 2336
Farber disease, 2830–2831, *2831*
Farber lipogranulomatosis, 2830–2831, *2831*
Farnsworth Panel D-15 test, 211–212, *212,* 407, *407*
in color vision testing, 156
Farnsworth-Munsell 100-Hue Test, 212, *213,* 407, *408,* 436, 437, 612, 745, 749, 756
Fascia, capsulopalpebral, 1512–1513
Fasciculus lenticularis, 1863
Fasciculus thalamicus, 1863
Fat emboli, 3377, 3379, *3379, 3380*
FAT scanning, 933
Fatal familial insomnia, 4595, 4598
cerebral metabolism, 4601–4602
clinical characteristics, 4598–4599
genetics, 4599–4600, *4601*
pathology, 4600–4601, *4601, 4602*
Fatigue
accommodative, 951
and multiple sclerosis, 5574
Fatty streak, 3332
Feedback control of saccades, 1113–1114, *1114*
Feeding center, 1814
Festinating gait, 5729
Fetal alcohol syndrome, 782
Fibrillary astrocytes, 1865, 1920
Fibrillary astrocytomas, 1922
Fibrinogen, 3774
Fibrinous iritis, 4901
Fibroblast, 853
Fibroblast growth factor (FGF), 3334
Fibroblastic meningiomas, 2027, *2028*
Fibromas
periungual, 2675, *2675*
soft, 2675, *2676*
subungual, 2675, *2675*
Fibromuscular dysplasia, *2982,* 2982–2983, *2983, 2984,* 2985, 3348, *3349*
Fibrosis, congenital, 1353–1354
Fibrous molluscum, 2649
Fibrous plaque, 3332
Filamentous fungi, 4281
Filaria, 4503
Filoviridae, 5166–5167
Filovirus hemorrhagic fever, 5166
Finger agnosia, 1841
Finger clubbing, 5374
Fingerprint body myopathy, 1358
Fisher's syndrome, 1029
Fisher's variant of Guillain-Barré syndrome, 5019
Fistulas. (*See* Carotid-cavernous sinus fistulas.)
Fixation, 1156
disorders of, 5599, *5602,* 5602–5603, 5728
and gaze-holding ability, 1171
general principles of, 1136–1137
neurophysiology of, 1137
nonorganic disease affecting, 1777, 1779, *1779*
Fixation neurons, 1115
FK-506 and headaches, 1718
Flaccid monoplegia, 5246
Flaccid motor paralysis, 5239, 5242
Flagella, 4613
Flatworms
cestodes, 4439–4440, *4440*
Coenurus cerebralis, 4440–4441, *4441, 4442, 4443*
Diphyllobothrium latum, 4441, 4443, *4444*
Diphyllobothrium nihonkaiense, 4441, 4443, *4444*
Echinococcus, 4443, *4445,* 4445–4447, *4446, 4447, 4448, 4449,* 4449–4453, *4450, 4451, 4453, 4454*
Spirometra species, 4453–4455, *4455, 4456, 4457, 4458, 4459,* 4460, *4460*
Taenia crassiceps, 4479
Taenia solium, 4460
clinical manifestations, 4462–4469, *4463, 4464, 4465, 4466, 4467, 4468, 4469, 4470,* 4471, *4471, 4472*
diagnosis, 4474–4477, *4475, 4476, 4477*
epidemiology, 4460
neuropathology, 4471–4474, *4473, 4474*
ocular pathology, 4474
pathogenesis, 4460–4461, *4461, 4462*
treatment, 4477–4479, *4478*
trematodes, 4479, *4480*
miscellaneous, of neuro-ophthalmologic significance, 4492, *4493,* 4494
Paragonium species, 4479, *4481,* 4481–4483, *4482, 4483, 4484,* 4485
Schistosoma species, 4485, *4485*
clinical manifestations, 4487–4489, *4488, 4489*
diagnosis, 4491–4492, *4493*
epidemiology, 4486
life cycle, 4485–4486, *4486*
pathogenesis and pathology, 4489–4491, *4490, 4491, 4492*
treatment, 4492
Flavimonas oryzihabitans, 4245
Flaviviridae, 5170
Flavobacteria, 4228
Flechsig's Field 16, 143
Fleurettes, 1993, 1996
Flicker perimetry, 207
Flight of colors test, 622
Flocculus, experimental lesions of, 1290
Flow void, 3132
Fluconazole
for candidiasis, 4353
for coccidioidomycosis, 4365
for fungal infections, 4286, *4286*
for histoplasmosis, 4404
Flucytosine
for allergic aspergillosis, 4317
for cryptococcosis, 4384–4385
for fungal infections, 4284, *4284*
Fluent aphasia, 1841
Fluid-attenuated inversion recovery (FLAIR), 5000
Fluorescein angiography, 159
Fluorescence antibody to membrane antigen (FAMA) in diagnosing varicella-zoster virus infections, 5075–5076

5-Fluorouracil, 2558–2560
neuro-ophthalmologic toxicity, 2559–2560
cytosine arabinoside, 2560–2562
neurotoxicity, 2558–2559
ocular toxicity, 2559
systemic toxicity, 2558
Foam cell, 3332
Focal dystonia, 1567, 1840–1841
Focal electroretinography, 159, 220–222
Focal encephalitis, 4394
Focal encephalopathy, 2599
Focal eyelid dystonia, 1539
Focal myasthenia, 1424
Focal neurologic deficits, 2717, 3958
Focal proliferative nephritis, 3817, *3817*
Focal seizures, 1570
Folic acid deficiency as cause of optic neuropathy, 670
Follicle-stimulating hormone (FSH), 2148
Follicular conjunctivitis, 4202
Fonsecaea compacta, 4353
Fonsecaea pedrosoi, 4353
Food poisoning, 4117. (*See also* Botulism.)
Food-borne botulism, 1438
Foods in inducing headache, 1718
Foramen lacerum, 2871
Foramen magnum
chordoma in, 2441
meningiomas in, 2054–2055
Forbes-Albright syndrome, 2152, 2155–2156, 2186–2187
Forced duction, 1173
Forced duction testing, 1171
Foreign body emboli, 3381–3383, *3383, 3384, 3385,* 3385–3386, *3386, 3387*
Foreign-body giant cells, 3989
Form, discrimination of, 395, *397*
Formalin-inactivated vaccines, 5196–5197
Formed visual hallucinations, 3473–3474
Fortification figure, 3667, *3668*
Fortification scotomas, 3667, *3668*
Foster Kennedy Syndrome, 296, 298, 498–499, *500,* 700, 1824, 1826, *1826,* 2044, 2060, 2063, 2176
Foveal avascular zone, 52
Foveation periods, 1482, 1483
Foville's syndrome, 1249
Francisella tularensis, 4228, 4228–4229, 5679
Frataxin, 2789
Freckles, 2649
Free-living amoebae
Acanthamoeba species, 4628–4630, *4630, 4631,* 4632, *4632, 4633, 4634,* 4635, *4635, 4636, 4637,* 4638, *4638*
Balamuthia mandrillaris (Leptomyxida), 4638, *4639, 4640,* 4640–4641, *4641*
Naegleria fowleri, 4623–4626, *4624, 4625, 4626, 4627,* 4628, *4628, 4629*
Frequency doubling perimetry, 208–209, *209*
Friedman Visual Field Analyzer, 612
Friedreich's ataxia, 762, 1292, 2787–2787*t*
etiology and genetics, 2789
laboratory and neuroimaging findings, 2789
neurologic manifestations, 2789
neuro-ophthalmologic manifestations, 2789
pathology, 2787, *2788,* 2789
prognosis, 2789–2790
treatment, 2789
Froehlich's syndrome, 1814
Frontal eye fields, 1130
in saccadic eye movements, 1114–1115, *1115, 1116, 1117*
Frontal lobe
abscess of, 3957, 3958, *3958, 3959*
intracerebral hemorrhage into, 3023–3024
lesions of, 1324–1325
tumors in, 1818–1825, *1819, 1820, 1821, 1823,* 3425
ocular symptoms and signs produced by, 1824–1825
Frontal nerve, 1613
Frontal sinus mucoceles, 4017, 4019, *4019, 4020*
Frontalis, 1513, *1513*
Frontopolar artery, 2897
Frontotemporal dementia
behavioral and psychiatric manifestations, 2760–2762
epidemiology, 2759
laboratory and neuroimaging findings, 2762, *2762*
neurologic manifestations, 2759–2760
pathology, 2759, *2760, 2761*
prognosis, 2762
Fukuyama congenital muscular dystrophy, 1361
Fulminant colitis, 4619
Functional MR imaging, 3533
Fundus examination, 158–159
Fungal aneurysms, *3003,* 3003–3004, *3004,* 3971–3973, *3972, 3973*
mycotic, 3113
Fungal infections, drugs used to treat, 4283
amphotericin B, *4283,* 4283–4284
fluconazole, 4286, *4286*
flucytosine, 4284, *4284*
imidazoles, 4284
itraconazole, 4286
ketoconazole, *4284,* 4284–4286, *4285*
triazoles, 4284
Fungal meningitis, 5421–5423
Fungi, 4281–4283, *4282,* 4282*t*
filamentous, 4281
in meningoencephalitis, 3987
Funnel-shaped dilations, 2980–2981, *2981*
Furadantin, 1263
Furaltadone, 1263
Fusarium, 4282, *4387,* 4387–4389, *4388, 4389,* 5422
Fuscoceruleus, 2649
Fusiform aneurysms, 2977
clinical manifestations, treatment, and prognosis according to site
of basilar artery and its branches, *3198,* 3198–3199, *3199, 3200, 3201,* 3201–3203, *3202, 3203*
of internal carotid artery and its branches, 3183–3186, *3184, 3185, 3187,* 3188–3192, *3189, 3190, 3191, 3192, 3193, 3194,* 3195, *3195, 3196*
of vertical artery and its branches, 3195–3198, *3197*
general considerations, *3180,* 3180–3183, *3181, 3182*
Fusional convergence, 948
Fusobacterium, 4229–4232, *4230*
in brain abscess, 3946
in intracranial abscess, 3947
Fusobacterium mortiferum, 4230–4232
Fusobacterium necrophorum, 4230–4232
in intracranial brain abscess, 3952
in sinusitis, 4025
Fusobacterium nucleatum, 4230–4232, 4231–4232
F-wave, 5689–5690

G

Gabapentin, 1496
Gag gene, 5364, 5365, 5434
Gagel's granuloma, 2407, *2409*
Gait, festinating, 5729
Gait apraxia, 1820
Gait ataxia, 5568
Galactorrhea, 2155–2156
Galactorrhea-amenorrhea syndrome, 2152, 2155–2156, 2186–2187
Galactose, 4616
Galen, vein of
aneurysms of, 2263–2266, *2264, 2265*
natural history of arteriovenous malformations (AVMs) of, 2278
Gallium, 5522–5523
Galvanic stimulation, peripheral vestibular nystagmus induced by, 1471–1472
Gametocytes, 4651
Gangliocytomas, 1975–1977, *1976*
dysplastic cerebellar, 1977, *1978*
Ganglioglioma, 689–690, 1975–1977, *1976*
disembryoplastic infantile, 1977
Ganglion cell tumors, 1975
central neurocytoma, 1977–1978, *1978*
disembryoplastic infantile gangliogliomas, 1977
dysembryoplastic neuroepithelial, 1978–1979, *1979*
dysplastic cerebellar gangliocytoma, 1977, *1978*
gangliocytomas, 1975–1977, *1976*
gangliogliomas, 1975–1977, *1976*
Ganglioneuromas, 690
Gangliosidoses, 2824–2828, *2825, 2826, 2828*
Gardner syndrome, 2735
Garin-Bujadoux-Bannwarth Syndrome, 4794–4795
Gasserian ganglion, 1618–1620, *1619, 1620*
Gastroenteritis, 4959
Gastrointestinal anthrax, 4106
Gastrointestinal involvement in neurofibromatosis type 1, 2662
Gastrointestinal mucormycosis, 4326–4327
and malnutrition, 4326–4327
Gaucher disease, 1326, 2828–2830, *2829, 2830*
Gaze deviations, 1327–1328
Gaze stability, normal mechanisms for, 1461–1462
Gaze velocity Purkinje cells, 1132
Gaze-evoked amaurosis, *1798,* 1798–1799
Gaze-evoked eyelid nystagmus, *1478,* 1478–1480, 1551
in familial paroxysmal ataxia, 1479–1480
Gaze-paretic nystagmus, 3900
in botulism, 4119
Gegenhalten, 1821
Gegenrucke, 1486
Gelastic seizures, 2129
Gelsemium sempervirens (yellow jasmine), 1262
Gemella haemolysans, 4091

Gemistocytic astrocytes, 1921, *1921*
Gender in relationship between optic neuritis and multiple sclerosis, 618
General paresis, 4889–4891
Generalized limitation of eye movements as sign of tumor, 1797–1798
Generalized tetanus, 4110, 4112–4113
Generalized vaccinia, 5152–5153
Genetic disorders, hypercoagulability states resulting from, 3888–3889
Genetic resistance, 4141
Geniculocalcarine tract. (*See* Optic radiations.)
Genital ulcers, 3803, *3804*
Genitourinary amoebiasis, 4620
Genitourinary tract blastomycosis, 4335–4336
Genitourinary tract coccidioidomycosis, 4360
Gennari, Francesco, 126
Gentamycin, 1002
Germ cell tumors, 2083–2085, *2084*
Germinal mutation, 1990
Germinomas, 2085
  clinical characteristics, *2087,* 2087–2088
  diagnosis and treatment, *2088,* 2088–2089
  nomenclature, 2085
  occurrence, 2085
  pathology, 2085–2087, *2086*
  prognosis, 2089
  suprasellar, 2085
Gerstmann's syndrome, 412, 449, 1841, 3485
Gerstmann-Sträussler-Scheinker disease, 4592, 4594
  clinical characteristics, *4593,* 4594
  pathology and genetics, *4594,* 4594–4595, *4595, 4596, 4597, 4598, 4599, 4600*
Giant aneurysms, 3141–3142
Giant cell arteritis, 3340, 3342, *3343,* 3424, 3727, 3755–3761, *3756, 3757, 3758, 3759, 3760*
  demographics, 3755
  diagnosis, 3775–3776, *3777, 3778,* 3778–3779, *3779, 3780*
  headaches associated with, 1712
  laboratory studies, 3772–3775, *3774*
  neurologic manifestations, 3757–3758, *3758, 3759*
  ocular and neuro-ophthalmologic manifestations, 3758–3761, *3760, 3761, 3762, 3763,* 3763–3769, *3764, 3765, 3766, 3767, 3768, 3769, 3771*
  pathogenesis, 3769, 3771
  pathology, 3771–3772, *3772, 3773, 3774*
  systemic manifestations, *3756,* 3756–3757, *3757*
  treatment and prognosis, 3779–3782
  vasculitides other than, 578, *579,* 580, *580, 581, 582*
Giant cell tumors, 2443–2444
Giant serpentine aneurysms, 3182
Gigantism, 2156–2160, *2157, 2159*
Gilles de la Tourette syndrome and tics, 1570
Gillespie syndrome, 2785, *2785*
Gingivostomatitis, 4981
Glands of Krause, 918
Glands of Wolfring, 918
Glandular tularemia, 4229
Glaucoma, 988, 2709–2710, *2710,* 3284, *3285,* 5040, 5292–5293
  acute angle closure, *1010,* 1010–1011, 1724–1725
  angle closure, 3424
  in children, 1012–1013
  chronic open angle, 253, *255,* 255–256, *256, 257*
  congenital, 2652
  open-angle, 2350
  secondary, 1997
Glaucoma Hemifield Test (GHT), 182
Glaucomatous optic neuropathy, 253, *255,* 255–256, *256, 257*
Glial cells, 43–44
Glial fibrillary acidic protein (GFAP), 1919
Glioblastoma multiforme (GBM), 1922, 1925–1930, *1926, 1927, 1928, 1929,* 2559
Gliofibromas, 1931–1932
Gliomas, 1920
  bilateral optic nerve, 1951
  brainstem, 2659–2660
  chiasmal, 2652–2654, *2653, 2654, 2655*
  malignant optic, 1957, *1958, 1959*
  optic chiasmal, 1945, 1951–1956, *1952, 1954*
  optic disc, *1956,* 1956–1957
  optic nerve, *1945,* 1945–1951, *1946, 1948, 1949*
Gliomatosis
  papilledema in cerebral and leptomeningeal, 518
  primary leptomeningeal, 1941, *1941*
Gliomatosis cerebri, 1932, *1933*
Gliosarcoma, 1925–1930, *1926, 1927, 1928, 1929*
Glissade, 1105
Globoid cell leukodystrophy, 2857–2859, *2858, 2859*
Globus pallidus, 1863
Glomerulonephritis, 4072
  poststreptococcal acute, 4085
Glomus jugulare bodies, 2462
Glomus jugulare paragangliomas, 2468, *2469,* 2470–2471
Glomus jugulare tumors, 2468, *2469,* 2470–2471
Glossopharyngeal neuralgia, 1722, 1745–1747, *1746*
Gnathostoma spinigerum, 4500
  clinical manifestations, 4501–4503, *4504, 4505*
  diagnosis, 4503
  epidemiology, 4500–4501
  intraocular, 4501–4503, *4504*
  life cycle, 4500, *4500, 4501*
  pathogenesis and pathology, 4501, *4502*
  subjunctival, 4501
  treatment and prognosis, 4503
Gnathostomiasis, 4500
  clinical manifestations, 4501–4503, *4504, 4505*
  diagnosis, 4503
  epidemiology, 4500–4501
  intraocular, 4501–4503, *4504*
  life cycle, 4500, *4500, 4501*
  pathogenesis and pathology, 4501, *4502*
  subjunctival, 4501
  treatment and prognosis, 4503
Goldenhar sequence, 788
Goldenhar syndrome, 782
Goldmann manual projection perimeter, 176–177, *177*
Goldmann perimeter, 156, 157
  for kinetic perimetry, 469
Goldmann-Weekers dark adaptometer, 214
Goltz focal dermal hypoplasia, 788
Gonadotropin-releasing hormone (GnRH), 2146
Gonadotropins, 2148
Gonococcal meningitis, 4102–4103
Gonorrhea, 4102
Gotton's papules, 2528
Gradenigo's syndrome, 1673, *1730,* 1730–1731, 3900, 4040
Gradient method, 952
Graft-versus-host disease (GVHD), 2626, 2627
  chronic, 2637
Gram-negative bacilli, 4192–4193, 4193*t*
  Actinobacillus species, 4193
  Bacteroides species, 4193–4195, *4194, 4195*
  Bartonella, 4196
    bacillary angiomatosis, 4208
    cat-scratch disease, 4196, *4196*
      clinical manifestations, 4199–4200
      diagnosis, 4207
      epidemiology, 4199
      etiology, 4196–4199, *4201*
      neurologic manifestations, *4201,* 4201–4202
      neuro-opthalmologic manifestations, 4202–4207, *4204, 4205, 4206*
      ocular manifestations, 4202, *4202, 4203*
      pathology, 4196, *4197, 4198, 4199, 4200*
      systemic manifestations, 4200–4201
      treatment, 4207–4208
  Bordetella species, 4208–4211
  Brucella species, 4211–4214, *4212, 4214*
  Campylobacter species, 4214–4217, *4215, 4216*
  clinical manifestations, 4199–4200
  Enterobacteriaceae, 4217–4218
    Citrobacter, 4218
    Edwardsiella, 4218
    Enterobacter, 4218–4219
    Escherichia coli, 4219
    Klebsiella, 4219–4220
    Proteus, 4220–4221
    Salmonella, 4221–4224, *4222, 4223*
      carrier state, 4223
      clinical manifestations, 4221–4223, *4222, 4223*
      prevention, 4223–4224
    Serratia, 4224
    Shigella, 4224–4225
    Yersinia, 4225, 4225–4228
  Flavobacteria, 4228
  Francisella tularensis, 4228, 4228–4229
  Fusobacterium, 4229–4232, *4230*
  Haemophilus, 4232, 4237
    Haemophilus influenzae, 4232–4234, *4233, 4235,* 4236, *4236*
  Helicobacter cinaedi, 4237
  Legionella, 4237, 4239–4240
    Legionella pneumophila, 4237–4239, *4238*
  miscellaneous, 4245
  Pasteurella, 4240
  Pseudomonas, 4240, 4243–4244
    Pseudomonas aeruginosa, 4240–4243
  Vibrio cholerae, 4244, *4244*
    central nervous system (CNS) infection, 4145
    cholera, 4244–4245

Gram-negative cocci, 4093, 4093*t*
Acetinobacter, 4104
Kingella, 4103–4104
Moraxella, 4103
Branhamella catarrhalis, 4103
species, 4103
Neisseria, 4093
Neisseria meningitidis, 4093–4094
Neisseria meningitis
Neisseria, 4103
diagnosis, 4100
meningococcal meningitis, 4094–4100, *4095, 4096, 4097, 4098, 4099, 4100*
meningococcal meningoencephalitis, 4100
prophylaxis, 4101
treatment and prognosis, 4100–4101
Neisseria gonorrhoeae, 4101, 4101–4103, *4102*
Veillonella parvula, 4104
Gram-positive bacilli, 4104–4105, 4105*t*
actinomycetales, 4136
atypical mycobacteria, 4176–4177
Actinomyces, 4177–4180, *4178, 4180, 4181*
Nocardia, 4189, 4189–4192, *4190, 4191*
Tropheryma whippelii, 4180–4189, *4182, 4183, 4184, 4185, 4186, 4187, 4188*
mycobacteria, 4136
Mycobacterium bovis, 4167–4168
Mycobacterium leprae, 4168–4176, *4169, 4170, 4171, 4172, 4174, 4175*
Mycobacterium tuberculosis, 4136, 4136–4167, *4137, 4138, 4139, 4140, 4141, 4142, 4143, 4144, 4145, 4146, 4147, 4148, 4149, 4150, 4151, 4152, 4153, 4154, 4155, 4156, 4157, 4158, 4159, 4160, 4161, 4162, 4163, 4164, 4165, 4166, 4167, 4168*
Arcanobacterium haemolyticum, 4105
Bacillus, 4105
Bacillus anthracis, 4105–4107, *4106*
other species, 4107–4109, *4109*
Clostridium, 4109
Clostridium botulinum (botulism), 4117, *4118, 4119,* 4119–4123, *4122*
clinical manifestations, 4117, *4118,* 4119, *4119*
diagnosis, 4119–4120
treatment, 4120
Clostridium botulinum (infant botulism), 4120–4121
Clostridium tetani, 4109, 4109–4117
diagnosis, 4115
epidemiology, 4111
general manifestations, 4111–4113, *4112, 4113*
neurological manifestations, 4114–4115
ocular and neuro-ophthalmologic manifestations, 4113–4114, *4114*
pathogenesis, 4109–4111, *4110, 4111*
prevention, 4116–4117
prognosis, 4116
treatment, 4115–4116
other species of, *4123,* 4123–4125, *4124, 4125*
Corynebacteria, 4125
Corynebacterium diphtheriae, 4125–4128, *4126, 4127*
other, 4128–4130, *4129*
Erysipelothrix rhusiopathiae, 4130, *4130*
lactobacilli, 4130
Listeria monocytogenes, 4130–4135, *4131, 4133, 4134, 4135*
propionibacteria, 4135–4136
Gram-positive cocci, 4068, 4068*t*
enterococci, 4090–4091
α-hemolytic streptococci, *4081,* 4081–4085, *4082, 4083, 4084, 4085, 4086*
β-hemolytic streptococci, 4085
group A, 4085–4086
group B, 4086–4087
group C, 4087–4088
group D, *4088,* 4088–4089
group F, 4089
group G, 4089
group H, 4089
group R, 4089–4090
other
Gemella haemolysans, 4091
micrococci, 4091–4092, *4092*
Peptostreptococci, 4092
other streptococci, 4080–4081
staphylococci, 4068
Staphylococcus aureus, 4068–4071, *4069, 4070, 4071, 4072*
Staphylococcus epidermidis and other coagulase-negative, 4071–4073, *4073, 4074*
streptococci, 4073–4075, *4074*
Streptococcus pneumoniae (pneumococcus), *4075,* 4075–4080, *4076, 4077, 4078, 4079, 4080*
Granular cell astrocytomas, 1932–1933
Granular cell myoblastoma, 2321–2322
Granulocytes, 2329
accumulation of, 3726
Granulocytic sarcomas, 2338–2339, 2341
Granuloma, 3989–3990, *3990, 3991, 3992*
cutaneous, 5480, *5481*
eosinophilic, 2405
Gagel's, 2407, *2409*
orbital, 3796
osteal, 5482, *5484*
plasma-cell, 2398
pulmonary, 5467–5468
Granulomatosis
conjunctival, 5487, *5488, 5489*
lymphomatoid, 703, *3786,* 3786–3788, *3787*
Granulomatous amoebic encephalitis (GAE), 4623, 4629–4630, 4632, *4632, 4633, 4634, 4635,* 5415–5416
Granulomatous angiitis, 5468
of central nervous system, 3727–3729, *3728, 3729, 3730,* 3731–3732
Granulomatous infiltration of optic disc, 5501, *5503, 5504*
Graphic representation of visual field data, 178, *180*
Graves' disease, 1399, *1402, 1403,* 1403–1404
radiation therapy in, 2598
Great cerebral vein (of Galen), 2952
Greater auricular neuralgia, 1749
Greater occipital neuralgia, *1748,* 1748–1749
Greisinger's sign, 3899
Groping reflex, 1821
Group A streptococcal meningitis, 4086
Group A streptococci, 4085–4086
Group B streptococci, 4086–4087
Group C streptococci, 4087–4088
Group D streptococci, *4088,* 4088–4089
Group F streptococci, 4089
Group G streptococci, 4089
Group H streptococci, 4089
Group R streptococcal meningitis, 4089–4090
Group R streptococci, 4089–4090
Growth hormone (GH), 2148–2149
deficiency in, 779–780
Growth hormone release-inhibiting hormone (GHRIH, somatostatin), 2146
Growth hormone-releasing factor (GHRF, somatocrinin), 2146
Growth retardation, alopecia, pseudoanodontia and optic atrophy (GAPO syndrome), 767
Guanethedine, 1005
Guanidine hydrochloride for botulism, 4120
Guarnieri bodies, 5148
Guillain-Barré syndrome (GBS), 631, 1176, 4128, 4552, 5019, 5058–5059, 5061, 5088, 5103, 5171, 5194, 5198, 5239, 5242–5243, 5248, 5539, 5677–5678
antecedent and associated events, 5678
miscellaneous associations, 5680–5681
and systemic infections, 5678–5680, *5679*
and vaccinations, 5680, *5681*
Central European and Russian spring-summer tick-borne encephalitis viruses (Tick-Borne encephalitis), *5186,* 5186–5188, *5188*
clinical manifestations, 5683
general neurologic, 5683–5685
neuro-ophthalmologic, 5685, *5686, 5687, 5688, 5689*
diagnosis, 5173–5174, 5690–5691
epidemiology, 5678
Fisher's variant of, 5019
hepatitis C virus, 5190
Kunjin virus, 5174–5175
Kyasanur Forest disease virus, 5188–5189
laboratory tests, 5687
electrophysiologic studies, 5688–5690
lumbar puncture, 5690
louping III virus, 5189
Murray Valley encephalitis, 5175–5176, *5177, 5178,* 5178–5179, *5179*
Negishi virus, 5189
nomenclature, 5678
pathogenesis and pathophysiology, 5682–5683
pathogenesis of zoster-associated, 5059, 5061
pathology, *5172,* 5172–5173, *5173,* 5681–5682, *5682, 5683, 5684*
Powassan virus, 5189–5190
prevention, 5174, *5175*
prognosis, 5174, 5693–5694
St. Louis encephalitis, 5179–5184, *5181, 5183*
site of lesion, *5693, 5694,* 5694–5695
treatment, 5174, 5691–5693
West Nile virus, 5184
yellow fever virus, 5184–5186, *5185*
Gummas, 4881
Gummatous iritis, 4901
Gummatous syphilis, *4892,* 4892–4895, *4893, 4894, 4896, 4897, 4898,* 4898–4900, *4899, 4900*
Gunn pupil, 939
Gustalacrimal reflexes, 930
Gustatory pathways, anatomy of, 1022, *1023*

Gustolacrimal reflexes
acquired, 1024–1025
congenital, 1024
general considerations concerning, 1024
types of, 1024
Gyrus subangularis, 143

H

Habituation of vestibulo-ocular reflex (VOR), 1147
Haemophilus, 4232, 4237
in intracranial abscess, 3950
Haemophilus aphrophilus, 4237
Haemophilus influenzae, 4232–4234, *4233, 4235,* 4236, *4236,* 5680
in bacterial meningitis, 3993, 3994, 3995
in meningitis, 4233–4234, *4235*
in sinusitis, 4025
in vasogenic cervical edema, 3981
Haemophilus parainfluenzae, 4237
Haemophilus paraphrophilus, 4237
Haemophilus pertussis in vasogenic cervical edema, 3981
Hallervorden-Spatz disease, 766
Hallervorden-Spatz syndrome, 1568
Hallucinations
auditory, 1831–1832
during eye closure, 467
formed visual, 3473–3474
migrainous, 463–464, *464, 465,* 466, *466*
peduncular, 463–464
visual, 1842, 1846–1848, 3765
and cyclosporine, 2634
as sign of tumors, 1794
Hallucinosis, peduncular, 1873
Halogenated hydroxyquinolines, 674
Hamartoma, 2083. (*See also* Intracranial hamartomas.)
astrocytic, 690, *691,* 2676, *2678, 2679, 2680*
of blood vessels, 2230
arteriovenous malformations, 2252
associations, 2274–2275
clinical manifestations, 2256–2261, *2258, 2259, 2260, 2261, 2262, 2263,* 2263–2274, *2264, 2265, 2266, 2267, 2268, 2269, 2270, 2271, 2272, 2273*
diagnosis of, 2275, *2276*
embryogenesis, 2252–2253
incidence, 2253, 2255
natural history of, 2275–2280, *2280, 2281,* 2282, *2283,* 2284
pathology, 2253, *2253, 2254, 2265, 2266*
capillary telangiectases, 2230–2231, *2231, 2232,* 2233, *2233*
cavernous angiomas
intracranial, *2233,* 2233–2236, *2234, 2235, 2236, 2237,* 2238, *2238, 2239, 2241, 2242,* 2242–2244, *2243*
orbital, *2243, 2244,* 2244–2245
retinal, *2245,* 2245–2246
venous angiomas, 2246, *2247, 2248, 2249, 2250,* 2250–2252, *2251, 2252*
conjunctival, 2658
retina, 2676, *2677,* 2678, *2678, 2679, 2680*
Hand-Schupller-Christian disease, 2405
Hangover headache, 1719
Hansen's disease, 4168–4176, *4169, 4170, 4171, 4172, 4174, 4175*
Haploscopic tests, 1180
Hardy-Rand-Rittler Pseudoisochromatic Plates, 330, 602, 1772–1773
Harmanella in encephalitis, 3987
Head, paragangliomas of, 2462–2464, *2463, 2464, 2465*
branchiomeric, 2464–2468, *2466, 2467, 2468, 2469, 2470,* 2470–2471
intravagal, 2471–2472, *2472*
Head position, nystagmus induced by change of, 1470–1471
Head tilt test, 1182–1183
Head tilts, 1177–1178
Head turns, 1177
Headaches, 1830. (*See also* Migraine headaches.)
with metabolic disorders, 1720–1721
with metabolic disturbances, 1721
with neck disease, 1722–1723
with noninfectious inflammatory disorders, 1716
with nonvascular intracranial disorders, 1714–1717
with ocular and orbital disease, 1723–1726, *1726t*
with acute ischemic cerebrovascular disease, 1706–1707
acute posttraumatic, 1705
with adrenal dysfunction, 1721
alcoholic beverages in, 1717
among patients with intracerebral hemorrhage, 3582–3583
analgesic-abuse, 1719
and aniline compounds, 1718
apresoline and, 1718
with arterial dissections, 1708
benign cough, 1702–1703, *1703*
benign exertional, 1703–1704, *1704*
caffeine in, 1719
calcium channel blockers in, 1718
carbon monoxide in, 1719
after carotid endarterectomy, 1713–1714
and cavernous sinus thrombosis, 1709
in chordomas, 2439
chronic daily, 1752
chronic posttraumatic, 1705–1706
classification of, 1693, *1694*
cluster, 970
cluster-tic, 1752
coital, 1704
cold stimulus, 1702
with cranial bone disorders, 1722
decompression, 1720
with decreased intracranial pressure, 1714–1716
with dialysis, 1721
with epidural hematomas, 1709
evaluation of patient with, 1696–1697
external compression, 1702
eyestrain, 1731–1732
and FK-506, 1718
following seizures, 1720
in giant cell arteritis, 3756
with giant cell (temporal) arteritis, 1712
hangover, 1719
high altitude, 1720
HIV-related, 5387–5389
hot dog, 1718
with hypercapnia, 1720–1721
with hypoglycemia, 1721
with hypoxia, 1720
ice cream, 1702
icepick, 1701
idiopathic stabbing, 1701
with increased intracranial pressure, 1714
with infections, 1716
in intracranial abscess, 3955
with intracranial infections, 1716
with intracranial neoplasms, 1716–1717
with intraparenchymal hemorrhage, 1709
with lacunar infarcts, 1708
lumbar puncture, 1714–1715
mechanisms of, 1693–1695
orgasmic, 1704
in patients with neurofibromatosis, 2660
postural suboccipital, 1704
psychogenic, 1698
related to intrathecal injections, 1716
relationship between episodic paroxysmal hemicrania, migraine and cluster, 3699–3701
role of radiation therapy in, 2612
sentinel, 1710
with sexual activity, 1704–1705
as sign of tumors, 1790–1791
sinus, 1732–1733
with subarachnoid hemorrhage, 1710
with subdural hematomas, 1709
with substance abuse, 1717–1720
swim-goggle, 1702
with systemic hypertension, 1713
with systemic hypotension, 1713
in systemic lupus erythematosus, 3819
tension-type, 1697–1698, 1790
thunderclap, 1710–1711, *1711*
before rupture of intracranial aneurysm, 3021
transmission of painful impulses, 1695–1696
with unruptured vascular malformations, 1711–1712
and venous sinus thrombosis, 1708–1709
vitamin A-induced, 1718–1719
warning leak, before rupture of intracranial aneurysm, 3021
Heat, sensations of, 1650
Heavy chain diseases (HCDs), 2389, 2401
Heerfordt's syndrome, 5478
Heerfordt-Waldenström syndrome, 5478–5479
Heidenhain's variant, 4572–4573
Helicobacter cinaedi, 4237
Heliobacter pylori, 5721
Heliotrope rash, 2528, 3839
Helminthic meningitis, 5423
Helminths. (*See also* Flatworms; Roundworms (nematodes).)
diseases caused by, 4439–4531, 5415
Hemangioblastomas, 2223–2226, *2224, 2225, 2226, 2227,* 2228, 2322, 2698, 2700, 2702–2704, *2704, 2705*
cerebellar, 2707
intracranial, 2226
optic nerve, 694, *695,* 696, *696*
posterior fossa, 2223, 2225, *2225*
relationship between hemangiopericytomas and, 2225
supratentorial, 2223–2224, 2225
Hemangioma calcificans, 2233–2234
Hemangiomas, 2322
capillary, 691–694, *692, 693, 694*
cavernous, 691–694, *692, 693, 694*
intraosseous, 2444, *2445*
Hemangiomatosis
congenital diffuse, 2234–2235, *2236, 2237*
diffuse congenital, *2731, 2732,* 2735

Hemangiopericytomas, 2027, 2228,	Hemisensory loss, 3434	thalamic-subthalamic, 3022, 3022-3023
2228–2230, 2229	Hemisomatagnosia, 1842	vitreous, 3025–3026, 3027, 3028
central nervous system, 2229	Hemodynamic processes in aneurysm	Hemorrhagic cerebritis, 4303, 4303
diagnosis of, 2229–2230 intracranial, 2229	formation, 2978	Hemorrhagic cerebrovascular disease,
relationship between hemangioblastomas	Hemoglobinopathies, $3357-3358$ α -Hemolysis, 4074	3581-3582 causes
and, 2225	β -Hemolysis, 4074, 4074	alcohol abuse, 3593
treatment of choice for, 2229	Γ -Hemolytic, 4074	amyloid angiopathy, 3586–3588
Hematoma, 1014	Hemolytic anemia, 5103	bleeding disorders, 3584–3585, <i>3585</i>
brainstem, 3611	α -Hemolytic patterns, 4089	exogenous agents, 3585-3586, 3586
epidural	α -Hemolytic streptococci, 4075, 4081,	hypertension, 3584, 3584
headaches associated with	4081–4085, 4082, 4083, 4084, 4085,	infective endocarditis, 3590, 3592, 3593
intraparenchymal, 1709	4086	intracranial aneurysm, 3589
papilledema from, 516	β -Hemolytic streptococci, 4075, 4085	migraine, 3593
intracerebral, 3611	group A, 4085–4086	trauma, 3588, 3589–3590, 3590
subcortical, 3611	group B, 4086–4087	tumor, 3590
subdural, headaches associated with intraparenchymal, 1709	group D. 4088 4088 4089	vascular malformations, 3587, 3588–358
Hematopoiesis, 2329	group D, 4088, 4088–4089 group F, 4089	diagnosis, 3609–3610 general symptoms and signs, 3582
medullary, 2330	group G, 4089	headache, 3582–3583
Hematopoietic system, classification of	group H, 4089	intraocular hemorrhage, 3583
neoplastic disease of, 2330, 2331t	group R, 4089–4090	loss of consciousness, 3583
Hematuria, 4139	Hemoptysis, 5479	other, 3583–3584
postmicturition, 4488	Hemorrhage	seizures, 3583
Hemiachromatopsia, 406	acute subarachnoid, 3348-3349	vomiting, 3583
Hemiakinetopsia, 438	anterior chamber, 3426	pathophysiology, 3582
Hemi-alexia, 428, 451	arteriovenous malformations (AVMs)	prognosis, 3611–3612
Hemianesthesia, hysterical, 1687	presenting with, 2277	signs and symptoms by location, 3593
Hemianopia	associated with aneurysmal rupture	brainstem, 3597–3598
altitudinal, 2170	intracerebral, 3033–3034, 3034 <i>t</i>	caudate, 3594, 3594
bilateral "checkerboard" altitudinal, 300,	intraventricular, 3034	cerebellar, 3604–3607, 3606
302, <i>302</i> bilateral homonymous, 357, <i>359</i> , 360	brainstem, 3597–3598 caudate, 3594, <i>3594</i>	of lateral basal ganglia, putamen, and
bilateral nasal, 302–304, 303, 304, 305, 306,	cerebellar, 3024, 3604–3607, 3606	internal capsule, 3593, 3593–3594 lateral geniculate, 3608–3609
307	cerebral, 2611–2612	medullary, 3604
bilateral nonsimultaneous homonymous, 360	headaches associated with intraparenchymal	mesencephalic, 3598, 3598–3601, 3599,
bilateral superior or inferior (altitudinal),	epidural, 1709	3600, 3601, 3602
299, 300, 300, 301	subdural, 1709	optic nerve and optic chiasmal, 3607,
bitemporal, 706, 756, 1794, 2171	headaches associated with subarachnoid,	3607–3608, <i>3608</i>
from optic chiasmal ischemia, 3692–3693	1710	pontine, 3601–3604, 3603, 3604
complete, 5640	intraocular, 3024–3025	primary intraventricular, 3597
crossed quadrant, 361, 364, 365–366, 367	intraretinal, 3025	subcortical (lobar, slit), 3596, 3596–3597
double, 357	lateral geniculate, 3608–3609	thalamic, 3594–3596, 3595
homonymous, 323–324, 1794, 2257 treatment and rehabilitation for, 375–376	medullary, 3604	treatment, 3610–3611
postgeniculate congenital homonymous, 989	meningeal, 2976 mesencephalic, 3598, 3598–3601, 3599,	Hemorrhagic cystitis, 4959 Hemorrhagic fever, viral, 5166
unilateral nasal, 302–304, 303, 304, 305,	3600, 3601, 3602	Hemorrhagic infarct, 5061
306, 307	occipital lobe, 3597	Henoch-Schönlein purpura, 3727, 3783
Hemianopic dyslexia, 432	within optic nerve, 3032, 3033	Hepadnaviridae, 4961–4962, 4962
Hemiballismus, 3518	optic nerve and optic chiasmal, 3607,	structure of, 4962–4963, 4963
Hemicholinium, 1002	3607–3608, <i>3608</i>	clinical syndromes caused by infection,
Hemichorea, 3518	optic nerve sheath, 3029, 3029, 3030, 3031,	4965–4972, 4966, 4968, 4969, 4970,
Hemicrania continua, 1701	3032	4971
Hemidecorticate patients, blindsight in,	orbital, 3024, 3025	epidemiology of infection, 4964
397–398, 398	perimesencephalic, 3131	extrahepatic disease caused by, 4972
Hemidyschromatopsia, 406	peripapillary, 812–813	prevention of infection, 4973–4975, 4974
Hemifacial atrophy, 783	pontine, 3023, 3601–3604, 3603, 3604	4975
Hemifacial microsomia, 1564 Hemifacial spasm, 1572–1575, 1573, 1574,	prepapillary, 812–813 preretinal, 3025	replication of, 4963, 4963–4964 routes of transmission, 4964–4965
1575, 1576	primary intraventricular, 3597	tropism of, 4964
Hemifield slide phenomenon, 432, 435, 2180,	putaminal, 3022, 3611	Heparin, 3557–3558
2180	recurrent, 3144–3145	Hepatic encephalopathy, 4969
Hemimasticatory spasm, 1670–1671	retinal, 2976	Hepatitis, 5104, 5288
Hemimicropsia, 468	retrobulbar, 716	as adverse effect of ketoconazole, 4285
Hemiparalexia, 431	after retrobulbar block, orbital, 716	as form of Q fever, 4768
Hemiparesis, 1860, 3434, 4128	spinal cord, 2607, 2608	in immunocompetent patients, 5102
transient, 3676-3677	subarachnoid, 2975, 3130, 3268	Hepatitis A virus, 5246, 5246-5250
from vertebrobasilar arterial disease, 3477	headaches associated with, 1710	Hepatitis B surface antigen (HBsAg),
Hemiparkinsonian stiffness, 3518	papilledema from, 516-517	4962–4963, 4963
Hemiplegia, 1860, 3433	subconjunctival, 3029	Hepatitis B virus (HBV), 4961–4962, 4962
Hemiplegia vegetative alterna, 3483 Hemi-seesaw nystagmus, 1477	subcortical (lobar, slit), 3596, 3596–3597 thalamic, 3594–3596, 3595	extrahepatic disease caused by, 4972 structure of 4962–4963, 4963
LIVIIII-SCOSAW IIVSIAZIIIUS, 14//	uiaiaiiiiし、フンプサーンファリ、コンダン	SUBCUIE OI, 4702-4901, 4901

clinical syndromes caused by infection, 4965–4972, *4966, 4968, 4969, 4970, 4971*
epidemiology of infection, 4964
extrahepatic disease caused by, 4972
prevention of infection, 4973–4975, *4974, 4975*
replication of, *4963,* 4963–4964
routes of transmission, 4964–4965
tropism of, 4964
vasculitis associated with, 3754–3755, *3755*
Hepatitis B virus type 2, 4963
Hepatocellular carcinoma, 4972
Hepatolenticular degeneration, 1319, 1326, 1331
Hepatorenal tyrosinemia, 2812
Hepatosplenic disease, 4488
Hepatosplenomegaly, 4392, 4393–4394
Hepatotoxicity, 4141
Herald hemiparesis, 3477
Hereditary anhidrotic ectodermal dysplasia, 1027
Hereditary ataxias, 762–763
Hereditary hemorrhagic telangiectasia, 2230, 2275, 3012
Hereditary optic atrophy
with other neurologic or systemic signs
autosomal-dominant progressive, with congenital deafness, 759
autosomal-dominant progressive, with progressive hearing loss and ataxia, 759
autosomal-recessive, with progressive hearing loss, spastic quadriplegia, mental deterioration, and death (opticocochleodentate degeneration), 760
complicated infantile, 761–762
dominant, deafness, ophthalmoplegia, and myopathy, 759–760
opticoacoustic nerve, with dementia, 760
progressive, with juvenile diabetes mellitus, diabetes insipidus, and hearing loss, 760–761
progressive encephalopathy with edema, hypsarrhythmia, and, 760
with progressive hearing loss and polyneuropathy, 759
sex-linked recessive, ataxia, deafness, tetraplegia, and areflexia, 760
with progressive hearing loss and polyneuropathy, 759
Hereditary optic neuropathies, 743–767
atrophy with other neurologic or systemic signs
autosomal-dominant progressive
with congenital deafness, 759
with progressive hearing loss and ataxia, 759
autosomal-recessive, with progressive hearing loss, spastic quadriplegia, mental deterioration, and death (opticocochleodentate degeneration), 760
complicated infantile, 761–762
dominant, deafness, ophthalmoplegia, and myopathy, 759–760
opticoacoustic nerve, with dementia, 760
progressive, with juvenile diabetes mellitus, diabetes insipidus, and hearing loss, 760–761
progressive encephalopathy with edema, hypsarrhythmia, and, 760
with progressive hearing loss and polyneuropathy, 759
sex-linked recessive, ataxia, deafness, tetraplegia, and areflexia, 760
classification of, 743–744
as manifestation of degenerative or developmental diseases
ataxias, 762–763
polyneuropathies, 763–764
storage, and cerebral degenerations of childhood, 764–767
monosymptomatic
apparent sex-linked atrophy, 758
congenital recessive, 758
dominant atrophy, 755–758, *757*
Leber's, 744–755
Hereditary polyneuropathies, 763–764
Hereditary spastic paraplegia (HSP), 2794, 2795*t*
complicated forms of, 2795
Heredoataxia cerebelleuse, 762
Heredopathia atactica polyneuritiformis, 2840–2841
Hering's law, 912, 1173, 1523, 1555
Herniation, syndrome of uncal, 997–998
Heroin, 1005
addiction to, 3363
Herpangina, 5235
Herpes B virus, 5128–5129
characteristics of, 5129
clinical manifestations, 5129–5131
diagnosis, 5131
epidemiology, 5129
pathogenesis and pathology, 5129
prevention, 5131
prognosis, 5131
treatment, 5131
Herpes simplex virus (HSV), 4979–4980, *4980,* 5417, 5721
in encephalitis
acyclovir for, 5011–5012
neuroretinitis associated with, 636
in endemic encephalitis, 3985
epidemiology, 4980
pathogenesis, 4980–4981, *4981*
primary infections, 4981–4984, *4982, 4983, 4984, 4985,* 4985–4987, 4986
Herpes zoster, 3340, 5025
epidemiology, 5025–5026
facial (geniculate) ganglion neuralgia from, *1742,* 1743–1745, *1745*
neurologic manifestations, 5029, 5031–5033, *5033, 5034,* 5035, *5035, 5036, 5037,* 5037–5039, *5038, 5040, 5041, 5042, 5043,* 5043–5047, *5044, 5045, 5046,* 5047, *5048, 5049, 5050, 5051,* 5051–5054, *5052, 5053, 5054, 5055, 5056,* 5056–5059, *5057, 5058, 5059, 5060,* 5061, *5062, 5063,* 5063–5064, *5064, 5065, 5066,* 5067–5068, *5068, 5069,* 5072
ocular manifestations, 5072, *5073, 5074, 5075, 5076*
systemic manifestations, 5028–5029, *5031*
in virus-induced vasculitis, *4029,* 4029–4030
Herpes zoster myelitis, 5056–5057
Herpes zoster ophthalmicus, 3973, 5033–5035
trigeminal pain during and after, 1729
Herpes zoster oticus, 1744–1745, *5033,* 5033–5035, *5034, 5035, 5036,* 5037–5038
Herpesviridae, 4975
cellular transformation, 4978–4979
classification and structure, *4976,* 4976–4977
cytomegalovirus, 5096–5097
acquired infection in immunocompetent children and adults, 5102–5104, *5103*
acquired infection in immunosuppressed persons, 5104–5113, *5105, 5106, 5107, 5108, 5109, 5110, 5111, 5112*
characteristics of, 5097
congenital infection, 5098–5100, *5099, 5101*
diagnosis, 5115, *5118–5119*
epidemiology, 5097–5098
pathology, *5113,* 5113–5115, *5114, 5115, 5116, 5117, 5118, 5119*
perinatal infection, 5100–5102, *5102*
prophylaxis, 5122
treatment, 5119–5122, *5120, 5121*
epidemiology and transmission, 4979
Epstein-Barr virus, 5081–5091, *5082, 5083, 5084, 5086, 5088, 5089, 5090, 5091, 5092,* 5094
characteristics of, 5081–5082
clinical manifestations, *5083,* 5083–5091, *5085, 5086, 5088, 5089, 5090, 5091, 5092, 5093,* 5093–5094, *5094*
diagnosis of, 5095–5096
epidemiology of, 5082
pathology of, *5094,* 5094–5095, *5095*
prevention, 5096
herpes B virus, 5128–5129
characteristics of, 5129
clinical manifestations, 5129–5131
diagnosis, 5131
epidemiology, 5129
pathogenesis and pathology, 5129
prevention, 5131
prognosis, 5131
treatment, 5131
herpes simplex virus, 4979–4980, *4980*
congenital and neonatal infection, 4990–4991, *4991, 4992, 4993*
diagnosis, *5009,* 5009–5011
encephalitis, 4991–4992, 4994–4997, *4995, 4996, 4997, 4998, 4999,* 4999–5002, *5000, 5001, 5002, 5003, 5004,* 5004–5005, *5005, 5006, 5007,* 5007–5008, *5008*
epidemiology, 4980
idiopathic neurologic syndromes, 5008–5009
pathogenesis, 4980–4981, *4981*
primary infections, 4981–4984, *4982, 4983, 4984, 4985,* 4985–4987, 4986
prophylaxis, 5012
treatment and prognosis, *5011,* 5011–5012
human herpesvirus type 6, *5122,* 5122–5127, *5123, 5124, 5125, 5126, 5127*
human herpesvirus type 7, 5127–5128, *5128*
human herpesvirus type 8, 5127–5128, *5128*
latency, 4978, *4978, 4979*
pathogenesis, 4979
replication, 4977, *4977*
tropism, 4977–4978
varicella-zoster virus, 5012–5013, *5013*
diagnosis of infections, 5075–5076
prevention of, 5081
treatment and prognosis of, 5076–5081, *5078, 5079*

Herpesviridae—*continued*
epidemiology, 5025–5026
neurologic manifestations, 5029, 5031–5033, *5033, 5034,* 5035, *5035, 5036, 5037,* 5037–5039, *5038, 5040, 5041, 5042, 5043,* 5043–5047, *5044, 5045, 5046,* 5047–5061, *5048, 5049, 5050, 5051,* 5051–5054, *5052, 5053, 5054, 5055, 5056,* 5056–5059, *5057, 5058, 5059, 5060, 5062, 5063,* 5063–5064, *5064, 5065, 5066, 5067,* 5067–5068, *5068, 5069,* 5070, *5071,* 5072
ocular manifestations, 5072, *5073, 5074, 5075, 5076*
systemic manifestations, 5028–5029, *5031*
varicella (chickenpox), 5013
clinical manifestations, 5014, *5015, 5016,* 5016–5025, *5018, 5020, 5021, 5022,* 5024
congenital and perinatal infection, 5025
epidemiology, 5013–5014, *5014, 5015, 5016,* 5016–5025, *5018, 5020, 5022, 5024*
pathogenesis, 5013
pathology, 5013, *5014*
Heschl's gyri, unilateral lesions of, 1830–1831
Hess test, 1180
Heterochromia iridis, 1009
Heterophoria, 952, 1181
Heterotropia, 1181
vertical, 1183
Hexaminidase A deficiency, 2785
High altitude headaches, 1720
High dose viral inoculation, 5376
High-pass resolution perimetry (HRP), 205–207, *207*
Hindbrain, developmental anomalies of, 1291–1292, 1292*t*
Hirano bodies, 2749
Hirsutism and Cushing's syndrome, 2160
Histiocytes, 2329, 2403
Histiocytoma, eruptive, 2421
Histiocytoses, 2330
diseases of, *2403,* 2403–2405, *2404*
neoplastic non-Langerhans cell, *2413, 2414,* 2414–2415
non-Langerhans cell, 2413, *2415,* 2415–2416, *2416, 2417,* 2418, *2418, 2419,* 2420, *2420*
reactive non-Langerhans cell, 2413–2414
Histiocytosis
Langerhans cell, 703, 2405–2413, *2406, 2407, 2408, 2409, 2410, 2412*
malignant, *2413, 2414,* 2414–2415
Histiocytosis X, 2405
Histochemistry of trigeminal corneal nerve fiber endings, 1600
extra-trigeminal (sympathetic) innervation, 1600–1601
Histoplasma, in encephalitis, 4394, *4395, 4396, 4397*
Histoplasma capsulatum, 4282, 4389, *4390*
in chronic basal meningitis, 4030
clinical manifestations, 4392
acute pulmonary histoplasmosis, 4392
chronic pulmonary histoplasmosis, 4392
disseminated histoplasmosis, 4393–4401, *4394, 4395, 4396, 4397, 4398, 4399, 4400, 4401*
isolated central nervous system histoplasmosis, 4401–4402, *4403*
demographics, 4389, *4391*
diagnosis, 4402, 4404, *4404*
in intracranial brain abscess, 3952
in neuritis, 4026
pathogenesis, 4389, 4391–4392
presumed ocular histoplasmosis syndrome, 4404–4406, *4405, 4406, 4407*
prevention, 4404
treatment, 4404
Histoplasmosis, 4281, 4394, *4397*
acute disseminated, 4393
acute pulmonary, 4392
association with neuroretinitis, 636
human immunodeficiency virus in, 5422
isolated central nervous system, 4401–4402, *4403*
ocular, 4397
Histotoxic hypoxia, 3324
HIV infections. (*See* Acquired immune deficiency syndrome (AIDS); Human immunodeficiency virus (HIV).)
HLA typing and relationship between optic neuritis and multiple sclerosis, 619
Hodgkin's disease, 2351, *2351*
general considerations, 2351
neurologic and ocular disorders in, 2352–2353, *2353, 2354, 2355,* 2355–2357, *2356, 2357, 2358,* 2359–2360
prognosis, 2360
systemic symptoms, 2352
treatment, 2360
Hollenhorst plaques, 3365–3367, *3366, 3367, 3368, 3369*
Holoprion, 4565
Holter monitor, 3548
Homocysteine and incidence of atherosclerosis, 3330
Homocystinuria, 3352
Homonymous hemianopia, 323–324, 1794, 2257, 3691
and cortical blindness, 4153–4154
treatment and rehabilitation for, 375–376
Homonymous hemioptic hypoplasia, 324
Homonymous quadrantanopsia, 3691–3692
Homonymous scotomas, 3667–3668
Homonymous visual field defects, 2717, *2717,* 3434, 3444, 3467, 3765, 3805, 4160, 4374–4375, 4907, 5433, 5728–5729
Homozygous sickle cell anemia, 3349
Hooper Visual Organization Test, 470
Horizontal angular vestibulo-ocular reflex (VOR), 1142–1143, *1144*
Horizontal cells, 36, *38,* 39
Horizontal diplopia, 2439
Horizontal eye movements, 1314
Horizontal gaze, 3599–3601
Horizontal gaze paresis, 3509, *3510,* 5433, 5603, 5727
Horizontal nystagmus, 1473
Horizontal saccades, brainstem generation of, 1110–1111, *1111*
Hormones, 2584
corticosteroids, 2586–2589
tamoxifen, 2584
Horner's syndrome, 936, 1542, *1544,* 1698–1699, 1701, 1893, 1986–1987, *1987,* 2352, 2561, 2990, 3037, 3465, *3465,* 3466, *3466, 3467,* 3767, 3797, 4375, 4451, 5033, 5053, 5433
acquired, in children, 971
alternating, 968
anisocoria in, 965
clinical characteristics, 964–966, *965*
congenital, 971–973, *972, 973*
diagnosis, 966–967
and headaches, 1708
historical background, 963–964
localization, 967–971
and Lyme disease, 4808
postganglionic, 2447–2448, 3043
preganglionic, 969
Horton's disease, 3755
Host cell binding sites, 4947
Hot dog headache, 1718
HOTV test, 161
H-reflex, 5690
HTLV-I infection
and miscellaneous neurologic diseases, 5441
and ocular inflammation, 5440–5441, *5441*
HTLV-I-associated myelopathy with CNS angiitis, 5438, 5440
HTLV-I-associated myelopathy/tropical spastic paraparesis, 5436–5438, *5439*
Hubel, David, 129, *130,* 131
Hughes-Stovin syndrome, 3888
Human diseases
Creutzfeldt-Jakob disease, 4568–4569
diagnosis, 4584, *4587,* 4587–4591, *4588, 4589, 4590, 4591*
epidemiology, 4569, 4571
familial, 4576–4577
Iatrogenic, *4578,* 4578–4579
pathology, 4580–4581, *4581, 4582, 4583,* 4584, *4584, 4585, 4586*
prevention of Iatrogenic, 4592
sporadic, 4571–4574, *4572, 4574, 4575,* 4576, *4576*
treatment, 4592
fatal familial insomnia, 4595, 4598
cerebral metabolism, 4601–4602
clinical characteristics, 4598–4599
genetics, 4599–4600, *4601*
pathology, 4600–4601, *4601, 4602*
Gerstmann-Sträussler-Scheinker disease, 4592, 4594
clinical characteristics, *4593,* 4594
pathology and genetics, *4594,* 4594–4595, *4595, 4596, 4597, 4598, 4599, 4600*
kuru, 4567, *4568*
clinical characteristics, 4568
diagnosis, 4568
neuro-ophthalmologic features, 4568
pathology, 4568, *4569, 4570, 4571*
treatment, 4568
Human herpesvirus type 6, *5122,* 5122–5127, *5123, 5124, 5125, 5126, 5127,* 5427–5428
Human herpesvirus type 7, 5123
Human herpesvirus type 8, 5123
Human homologues of Area V5, 1127–1128
Human Immune Globulin (HIG)
for Lambert-Eaton myasthenic syndrome, 1437
for myasthenia gravis, 1430
Human immunodeficiency virus (HIV), 5721. (*See also* Acquired immune deficiency syndrome (AIDS).)
clinical manifestations of
advanced immune deficiency, 5374, 5374*t, 5375*
early immune deficiency, 5373
intermediate immune deficiency, 5373–5374

primary (seroconversion illness), 5372–5373
culture of, 5380
pathogenesis of, 5369–5372, *5370, 5371*
peripheral neuropathies associated with, 5386–5387
progressive encephalopathy of childhood associated with, 5403–5407, *5405, 5406, 5407*
vacuolar myelopathy associated with, 5386
Human immunodeficiency virus (HIV) encephalitis, 5389
Human immunodeficiency virus (HIV) encephalopathy, 5389
Human immunodeficiency virus (HIV) histoplasmosis, 5422
Human immunodeficiency virus (HIV) infection, 4916, 4918, *4919, 4920, 4921, 4922,* 4922*t*, *4923, 4924, 4925,* 4925–4929, *4926,* 4928*t*
and encephalitis, 3985
testing for, in patients with syphilis, 4929
Human immunodeficiency virus (HIV)-induced dementia, 5373, 5389–5390
Human immunodeficiency virus (HIV)-induced neurocognitive disorders, 5383
Human immunodeficiency virus (HIV)-related headache, 5387–5389
Human immunodeficiency virus type 1 (HIV-1), 5361, 5363
life cycle, 5365–5368, *5367, 5368*
neurologic complications of, 5385, *5386,* 5386*t*
myopathic, 5386–5387
peripheral nervous system, 5386–5387
primary spinal cord, 5386–5387
neurologic complications of, primary intracranial, 5387–5395, *5388, 5389,* 5390*t*, *5391, 5392, 5393, 5394, 5395, 5396, 5397,* 5397–5399, *5398, 5399, 5400, 5401,* 5401–5407, *5402, 5403, 5404, 5405, 5406, 5407, 5408*
prevention of, 5384–5385
screening for, 5384
structure, 5363–5365, *5364, 5366*
variability, 5368
Human immunodeficiency virus type 1 (HIV-1) associated cognitive/motor complex, 5390
Human immunodeficiency virus type 1 (HIV-1) associated mild neurocognitive disorder (MND), 5390
Human immunodeficiency virus type 1 (HIV-1) associated minor cognitive/motor disorder, 5390
Human immunodeficiency virus type 1 (HIV-1) associated neurocognitive disorders, 5389–5395, 5390*t*, *5391, 5392, 5393, 5394, 5395, 5396, 5397,* 5397–5399, *5398, 5399, 5400, 5401,* 5401–5403, *5402, 5403, 5404*
Human immunodeficiency virus type 2 (HIV-2), 5361, 5368–5369
Human leukocyte antigens (HLA) and development of multiple sclerosis, 5542
Human spumaretrovirus, 5362
Human syncytium-forming virus, 5362
Human T-cell leukemia/lymphoma virus type I (HTLV-1), 5361, 5434
diagnosis, 5435
diseases associated with, *5433,* 5435–5438, *5436, 5437, 5438, 5439, 5440,* 5440–5442, *5441*
epidemiology, 5434
transmission, 5434
Human T-cell leukemia/lymphoma virus type II (HTLV-II), 5361, 5441–5442
counseling, 5442
Human tetanus immune globulin (TIG), 4115–4116
Humoral immunity, abnormalities in, 5372
Humphrey Field Analyzer, 177, 182, 206, 469, 612
Hunter syndrome, 520, 2819–2820
Huntington's disease, 1318–1319, 1326, 1568, 2748, 2780
diagnosis, 2783–2784
epidemiology, 2780–2781
etiology, 2781–2782
genetic testing, 2784
laboratory and neuroimaging studies, 2783
neurologic manifestations, 2782–2783
ocular motor manifestations, 2783
pathology, 2781, *2782*
pathophysiology, 2782
prognosis, 2784
treatment, 2784
visual sensory manifestations, 2783
Hurler syndrome, *2816,* 2816–2819, *2817, 2818*
Hurler-Scheie compound, 2819
Hutchinson's sign, 5035
Hutchinson's triad, 4903
Hyaluronidase, 4075
Hydatid cyst, 4445
Hydatidosis, 4443, 4445, *4445,* 4445–4447, *4446, 4447, 4448, 4449,* 4449–4453, *4450, 4451, 4453, 4454*
Hydrocephalus, 519, 4167, 4686
communicating, 1568
as complication of meningococcal meningitis, 4095–4096
otitic, 4040
after rupture of intracranial aneurysm, *3035,* 3035–3036
as sign of tumors, 1792–1794, *1793*
traumatic, 3908
Hydroxyamphetamine hydrobromide, 1003
Hydroxyurea
neurotoxicity, 2563
ocular toxicity, 2563
systemic toxicity, 2563
Hyperactivity
of ocular motor nerves, 1259
neuromyotonia, 1259, *1260*
superior oblique myokymia, 1259–1261
sympathetic, *973,* 973–974
Hyperbaric oxygen, 3175
for mucormycosis, 4331–4332
for radionecrosis, 591–592
for radionecrosis of bone, 2622
Hypercapnia, headaches associated with, 1720–1721
Hypercoagulability, 3357–3359, *3358, 3359, 3360, 3361,* 3361–3362, *3362,* 3426, 3888–3889
of blood, 3889, 3890
Hypercoagulable syndrome, 3359
Hypercolumn, 135, *135, 136*
Hypercomplex cells, *130,* 130–131, *131*
Hyperemia of optic disc, 487
Hyperfractionation, 2595, 2604
Hyperhidrosis, 2158
Hyperhomocystinemia, 3889
Hyperinfection syndrome, 4512
Hyperkalemic periodic paralysis, 1377, *1378*
Hyperlipidemia
and incidence of atherosclerosis, 3329
as risk factor for stroke, 3567
Hypernatremia, 1871
Hyperoxaluria type 1, 2848
Hyperplasia, adrenal, 2197
Hyperprolactinemia, 2159
and radiation damage, 2597
Hyperprolactinemia syndrome
in men, 2156
in women, 2155–2156
Hyperreflexia
autonomic, 1029
and bilateral extensor plantar responses, 5700–5701
Hypersensitivity of pupils, 974
Hypersensitivity vasculitis, *3782,* 3782–3783, *3783*
Hypertension, 529, 2662, *3335,* 3335–3336, *3336, 3337, 3338,* 3567
in aneurysm formation, 3007–3008
headaches associated with systemic, 1713
and incidence of atherosclerosis, 3330
in intracerebral hemorrhage, 3584
systemic, 1713
Hypertensive encephalopathy, headaches associated with, 1713
Hyperthyroidism, 2163–2164
and papilledema, 521
pituitary, 2163–2164
Hyperviscosity, 3426
Hyperviscosity syndromes, 2332
Hypervitaminosis
acute, 1718
chronic, 1718–1719
Hypesthesia, 4172
corneal, 1666, 1844
congenital, 1666
due to acquired disease, 1664–1666, *1665*
inherited, 1666
iatrogenic corneal, 1664
Hypesthetic ataxic hemiparesis, 3517–3518
Hyphae, 4281
Hyphema, 3029
Hypnozoites, 4650
Hypocalcemia, 4139–4140
Hypochondriasis, 1766
Hypochromia iridis, 966
Hypoglycemia, headaches associated with, 1721
Hypogonadism, 2164–2165
Hypokalemic periodic paralysis, 1377, *1377*
Hypometria, 1106
saccadic, 2722
Hypometria saccade, 1106
Hyponatremia, 4139
Hypophyseal portal system, 2145, *2145*
Hypophysis, 2141
Hypophysitis, lymphocytic, *2207,* 2207–2208, *2208*
Hypopigmented spots, 2649
Hypopituitarism, 2165
role of radiation therapy in, 2597
Hypoplasia
homonymous hemioptic, 324
segmental optic nerve, *783,* 783–784, *784*
Hypoprolactinemia and radiation damage, 2597

Hypotension
spontaneous intracranial, 1252–1253, 1715–1716
systemic, 1713
causes of, 3407, *3408,* 3409–3413
general considerations, 3407
headaches associated with, 1713
Hypotensive retinopathy, 3453–3454, *3454, 3455, 3456,* 3457, *3457*
Hypothalamic dysfunction, 5493, *5573,* 5573–5574
Hypothalamic inhibition of pupillary constriction, 878–879
Hypothalamic syndromes, 1812–1814, 2165
Hypothalamus, 879
anatomy of, 828–830, *829, 830, 831,* 832, 2141, *2142*
astrocytomas of, 1936–1937, *1937*
endocrine functions of, 2145
neurohypophyseal system, 2145–2146
tuberohypophyseal system, 2146, 2147*t*
fiber connections, *832,* 832–835, *834*
function of, *835,* 835–837
hamartomas of, 2126–2127, *2129,* 2129–2130
neuromediators, 832
Hypothyroidism
primary, 2163–2164
secondary, 2163
Hypotony, 265
Hypovitaminosis A, 32
Hypoxia, 3323–3326, *3325, 3326*
anemic, 3324
headaches associated with, 1720–1721
histotoxic, 3324
hypoxic, 3324
of occipital lobes, 363
stagnant, 3324
Hypoxic hypoxia, 3324
Hysteric rabies, 5273
Hysterical hemianesthesia, 1687

I

Iatrogenic blood loss as causes of decreased cerebral perfusion, 3411–3413, *3413*
Iatrogenic corneal hypesthesia, 1664
Iatrogenic Creutzfeld-Jakob disease, *4578,* 4578–4579
Iatrogenic trauma, 1013
Ice cream headache, 1702
Ice test, 1419, *1419*
Icepick headache, 1701
Icteric leptospirosis, 4842, *4843*
Ideation, 1765
Identification acuity, 160
Idiopathic CD4+ T-lymphocytopenia, 5098
Idiopathic central visual loss, 812
Idiopathic hypertrophic cranial pachymeningitis, 5529–5533, *5530, 5531, 5532*
Idiopathic inflammatory pseudotumor, 651
Idiopathic late-onset cerebellar ataxias, 2794
clinical manifestations, 2794
diagnosis and investigations, 2794
pathology, 2794
Idiopathic myelofibrosis, 2335–2336
Idiopathic myositis
dermatomyositis, 1395, 1397
myositis limited to, 1393, 1395, *1395, 1396*
systemic, 1395, 1397
Idiopathic neurologic syndromes, 5008–5009
diagnosis, *5009,* 5009–5011
prophylaxis, 5012
treatment and prognosis, *5011,* 5011–5012
Idiopathic opsoclonus, 1489–1490
Idiopathic Parkinson's disease (IDP), 2764
differential diagnosis, 2770–2771
epidemiology, 2764
etiology, 2767–2768
laboratory and neuroimaging findings, 2770
neurologic manifestations, 2768–2769
ocular motor manifestations, 2770
pathology and neurochemistry, *2764,* 2764–2767, *2765, 2766, 2767*
pathophysiology, 2768, *2769*
prognosis, 2772
treatment, 2771–2772
visual sensory manifestations, 2770
Idiopathic perioptic neuritis, 709
Idiopathic retinal vasculitis, *3864,* 3864–3865
Idiopathic stabbing headache, 1701
Idiopathic trigeminal neuralgia, 1750
IFA test in diagnosing toxoplasmosis, 4692
Ifosfamide
neurotoxicity, 2567
ocular toxicity, 2567–2568
systemic toxicity, 2567
IgE antibodies, 3726
Illusory visual spread, 454
Imidazoles for fungal infections, 4284
Imitation behavior, 1822
Immune adherence hemagglutination in diagnosing varicella-zoster virus infections, 5075
Immune complexes, 3726
Immune enhancement, 5169
Immune globulin in treatment of acute Guillain-Barré syndrome (GBS), 5692–5693
Immune-based therapies, 5384
Immune-mediated damage to central nervous system, 2637
Immune-mediated disorders, remyelination in, 3981
Immune-mediated poststreptococcal nephritis, 4086
Immunity and infectious disease
barriers to, 3941–3942
cerebral edema, *3942,* 3942–3943, *3943*
interstitial cerebral edema, 3943
routes of invasion, 3943
Immunization. (*See* Vaccine.)
Immunocompetent patients, acquired infection in, 5102–5104, *5103*
Immunocompromised patients
bacterial meningitis in, 3995
measles in, 5207–5208, *5209*
Immunologic responses to malaria, 4653
Immunoprophylaxis, 4101
Immunostains, 1
Immunosuppressed patients, 4294
acquired infection in, 5104
bacterial meningitis in, 3995
Immunosuppression
in bone marrow transplantation, 2627–2630, *2628, 2629*
complications of, 2626–2627
Immunosuppressive therapy, 3175
for myasthenia gravis, 1425–1429, 1426*t*
Immunotherapy
for Lambert-Eaton myasthenic syndrome, 1437
for nasopharyngeal carcinoma, 2449
short-term, 1429–1430
Impotence, 2156
and multiple sclerosis, 5573
Impulsive rotation, 1142
Inappropriate secretion of antidiuretic hormone, 3144
Inattention, 1841
Incisura tentorii, 2018
Incisural meningiomas, 2055–2056
Incontinence, 3434
Increased ICP and ventricular dilation, 2717–2718
Increased intracranial pressure, 3424, 3957
headache associated with, 1714
Indirect arterial trauma, 2990
Indirect immunofluorescence assay (IFA), 5379
Indirect optic nerve injuries, 715
Indirect optokinetic pathway, 1151–1153
Indirect vestibulo-ocular reflex (VOR), 1143
Indocyanine green angiography (ICG), 159
Indomethacin
for coital headaches, 1705
for cough-induced headache, 1703
for icepick headaches, 1701
Induced tears, 926
Infant, accommodation in, 912–914
Infant botulism, 4117, *4118, 4119,* 4119–4123, 4120–4121, *4122.* (*See also* Botulism.)
clinical manifestations, 4117, *4118,* 4119, *4119*
diagnosis, 4119–4120
in neuritis, 4026
treatment, 4120
in vasogenic cervical edema, 3981
Infantile desmoplastic astrocytomas, 1933–1934
Infantile neuroaxonal dystrophy (INAD), 766
Infantile neuronal ceroid lipofuscinoses, 2850
Infantile Refsum disease, 2843–2844
Infarction, *3326,* 3326–3328, *3327, 3328*
inferolateral, 3483
myocardial, 3568–3569
paramedian, 3483
posterior choroidal artery, 3483
of thalamus, 3483
tuberothalamic, 3483
ventral pontine, 3512
Infections
aneurysms caused by, 2998–3005, *3000, 3001, 3002, 3004*
as cause of aneurysms. (*See* Mycotic aneurysms.)
headaches associated with, 1716
neurologic, in bone marrow transplantation, 2630
systemic
with bone marrow transplantation, 2627
headaches associated with, 1716
Infectious arteritis, 3339–3340, 4028–4031, *4029*
Infectious mononucleosis
complications, 5084–5091, *5085, 5086, 5088, 5089, 5090,* 5091
symptoms and signs of, 5083–5084
Infective endocarditis, *3393,* 3393–3395, *3394, 3395, 3396, 3397,* 3590, *3592,* 3593
Infective metacyclic trypomastigotes, 4702
Infective myositis, 1392–1393, *1394*
Inferior alveolar artery, 2945
Inferior cavernous sinus, artery of, 2874, 2876
Inferior cervical ganglion, 838
Inferior hypophyseal artery, 2873
Inferior medullary velum, 1884

Inferior olivary nucleus, lesions of, 1284
Inferior parietal arteries, 2897
Inferolateral infarction, 3483
Infertility, decreased, 2156
Infiltrative optic neuropathies, 681–710
general considerations, 681, 682*t*
specific lesions, 681
inflammatory and infectious infiltrative, 705
disorders, 709–710
idiopathic perioptic neuritis, 709
sarcoidosis, *705,* 705–706, *706, 707, 708,* 709
tumors, 681
astrocytic hamartoma, 690, *691*
capillary and cavernous hemangiomas, 691–694, *692, 693, 694*
ganglioglioma, 689–690
lymphoma, 701–702, 701–703, *702*
lymphoreticular malignancies, 701
malignant teratoid medulloepithelioma, 691
melanocytomas, *696,* 696–697, *697, 698*
meningeal carcinomatosis, 700–701
metastatic and locally invasive tumors, 698–700, *699, 700*
nerve glioma, 681–689, *682, 683, 684, 685, 686, 687, 688, 689*
optic nerve hemangioblastoma, 694, *695,* 696, *696*
Infiltrative optic neuropathy, 266, *269*
Inflammation, 1009
intraocular, 1997
Inflammatory bowel disease, 3358–3359
Inflammatory giant cells, 3989
Inflammatory myopathies
idiopathic myositis, 1393
limited to orbit, 1393, 1395, *1395*
systemic, 1395, 1397
infective myositis, 1392–1393, *1394*
Influenza vaccine
complications following, 5197
and multiple sclerosis, 5544
Influenza viruses
clinical manifestations, 5192
diagnosis, 5196
epidemiology, 5190–5192
nonpulmonary complications of, 5193–5196, *5195*
prevention, 5196–5198
prognosis, 5196
pulmonary complications of, 5192–5193
treatment, 5196
uncomplicated, 5192
Infranuclear gaze disturbances, 4078
Infranuclear lesions, 5605–5606, *5607, 5608,* 5608–5609, *5609*
Infranuclear ophthalmoplegia, diagnosis of, 1258–1259
Infraorbital artery, 2945–2946
Infrared video pupillometry, 934
Infratentorial angiomas, 2235
Infratentorial arachnoid cysts, 2120–2121, *2121, 2122*
Infundibulum, 2018, 2141
Inhalation anthrax, 4106
Inhibitory pathways, 109, *109*
Injury-healing theory, 3333–3334
Inner ear, microangiopathy of, *3732,* 3732–3734, *3733*
Inner plexiform layer, 44–45
Innominate artery, 2869
collateral circulation with occlusion of, 3417
and left subclavian artery, occlusion of, 3522, *3522*
Innominate steal syndrome, *3521,* 3521–3522
Insular and striate veins, 2949–2950, *2950*
Intact septum pellucidum, 780
Integrase, 5363, 5365
Integrated DNA, 4950
Integrative agnosia, 5138
Intention tremor, 5568
Intercavernous sinuses, 2964
Interdigitating cells, 2404
Interfascicular oligodendrocyte, 21, 3974
α-2A-Interferon, 1263
Interferonbeta for multiple sclerosis, 5629–5630
Interior carotid arteries. (*See also* Carotid arteries.)
aneurysms arising from junction with anterior choroidal arteries, 3084, *3085, 3086*
Interleukin-1, 3996
Intermediate dendritic cells, 2404
Intermediolateral mesencephalic syndrome, 3506
Intermittent claudication in giant cell arteritis, 3756
Intermittent deviation, 1328
Intermittent proptosis, 2252
Internal auditory (labyrinthine) arteries, 2916–2917, 2917
Internal capsule lesions, 337, *337, 338,* 339
Internal carotid arteries, 2869. (*See also* Carotid arteries.)
aneurysm arising from bifurcation of, 3085, *3087,* 3087–3091, *3088, 3089, 3090, 3091, 3092, 3093*
aneurysms arising from cavernous portion of, 3040–3041, *3041, 3042, 3043, 3044, 3045, 3046,* 3046–3047, *3047, 3048, 3049,* 3050, *3050, 3052, 3053,* 3054, *3054*
aneurysms arising from clinoid segment of, *3055, 3056,* 3056–3059, *3057, 3058*
aneurysms arising from extracranial portion of, 3037–3038, *3038, 3039*
aneurysms arising from intradural portion of, 3054, 3056
aneurysms arising from junction with opthalmic artery and, *3059,* 3059–3060, *3060, 3061, 3062,* 3062–3063, *3063, 3064, 3065,* 3065–3066, *3066, 3067*
aneurysms arising from junction with posterior communicating arteries, *3075,* 3075–3083, *3076, 3077, 3078, 3079, 3081, 3082, 3083*
aneurysms arising from junction with superior hypophyseal artery, 3059
aneurysms arising from portion of, 3038, *3039, 3040*
aneurysms arising from proximal supraclinoid portion of, 3075
dissecting aneurysms of branches of, 3216
dissecting aneurysms of extracranial portion of, 3210–3215, 3211*t, 3212, 3213*
dissecting aneurysms of intracranial portion of, 3215–3216
fusiform aneurysms of, 3183–3186, *3184, 3185, 3187,* 3188–3192, *3189, 3190, 3191, 3192, 3193, 3194,* 3195, *3195, 3196*
and its branches, 2869–2870, *2871*
cavernous segment of, *2873,* 2873–2874, *2874, 2875, 2876*
cervical segment of, 2870–2871
clinoid segment of, 2877
communicating segment of, 2884, 2886, 2889, *2890*
lacerum segment of, 2871, *2871,* 2873, *2873,* 2876–2877
ophthalmic segment of, 2877, *2878, 2879, 2880,* 2880–2881, *2881, 2882, 2883,* 2884, *2884, 2885, 2886, 2887, 2888*
petrous segment of, 2871, *2871, 2872*
terminal branches of, 2889, 2891, *2892, 2893, 2894, 2895, 2896, 2897,* 2897–2899, *2898, 2899, 2900, 2901,* 2902, *2902, 2903,* 2904
ligation of, 3150–3152
meningeal branches of, 3297–3298
occlusion of, 3428–3432, *3429, 3430*
occlusive disease of, 3010–3011, *3011*
signs of, 3428
Internal carotid artery, 15
occlusion and stenosis, ocular symptoms and signs of, 3444–3446
ophthalmic division pain associated with occlusion of, 1707
Internal carotid posterior communicating aneurysms, *3075,* 3075–3083, *3076, 3077, 3078, 3079, 3082, 3083*
Internal carotid-basilar anastomoses, 2934
anterior-posterior circulation, 2936, 2940
persistent primitive acoustic (otic) artery, 2936, *2940*
persistent primitive hypoglossal artery, 2936, *2939, 2941, 2942*
persistent primitive trigeminal artery, 2935, *2939*
Internal frontal arteries, 2897
Internal maxillary artery, 2944–2946, *2945*
Internal ophthalmoplegia, 974, 5248
International Headache Society (IHS), Headache Classification Committee on, 3658
International Society for Clinical Electrophysiology of Vision (ISCEV) standards, 224
Internode, 3974
Internuclear gaze pareses, 5729
Internuclear lesions, 5603–5605, *5604, 5605, 5606*
Internuclear ophthalmoplegia (INO), 1289, 1294, *1301,* 1301–1303, *1302,* 1794, 2558, 3023, 3500, *3501,* 4375, 5256, 5433, 5603, 5703
bilateral, 3766–3767, *3768*
unilateral, 3766–3767
Internuclear system, 1080, *1080*
Interphotoreceptor retinol binding protein, 26, *31*
Interplexiform cells, 42–43
Interstitial brachytherapy, 1902
Interstitial cerebral edema, 3943, 3982
Interstitial keratitis, 3733, 4901
Interstitial nucleus of Cajal, 1308, 1310
Interstitial pneumonitis in immunocompetent patients, 5102
Interstitial radiation, 2595
Intestinal schistosomiasis, 4488
Intima, 3332
Intorsion, 1172
Intracanalicular optic nerve, 7

Intracellular gram-negative rods, 4067
Intracerebral abscesses, *3944*, 3944–3945, *3945*
Intracerebral hematomas, 3611
Intracerebral hemorrhage
  associated with aneurysmal rupture, 3033–3034, 3034*t*
  into frontal lobe, 3023–3024
Intracranial abscesses, 3943–3945, *3944*, 4068–4069, *4069*, 4073, 4083, 4620
  aspergillosis in, 4305–4306, 4308
  caused by *Haemophilus influenzae*, 4234–4236
  diagnosis, 3960–3962, *3961, 3962, 3963*
  and empyemas, 4029
  etiology, 3950–3952, *3953*, 3954, *3954*
  general and neurologic manifestations, 3955–3958
  Listeria monocytogenes in, 4133
  neuro-ophthalmologic manifestations, *3958*, 3958–3960, 3959
  pathogenesis, 3945–3950, *3946, 3947, 3948, 3949, 3950, 3951, 3952*
  pathology, *3954*, 3954–3955, *3955, 3956, 3957*
  prognosis, 3963–3965
  treatment, 3962–3963, *3964, 3965*
Intracranial aneurysms, 2611–2612, 2983, *2983*, 2985, 3589
  warning signs and symptoms before major rupture, 3021
Intracranial arteriovenous malformations (AVMs), 3008–3010, *3009*
  management of patients with, 2279–2280, *2280, 2281*, 2282, *2283, 2284*
Intracranial aspergillomas, 4292–4293, *4293*
Intracranial cavernous angiomas, 2236–2237, *2240*
Intracranial chordomas, 2438–2439
Intracranial echinococcal cysts, 4452
Intracranial hamartomas
  arachnoid cysts, 2117–2118
    infratentorial, 2120–2121, *2121, 2122*
    in other locations, 2123, *2124*
    suprasellar, 2123–2125
    supratentorial, 2118–2120, *2119, 2120*
  cysts of septum pellucidum, 2124–2126, *2128*
  ectopias of neural tissue, 2130, *2130*
  ependymal cysts, 2123–2124, *2125*, 2126, *2127, 2128*
  of hypothalamus, 2126–2127, *2129*, 2129–2130
Intracranial hemangioblastomas, 2226
Intracranial hemangiopericytomas, 2229
Intracranial infections, headaches associated with, 1716
Intracranial lesions, pituitary adenomas associated with other, 2203
Intracranial masses, papilledema from, 515
Intracranial mycotic aneurysm, 4088
Intracranial neoplasms, headaches associated with, 1716–1717
Intracranial optic nerve, 7–8, 717
Intracranial pathology in tuberous sclerosis, 2684
Intracranial plasmacytomas, 2391
Intracranial pressure, measurements of, 486–487, *487*
Intracranial schistosomiasis, 4488–4489
Intracranial schwannomas, 2300–2302, *2301, 2302*, 2660
Intracranial steal phenomenon, 3120
Intracranial subdural or epidural empyema, 4069
Intracranial tuberculomas, 4167
Intracranial tumors, imaging of, 1898–1902, *1899, 1900, 1901*
Intracranial vertebral artery endarterectomy, 3575
Intracytoplasmic inclusion bodies, congenital myopathies with, 1358–1359
Intradural extramedullary disease, 4467
Intraocular angiostrongyliasis, 4496–4497, *4498*
Intraocular aspergillosis, 4297–4298
Intraocular cryptococcosis, 4378–4381, *4379, 4380, 4381*
Intraocular cysticercosis, *4471, 4472*
Intraocular echinococcosis, 4446–4447, *4448*
Intraocular gnathostomiasis, 4501–4503, *4504*
Intraocular hemorrhages, 3024–3025
Intraocular inflammation, 1997
Intraocular schwannomas, 2656
Intraocular toxocariasis, 4516, 4522–4523
Intraocular tuberculosis, *4145, 4146, 4147*
Intraosseous hemangiomas, 2444, *2445*
Intraparenchymal angiomas, 2235–2236
Intraparenchymal hemorrhage, headaches associated with, 1709
Intraretinal hemorrhages, 3025
Intrathecal injections, headaches related to, 1716
Intrauterine cytomegalovirus (CMV) infection, 5097
Intravagal paragangliomas, 2471–2472, *2472*
Intravenous human immune globulin (HIG) for myasthenia gravis, 1430
Intravenous neurocysticercosis, 4466–4467, *4467, 4468*
Intraventricular cysticercus, 4476
Intraventricular echinococcus cyst, 4447, *4450*
Intraventricular hemorrhage associated with aneurysmal rupture, 3034
Intrinsic tumors of brainstem, 1871–1875, *1872, 1874, 1876, 1877*, 1877–1878
Intussusception, 4959
Invasive aspergillosis, 4294–4299, *4295, 4296, 4297, 4298, 4299, 4300, 4301*, 4301–4306, *4302*, 4302–4303, *4303, 4304, 4305, 4306, 4307, 4308*, 4308–4310, *4309, 4310, 4311*, 4312, *4312, 4313, 4314, 4315, 4316*, 4316–4317
Invasive pituitary adenomas, 2203–2204
Inverse Anton's syndrome, 3486–3487
Inverse Argyll Robertson pupils, 993
Inverse bobbing, 1328
Inverse Marcus Gunn phenomenon, 1541, *1541*
Inverse ocular bobbing, 3512
Inverse Uhthoff's symptom, 5577
  of multiple sclerosis, 5577
Involuntary ocular deviations, 5602–5603
Ion channel disorders, 1376
  myotonia, 1376
    congenita, 1376
    paramyotonia congenita, 1376
    periodic paralysis, 1376–1377, *1377*
    Schwartz-Jampel syndrome (chondrodystrophic myotonia), 1377
Ipsilateral Horner's syndrome, 2996, *2997*
Ipsilateral medial rectus subnucleus, 1142
Ipsilateral relative afferent pupillary defect, 653
Ipsipulsion, 1123
  of saccades, 1286
Iridis
  heterochromia, 1009
  rubeosis, 1997
Iridocyclitis, 5226
Iris, 847
  abnormalities in, 3466
  anterior border layer, 852, *852*
  assessment of, 934
  atrophy, 1011, *1011*
  blood vessels of, 858, *858*
  crypts, 855
  effect of radiation therapy on, 2615
  embryology of, *848*, 848–850, *849, 850*
  gross and microscopic anatomy of, 850, *851*
  leukemic involvement of, 2349
  nerves of, 858–860, 860*t*
  pain associated with, 1724–1725
  physiology of, 860
    integrated activities of sphincter and dilator muscles, 883–887, *884, 885, 886*
    motor control of dilator muscle, 879–883, *881, 882*
    sphincter muscle, 860–879, *861, 862, 863, 864, 865, 866, 867, 869, 870, 871, 872, 873, 874, 875, 876, 877, 878*
  structural defects of
    acquired
      acute angle closure glaucoma, *1010*, 1010–1011
      atrophy, 1011, *1011*
      inflammation, 1009
      ischemia, 1009–1010
      postoperative mydriasis, 1011
      trauma, 1010
      tumor, 1010
    congenital
      abnormalities of color, 1009
      aniridia, 1006, *1007*
      cat-like (elliptic) pupils, 1006
      coloboma of, 1006
      ectopic (misplaced) pupils, 1008
      miosis, 1008–1009
      mydriasis, 1009
      peninsula pupils, 1008
      persistent pupillary membrane remnants, 1008
      polycoria, 1008
      pseudopolycoria, 1008
      scalloped pupils, 1008
      square pupils, 1006
  vascular abnormalities of, 1367
Iris dilator muscle
  cortical and subcortical influences on, 883
  pharmacologic stimulation of, 974
Iris heterochromia, 2712
Iris pigment and pupillary responses to drugs, 1006
Iris sphincter muscle
  aberrant regeneration after damage to innervation of, 994
  damage to, 983–984, *985*
  damage to parasympathetic outflow to, 974–983, *975, 976, 977, 979, 980, 981, 983, 984*
  pharmacologic stimulation of, 974
Iris stroma, 853, *853*
Iritis, 1724, 4864, 4866, 4901–4902, 5226
  fibrinous, 4901
  of meningococcal meningitis, 4096–4097

Iritis papulosa, 4901
Irradiation for nasopharyngeal carcinoma, 2449
Irvine-Gass syndrome, 631
Isaacs' syndrome, 2532
Ischemia, 1009–1010, 3324
choroidal, 3463, *3465*
delayed cerebral, 3145–3147, *3146, 3147*
Ischemic cerebrovascular disease
collateral circulation to brain and orbit, 3413–3414
aortic arch syndromes, *3519*, 3519–3524, *3520, 3521, 3522, 3523*
between cerebral vessels, 3414
channels to carotid siphon, 3415–3416
circle of Willis, 3414, *3414, 3415*
generalized disease of carotid and vertebrobasilar arteries, 3518–3519
neurologic and ocular signs of occlusive disease of vertebrobasilar arterial system, *3475*, 3475–3477, *3476, 3477, 3478, 3479*, 3479–3480, *3480, 3481, 3482*, 3482–3487, *3486, 3487, 3488, 3489*, 3489–3492, *3490, 3491, 3492, 3493*, 3494–3497, *3495, 3496, 3497*, 3498, *3498, 3499*, 3499–3502, *3500, 3501, 3502, 3503, 3504, 3505*, 3506, *3506, 3507, 3508, 3509*, 3509–3516, *3510, 3511, 3513, 3514*
with occlusion of common carotid artery, 3417
with occlusion of innominate artery, 3417
with occlusion of internal carotid artery, 3414–3415, *3416*
with occlusion of vertebral artery, 3417–3418, *3418*
ophthalmic collateral circuit, 3415–3416
with proximal occlusion of subclavian artery, 3417
rete mirabile, 3417
signs of occlusive disease in internal carotid arterial system, 3428
extracranial signs, 3428
neurologic signs, 3428–3444, *3429, 3430, 3432, 3433, 3435, 3436, 3437, 3438, 3439, 3440, 3441, 3442, 3443*
ocular signs, 3444–3450, *3445, 3446, 3447, 3448, 3449, 3450, 3451, 3452, 3453*, 3453–3454, *3454, 3455, 3456, 3457*, 3458, *3458, 3459, 3460*, 3460–3467, *3461, 3462, 3463, 3464, 3465, 3466, 3467, 3468, 3469*, 3469–3470, *3470, 3471*
signs of occlusive disease of common carotid artery, *3427*, 3427–3428
symptoms and signs of, 3418–3419
of aortocranial disease, 3518
of carotid arterial system ischemia, historical review, 3419
of lacunar infarction, 3516–3518
of vertebrobasilar artery system ischemia, 3471, *3471*
transient attacks from intermittent insufficiency in internal carotid artery, 3419–3426, *3421, 3422, 3425, 3426*
transient ischemic attacks from intermittent insufficiency of vertebrobasilar arterial system, 3471–3475
definitions, 3323–3324
diagnosis, 3524–3525
direct noninvasive assessment of carotid arterial system, 3533–3536, *3534, 3535*
imaging studies, 3525–3530, *3526, 3527, 3528, 3529*
indirect noninvasive assessment of carotid arterial system, 3536–3541, *3537, 3538, 3539, 3540*
invasive testing of extracranial and intracranial vascular disease, 3544–3545, *3547, 3548*, 3548–3549, *3549*
miscellaneous tests in patients with, 3549–3550
noninvasive tests of, 3533, *3541*, 3541–3544, *3542, 3543, 3544*
tests of cardiac function, 3546, 3548–3549, *3549*
tests that measure cerebral blood flow or metabolism, 3530, *3531, 3532*, 3532–3533, *3533*
management, 3556
medical therapy, *3557*, 3557–3562, *3559, 3561*
of patients with acute stroke, 3577–3581
of patients with asymptomatic cervical bruit, asymptomatic carotid disease, 3569–3570
of patients with retinal stroke, 3577
of patients with transient ischemic attacks, 3570–3576
of patients with transient monocular visual loss, 3576–3577
of risk factors, 3567–3569
surgical therapy, 3562–3567, *3564, 3565*
therapeutic options, 3556
pathology
hypoxia, 3324–3326, *3325, 3326*
infarction, *3326*, 3326–3328, *3327, 3328*
pathophysiology
decreased cerebral perfusion (systemic hypotension)
causes of, 3407, *3408*, 3409–3413
general considerations, 3407
embolism
air, 3379
appearance of, 3365
calcium, 3372–3373, *3374, 3375, 3376*
causes of, 3386–3396, *3389, 3390, 3391, 3392, 3393, 3394, 3395, 3396, 3397*, 3398, *3398, 3400*, 3400–3406, *3401, 3402, 3403, 3404, 3405, 3406*
cholesterol, 3365–3367, *3366, 3367, 3368, 3369*
fat, 3377, 3379, *3379, 3380*
foreign body, 3381–3383, *3383, 3384, 3385*, 3385–3386, *3386, 3387*
general considerations, 3364–3365, 3365*t*
organism, 3379, *3382*
platelet-fibrin, 3367, *3370*, 3370–3371, *3371, 3372*
tumor, 3376–3377, *3378, 3379, 3380*
thrombosis
amyloid angiopathy, 3351, *3353*
arterial wall constriction and compression, 3353–3355, *3354, 3355, 3356, 3357*
arteritis, 3339–3340, *3340, 3341*, 3342, *3343*, 3344, *3345, 3346*, 3346–3348, *3347*
atherosclerosis, 3329–3330, *3331*, 3332–3335, *3333, 3334*
causes, 3328–3329
drug abuse, 3363–3364
fibromuscular dysplasia, 3348, *3349*
general considerations, 3328
hypercoagulability, 3357–3359, *3358, 3359, 3360, 3361*, 3361–3362, *3362*
hypertension, *3335*, 3335–3336, *3336, 3337, 3338*
migraine and vasospasm, 3336–3339, *3338*
miscellaneous systemic disorders affecting arterial wall, 3351–3353
miscellaneous vasculopathies, 3362–3363
Moyamoya, 3348–3349, *3350*
neoplastic angiopathy, 3351
radiation angiopathy, 3350–3351, *3352*
sickle cell disease, 3349–3350
spontaneous and traumatic dissection, 3348
prognosis, 3550
of patients after initial stroke, 3555–3556
of patients with asymptomatic carotid artery disease, 3550–3552
of patients with asymptomatic cervical bruit, 3550
of patients with transient ischemic attacks, 3552–3553
of patients with transient monocular loss of vision (amaurosis fugax), 3553–3555
Ischemic myopathy, 1405
Ischemic ocular inflammation, 3457–3458, *3458, 3459, 3460*, 3460–3462, *3461, 3462, 3463*
Ischemic optic neuropathies, 259–260, *263, 264*, 549–592, 813
historical perspective, 549
papillophlebitis, 583, *584*
posterior (retrobulbar) ischemic neuropathy (PION), 583
arteritic, 583–585, *585*
nonarteritic, 585, *586, 587, 588, 589*, 592
terminology and nosology, 549
nonarteritic anterior
bilateral, 565–566, *566*
clinical characteristics, 557–559, *558, 559, 560, 572*, 572–573, *573*
appearance of disc, 559, *559, 560*
color vision, 557
fluorescein angiography, 559
initial symptoms, 557
initial visual acuity, 557
pain, 557
pupils, 559
visual field, 557–559, *558*
course, 559–560, *561, 562*, 563, 573, *574*
demographics, 550
diabetic papillopathy, *16*, 564–565
diagnosis and ancillary tests, 576–578
disc swelling preceding visual loss, 564
pathogenesis, 566–568, 573, *574*
pathology, 568–570, *569, 570*, 573, *575*, 576, *576, 577*
prevention, 571
arteritic anterior, 571–572
recurrent, 562–563
risk factors and associated conditions, 550–557

Ischemic optic neuropathies—*continued*
acute blood loss, anemia, and hypotension, 553–555
cardiac disease, 551–552
carotid artery disease, 552
cataract surgery, 556
cerebrovascular disease, 551
coagulopathies, 551
diabetes mellitus, 551
elevated intraocular pressure, 555–556
embolism, 552–553
favism, 555
hypertension, 551
migraine, 556
miscellaneous associations, 556–557
nocturnal hypotension, 555
treatment
medical, 570
surgical, 570–571
vasculitides other than giant cell arteritis, 578, *579,* 580, *580, 581, 582*
visual outcome, 560
vascular disc swelling without visual loss, 580–581, 583
Ischemic optic neuropathy, 3447–3448
management of patients with, 3577
permanent visual defects from, 3693–3694, *3694*
Ischemic retinal disturbances, 5040
Ischemic stroke, 3142
in patients with sickle cell disease, 3349–3350, *3351*
Ishihara Color Plates, 1772–1773
Isolated abducens nerve paresis, 3118, 3509
Isolated accommodation insufficiency, 1012
Isolated angiitis of central nervous system, 3342, *3345*
Isolated central nervous system (CNS) histoplasmosis, 4401–4402, *4403*
Isolated facial nerve paresis, 5023
Isolated intraocular large-cell lymphoma, 2375
Isolated oculomotor nerve palsy, 3118
Isoniazid (INH), 1263
Isonicotinic acid hydrazide, 4141
Isopter, 175
Itraconazole
for allergic aspergillosis, 4317
for coccidioidomycosis, 4365
for fungal infections, 4286
for histoplasmosis, 4404

J

Jakob-Creutzfeldt disease, 469. (*See also* Creutzfeldt-Jakob disease.)
Jamestown Canyon virus, 5159
Japanese encephalitis, 5170
clinical manifestations, *5171,* 5171–5172
epidemiology, 5170–5171
Japanese encephalitis type A, 5722
Japanese encephalitis type B, 3985–3986, 5722
Jarisch-Herxheimer reaction, 4830, 4835
Jaw jerk reflex, 1658–1659
Jaw movement, paradoxic eyelid retraction evoked by, 1553–1554, *1554*
JC virus, *5133,* 5133–5139, *5134, 5135, 5136, 5137, 5138, 5139, 5140, 5141,* 5141–5142, *5142*
Jerk nystagmus, 1107, 1462, *1462*
Jerk seesaw nystagmus, 1477
Jerk-waveform divergence nystagmus, 1481
Joubert's syndrome, 1326, 2784–2785
Judgment of Line Orientation (BVRT), 470, 471
Jugular bulb, 2967
Jugular foramen syndrome, 2448
Jugular vein, 2967
lesions of, 970
thrombosis of, 3926–3927
Junction, 841
Junctional syndrome, 2171
Jungle yellow fever, 5184
Juvenile dystonic lipidosis, 1319
Juvenile motor neuron disease, 2799
Juvenile neuronal ceroid lipofuscinoses, 2851
Juvenile rheumatoid arthritis, 3850–3852, *3852*
Juvenile xanthogranuloma, 2416, 2418, *2418, 2419, 2420, 2421*

K

Kallikrein, 727
Kaposi's sarcoma-associated herpesvirus (KSHV), 5128–5129
Katayama fever, 4487
Kawasaki's disease, 5722
cause, 5740–5741
clinical manifestations, 5735, *5736*
neurologic, 5738, *5738, 5739*
ocular, 5735–5736, *5736, 5738*
systemic, 5735, *5736, 5737*
diagnosis, 5738–5739, 5739*t*
epidemiology, 5733
laboratory findings, 5738
pathology, 5733, *5734,* 5735
prognosis, 5740
treatment, 5739–5740
Kearns-Sayre syndrome (KSS), 1381, *1383,* 1383–1385, *1384, 1385, 1386, 1387,* 1387–1388, 1388
cardiac involvement, 1384–1385
endocrine involvement, 1388
neurologic abnormalities, 1387–1388, *1388*
retinal involvement, 1383–1384, *1384, 1385*
treatment, 1388
weakness of somatic muscles, 1387, *1387*
Keratitis, 3855, 4090, 4182, *4185,* 5226–5227
Acanthamoeba, 4635, *4637,* 4638, *4638*
bilateral punctate, 5207
dendritic, 5023
epithelial, 5289
interstitial, 4901
neuroparalytic, *1676,* 1676–1677
neurotrophic, *1676,* 1676–1677, 5040
punctate, 4509
Keratitis linearis migrans, 4901
Keratitis pustuliformis profunda, 4901
Keratoconjunctivitis, 4145
epidemic, 4956
Keratoconjunctivitis sicca, 3841–3842
Keratopathy, neuroparalytic, 4172
Keratouveitis, chronic relapsing herpes zoster, 5080
Kernig's sign, 4201
positive, 1716
Kestenbaum test, 944
Kestenbaum's number, 944
Ketoconazole
for blastomycosis, 4342
for coccidioidomycosis, 4365
for fungal infections, *4284,* 4284–4286, *4285*
for histoplasmosis, 4404
Kidney disease
in patients with tuberous sclerosis, *2690,* 2690–2692, *2691, 2692, 2693, 2694*
polycystic, and development of aneurysms, 3010, *3011*
Kinesin, 49
Kinetic testing, 177
Kingella, 4103–4104
Kingella kingae meningitis, 4103–4104
Kjellin syndrome, 2795
Kjer's neuropathies, 666
Klebsiella, 4219–4220
Klebsiella ozaenae, 4220
Klebsiella pneumoniae, 4220
in intracranial abscess, 3950
in sinusitis, 4025
Klinefelter's syndrome, 2165, 2336
Klippel-Trénaunay-Weber syndrome, 782, 2275, *2728, 2729,* 2729–2730, *2730, 2731,* 2733, 3012
Klüver-Bucy syndrome, 3492
Knochenschädel, 3523
Koenen's tumor, 2675, *2675*
Koerber-Salus-Elschnig syndrome, 1868
Kollner's rule, 156
Koniocellular layer, 108
Koplik spots, 5201, *5201*
Korsakoff's syndrome, 3487
KPN virus, 5744
Krabbe disease, 765, 2857–2859, *2858, 2859*
Krabbe leukodystrophy, 2857
Krause, glands of, 918
Kunjin virus, 5174–5175
Kupffer cells, 2329, 2403
Kuru, 4567, *4568*
clinical characteristics, 4568
diagnosis, 4568
neuro-ophthalmologic features, 4568
pathology, 4568, *4569, 4570, 4571*
plaques in, 4568, *4570*
treatment, 4568
Kveim reaction, diagnostic testing for, 5526
Kyasanur Forest disease, 5188–5189

L

Labbé, vein of, 2947
Laboratory monitoring of HIV infection and quantitation of viral load, 5381–5382, 5382*t*
Laboratory-supported definite multiple sclerosis, 5627
Laboratory-supported probable multiple sclerosis, 5627
Lacerum segment of internal carotid artery, 2871, *2871,* 2873, *2873,* 2876–2877
Lacrimal flow, testing, 956
Lacrimal glands
anatomy of reflex tear secretion by, 917–918, *918*
parasympathetic pathway to, 2–3, *3, 4,* 5, *5, 6,* 7–8, 228, *1175*
sympathetic pathway to, 924–925
Lacrimal nerve, 1613
Lacrimal scintillography, 956
Lacrimal system, effect of radiation therapy on, 2614
Lacrimation
assessment of, 953
examination, 953–956, 954*t, 955*
history, 953
disorders of
brainstem lesions, 1018

denervation supersensitivity, 1021
drug effects, 1025
lesions affecting greater superficial petrosal nerve, 1019, *1020, 1021*
lesions affecting nervus intermedius, facial nerve trunk, and geniculate ganglion, 1018–1019, *1019, 1020*
lesions affecting sphenopalatine ganglions, 1019–1021, *1022*
lesions of zygomaticotemporal nerve, 1021
paradoxic gustolacrimal reflexes, crocodile tears, 1022–1025, *1023*
supranuclear lesions, 1018
drug effects on, 1025
nonorganic disturbances of, 1784–1785
reflexes associated with, 930
LaCrosse encephalitis, 5158–5162
characteristics of, 5159–5160, *5160*
clinical manifestations, 5160–5161
diagnosis, 5161
epidemiology of, 5160, *5161*
pathology, 5161, *5162*
prevention, 5162
treatment, 5161
Lactic acid in diagnosing bacterial meningitis, 4010
Lactic acidosis, 366, 767
in MELAS syndrome, 2854
Lactobacilli, 4130
Lacunae, 2956
Lacunar disease, 3427
Lacunar infarction
headaches associated with, 1708
symptoms and signs of, 3516–3518
Lacunar strokes, 3335–3336
Lacunes, 3335–3336
Laetrile, 2592–2593
Lagochilascaris, 4529, 4531
Lagophthalmos, 4171
Lambert-Eaton myasthenic syndrome
clinical features, 1434–1435
ocular manifestations, 1436
pathophysiology, 1436
therapy, 1436–1437
Lamina cribrosa, 57–58, *60*
Lamina ganglionaris of Brodmann, 128–129
Lamina granularis externa, 128
Lamina granularis interna, 128
Lamina multiformis of Brodmann, 129
Lamina pyramidalis, 128
Lamivudine (3TC), 5365
Lancaster test, 1180
Lancefield grouping system, 4075
Landry-Guillain-Barré syndrome, 1550
papilledema in, 518–519, *519*
Langerhans cell, 2404
Langerhans cell histiocytic system, 2404
Langerhans cell histiocytosis, 703, 2405–2413, *2406, 2407, 2408, 2409, 2410, 2412*
Langerhans giant cells, 3989, *3991*
Language, disturbances in, 1860
Lanreotide for pituitary adenomas, 2192, 2196
Lantern jaw, 2157, *2157*
Lantern tests, 212
Lanthony New Color Test, 407
Laplace's law, 3141
Large-cell lymphoma
isolated intraocular, 2375
primary central nervous system (CNS), 2364–2366, *2366, 2367, 2368,* 2368–2370, *2369, 2370, 2371, 2372,* 2372–2375, *2373, 2374*
systemic diffuse, 2361–2364, *2362, 2363, 2365*
Larynx, paralysis of, 4127
L-asparaginase, 2593
neuro-ophthalmologic toxicity, 2594
neurotoxicity, 2593–2594, *2594*
systemic toxicity, 2593
Late delayed encephalopathy, 2599–2602, *2600, 2601, 2603,* 2604, *2605*
Late delayed radiation myelopathy, 2605–2606, *2607*
Late infantile neuronal ceroid lipofuscinoses, 2851, *2852*
Latent nystagmus, 1484
Late-onset inherited ataxic disorders, 2790*t*, 2790–2795, *2791, 2793*
Lateral gaze, anisocoria in, 885
Lateral geniculate body
embryology of, 16–17, *17, 18, 19,* 29
lesions in, 333–334, *334, 335,* 336, *336*
tumors involving, 1815, 1818, *1818*
Lateral geniculate hemorrhage, 3608–3609
Lateral geniculate nucleus (LGN), 57, 101
afferent pathways to, 107–108
retinal ganglion cells, 107–108
anatomy of, *103,* 104–107, *105, 106, 107*
control of information flow through, 112–113
tier 1, global neuromodulatory control, 113
tier 2, specific neuromodulatory control, 113
tier 13, focal specific excitatory control, 113–114
nonretinal afferents to, 108
output from, 115–116, *118*
parallel pathways, 116–117
binocular vision, 117–118
on-off channels, 118
X, Y, W, *118,* 119
projection of visual field on, *113, 114,* 114–115, *115, 116, 117*
signal transmission properties of cells and visual sensory fibers, 108
center-surround organization, 110
contrast gain control, 110
inhibitory pathways, 109, *109*
lagged cells in, 112
magnification, 111–112, *112*
responses of to other stimuli, 112
spatial properties of, 110–111, *111*
temporal properties of, 111
transfer ratio, 109–110
Lateral inferior pontine syndrome, 3512
Lateral medullary infarction, *1285,* 1285–1287, *1286, 1287*
Lateral medullary syndrome, 3513
Lateral midpontine syndrome, 3512
Lateral pontine syndromes, 3512
Lateral sinus, 2959, *2962*
thrombosis of, *3899,* 3899–3903, *3900, 3901, 3902, 3903, 3904, 3905*
septic, *4039,* 4039–4041, *4040*
Lateral superior pontine syndrome, 3512
Laterality in incidence of saccular aneurysms, 3015, *3016, 3017*
Lateropulsion, 1286
of eye movement, *3514,* 3514–3515
of saccades, 1122–1123
Latex agglutination (LA) test, 4100, 5379
in diagnosing bacterial meningitis, 4009
Lead, 1263
Learning, motor, 1147
Leber's idiopathic stellate neuroretinitis, 634
Leber's optic neuropathy, 666, 744–755
ancillary testing, 749–750
associated findings, 746, 749
clinical features, 744–746, *747, 748*
determinants of expression, 753–755
hereditary, 987
inheritance and genetics, 750–751, *752,* 753
treatment, 755
"Leber's Plus," 749, 750
Leber's stellate maculopathy, 634
Lebombo virus, 5261
Left common carotid artery, 2869
Left subclavian artery, 2869
Leftward horizontal gaze, paralysis of, 4127
Legionella, 4237, 4239–4240
ibacterial encephalitis, 3986
Legionella bozemanii, 4239
Legionella dumoffii, 4239
Legionella longbeachae, 4239
Legionella micdadei, 4239
Legionella monocytogenes, 5419
Legionella pneumophila, 4237–4239, *4238,* 4550
in bacterial encephalitis, 3986
Legionellaceae, 4237
Legionnaires' disease, 4237
Leigh's syndrome, 767, 1331
Lemierre's syndrome, 4229–4230
Lens, effect of radiation therapy on, 2614
Lens capsule, 907
Lentiform nucleus, 1862–1863
Lentiviruses
acquired immune deficiency syndrome, 5375–5376
epidemiology, *5377,* 5377–5379, *5378*
history, 5376*t*, 5376–5377
adnexal complications of HIV infection, 5430
clinical manifestations of human immunodeficiency infection, 5372
advanced immune deficiency, 5374, 5374*t*, *5375*
early immune deficiency, 5373
intermediate immune deficiency, 5373–5374
primary infection (seroconversion illness), 5372–5373
diagnosis of human immunodeficiency virus infection, 5379
antibody detection, 5379–5380
antigen detection, 5380
CD4 + T-cell quantitation, 5380–5381
culture, 5380
laboratory monitoring of, and quantitation of viral load, 5381–5382, 5382*t*
molecular genetic techniques, 5380
human immunodeficiency virus type 1, 5363
life cycle, 5365–5368, *5367, 5368*
structure, 5363–5365, *5364, 5366*
variability, 5368
human immunodeficiency virus type 2, 5368–5369
neurologic complications of HIV-1 infection, 5385, *5386,* 5386*t*
myopathic complications, 5386–5387
parenchymal central nervous system (CNS) disease, 5409–5424, *5410, 5412, 5413, 5414, 5418, 5420*
peripheral nervous system, 5386–5387

Lentiviruses—*continued*
primary intracranial, 5387–5395, *5388, 5389,* 5390*t, 5391, 5392, 5393, 5394, 5395, 5396, 5397,* 5397–5399, *5398, 5399, 5400, 5401,* 5401–5407, *5402, 5403, 5404, 5405, 5406, 5407, 5408*
primary spinal cord, 5386–5387
neuro-ophthalmologic complications of HIV infection, 5431–5433
ocular complications of HIV infection, 5424, *5425*
anterior segment disease, 5429–5430
retinal microangiopathy, 5424–5426, *5426*
retinitis and chorioretinitis, *5426,* 5426–5429, *5427, 5428, 5429*
orbital complications of HIV infection, *5430,* 5430*t,* 5430–5431, *5431*
pathogenesis of human immunodeficiency virus infection, 5369–5372, *5370, 5371*
prevention, 5384–5385
screening for asymptomatic HIV-1 infection, 5384
treatment, 5382–5384
vaccine development to prevent HIV infection, 5385
Lepromatous leprosy, 4169
Leprosy, 4168–4176, *4169, 4170, 4171, 4172, 4174, 4175*
cardinal signs of, 4169–4170
clinical features of, 4169
diagnosis of, 4173
epidemiology of, 4169
lepromatous, 4169
neurologic complications of, 4172–4173, *4174, 4175*
ocular complications of, 4171–4172
pathologic changes in, 4173
treatment of, 4173–4176, *4175*
tuberculoid, 4169
Leptomeningeal arterioles, 2932
Leptomeningeal cysts, 4452
Leptomeningeal infiltration, 2338–2339, *2339*
Leptomeninges, 73, 2018
CSF dissemination or metastases to, 1929
local infiltration of, 1928
Leptomeningitis, 3990, 4337, 4369, *4369, 4370,* 4498. (*See also* Acute bacterial meningitis; Acute nonbacterial meningitis.)
Leptomyxida, 4638, *4639, 4640,* 4640–4641, *4641*
Leptomyxida amoeba, 4638, *4639,* 5416
Leptospira
association with neuroretinitis, 636
clinical manifestations, 4837–4842, *4840, 4841, 4842, 4843*
diagnosis, 4842–4843
epidemiology, 4836–4837
pathology and pathogenesis, 4837, *4838, 4839, 4840*
treatment, 4843
Leptospirosis, icteric, 4842, *4843*
Lesions
bone, in cryptococcosis, 4381–4382, *4383*
infranuclear, 5605–5606, *5607, 5608,* 5608–5609, *5609*
internuclear, 5603–5605, *5604, 5605, 5606*
nuclear, 5603
petechial, 4098
punctate inner retinal, 4682
punctate outer, 4682
supranuclear, 5603, *5604*
Lethal midline granuloma, 3802, *3803*
Lethargic encephalitis, 5213
Lethargica, encephalitis, 1568
Letterer-Siwe disease, 2405
Leukemia, *703,* 703–705, *704*
acute, 2337
central nervous system, 2337
chronic, 2337
general considerations, 2336
meningeal, 2337–2338
pathology, 2336–2337
symptoms and signs
involvement of vitreous, 2348–2350, *2349, 2350*
neurologic complications, 2337–2340, *2338, 2339*
ocular manifestations, *2340,* 2340–2348, *2341, 2342, 2343, 2344, 2345, 2346, 2347, 2348*
systemic, 2337
therapy and prognosis, 2350–2351
Leukemic retinopathy, *2344,* 2344–2348, *2345, 2346, 2347, 2348*
Leukocyte scintigraphy in diagnosing abscess, 3962, *3963*
Leukocytes, polymorphonuclear, 2329
Leukodystrophy
globoid cell, 2857–2859, *2858, 2859*
Krabbe, 2857
metachromatic, 765, 2837–2840, *2838, 2839, 2840*
Leukoencephalitis
acute hemorrhagic, 5653, *5654, 5655,* 5656
multifocal, 5064, 5067–5068
subacute sclerosing, 5213
clinical manifestations, *5214,* 5214–5216, *5215, 5216, 5217*
diagnosis, 5217, 5220, *5223, 5224*
epidemiology, 5213–5214
pathogenesis, 5217
pathology, 5216–5217, *5218, 5219*
treatment and prognosis, 5220, *5224*
Leukoencephalopathy, 2555
multifocal, 2631
progressive multifocal, 2339–2340, 3978, *5133,* 5133–5139, *5134, 5135, 5136, 5137, 5138, 5139, 5140, 5141,* 5141–5142, *5142,* 5409, 5412–5413, *5413*
Leukopenia, 3816–3817
Levallorphan, 1005
Levator aponeurotic defects, 1543
Levator aponeurotic ptosis, 1542–1543, *1544,* 1545
Levator palpebrae superioris, 1052, *1053,* 1075, *1078,* 1509, 1511–1512, *1512*
dysfunction of, 3077
innervation of, 1520–1522, *1521*
ptosis and other signs of, *1410,* 1410–1411, *1411*
Levator palpebrae synkinesias, 1553
Levator slow-twitch fiber, 1512
Levator tonus, 1550
Levodopa for pituitary adenomas, 2196
Lewy bodies, 2765–2767, *2766*
dementia with, 2756–2759, *2757,* 2758*t*
Lhermitte-Duclos disease, 1977, *1978*
Lhermitte's symptom, 154, 2574, 2604–2605, 5569, *5569*
Libido, decreased, 2156
Lid nystagmus, 1873
Lid-lag
myopathic eyelid retraction and, 1556–1559, *1557, 1558*
neuromuscular eyelid retraction and, 1555–1556, *1556*
neuropathic eyelid retraction and, 1550–1551, *1551, 1552*
Lidocaine, 1003
Light
paradoxical reaction of pupils to, 990
pupil reaction to, *887,* 887–892, *889, 890, 891, 892*
testing consensual response to, 937
testing pupillary reaction to, *936,* 936–937
Light-brightness sense in optic neuritis, 613
Light-near dissociation, 990, 5433
Argyll Robertson, *991,* 991–993
inverse, 993
lesions of afferent pathway, 994
mesencephalic lesions, 993–994, *994*
testing for, 938
Light-near pupillary dissociation, 3767
Lightness Discrimination Test, 407
Limb dysmetria, 5568
Limbic cortex and pupillary dilation, 883
Limbic system, 828, *829*
Limbus, sensory nerve endings in, 1601
Limulus amebocyte lysate test, 4100, 4739
in diagnosing bacterial meningitis, 4009–4010
Line bisection task, 470
Linear energy transfer (LET), 2595
Linear sebaceous nevus syndrome, 782, 788
Linear vestibulo-ocular reflex (VOR), 1139
Lingual artery, 2940
Lingula, 1884
Lining cells, 2404
Lipid, 4065
Lipid A moiety of *Pseudomonas* endotoxin, 4241
Lipid envelope, 4946
Lipid hypothesis of atherosclerosis, 3334–3335
Lipid metabolism disorders
metachromatic leukodystrophy, 2837–2840, *2838, 2839, 2840*
Refsum disease, 2840–2841
Lipid peroxidation and optic nerve injury, *726,* 726–727
Lipid storage disease, 1330–1331
Lipidosis, 764
juvenile dystonic, 1319
Lipofuscinoses
infantile neuronal ceroid, 2850
juvenile neuronal ceroid, 2851
late infantile neuronal ceroid, 2851, *2852*
neuronal ceroid, 2848–2850, *2849, 2850, 2851*
Lipogranulomatosis, farber, 2830–2831, *2831*
Lipomas, 2095–2098, *2096, 2097, 2098*
Lipomatosis, epidural, 2588
Lipomucopolysaccharidosis, 2822
Lipopolysaccharide molecules, 3996
Liposomes, 4283
β-Lipotropin hormone (β-LPH), 2147–2148
Lisch nodules, *2650, 2651,* 2652
Listeria brainstem encephalitis, 4132
Listeria meningitis, 4131
Listeria monocytogenes, 4130–4135, *4131, 4133, 4134, 4135,* 5679
in bacterial encephalitis, 3986
in bacterial meningitis, 3993, 3994
in brain abscess, 3946
in granuloma, 3990

in intracranial abscess, 3950, 3952
in meningoencephalitis, 4132–4133
Listing's law, 1103
Listing's plane, 1103
Lisuride, 2192
Lithium, impact of, on postsynaptic neuromuscular transmission, 1443
Liver
abscess of, 4619–4620
echinococcosis of, 4452
Loa loa, 4503, 4505–4507, *4506, 4507, 4508*
treatment of, 4507
Lobar degenerations, 2759–2764, *2761, 2762, 2763*
Local embolism, 3401
Local malignancy, invasion of brain, 2067–2068
Local tonic pupils, 977–978
Localized central chorioretinitis, 4867–4868, *4868, 4869, 4870, 4871,* 4871–4872
Localized *Salmonella* infection, 4222–4223
Localized tetanus, 4111, 4113
Locally invasive tumors, 698–700, *699, 700*
Location and residency and relationship between optic neuritis and multiple sclerosis, 618
Location in incidence of saccular aneurysms, 3015, *3016, 3017*
Locked-in syndrome, 1329, 3217–3218, 3506, 3512–3513, 5574
Lockjaw, 4112
Lockwood's ligament, 1512
Loiasis, 4503, 4505–4507, *4506, 4507, 4508*
central nervous system (CNS), 4505–4506
diagnosis of, 4506–4507
ocular, 4505, *4506, 4507*
subconjunctival, 4505, *4506*
treatment of, 4507
Long posterior ciliary arteries, 2884
Long terminal repeats (LTR), 5365
Lorenzo oil therapy for adrenomyeloneuropathy, 2847
Loss Variance (LV) on Octopus perimeter, 180
Louis-Bar syndrome, 1326
Louse-borne relapsing fever, 4833
Louse-borne typhus, 4752
Lovibond Color Vision Analyzer, 212
Low-density lipoprotein (LDL), 3335
Low-dose immunization, 5376
Lowe syndrome, 2814–2815
Lower cranial nerves, radiation damage to, 2613, *2613*
Lower cranial neuropathies, 5052
Lower eyelid retractors, 1512–1513
Lower motor neuron syndrome, 2606–2607
Lower Sonoran Life Zone, 4355
Lown-Ganong-Levine syndrome, 746
Lues, 3973
Lumbar puncture headache, 1714–1715
Lumbar puncture in diagnosing meningitis, 4007–4009
Lumbosacral plexopathy, 2607–2609
Luminal infection, noninvasive, 4619
Luminal stenosis, 3205
Lung cysts in patients with tuberous sclerosis, 2692
Lupus. (*See also* Systemic lupus erythematosus (SLE).)
drug-induced, 3830
Lupus panniculitis, 3815
Lupus pernio, 5480, *5482*
Lupus profundus, 3815
Luteinizing hormone (LH), 2148
Lutz, posterior internuclear ophthalmoplegia of, 1297–1298
Lyme borreliosis antigen test, 4828
Lyme disease, 637, 3339, 4779–4780, 4783, 5721
arthritis, 4809, *4810*
association with neuroretinitis, 636
cardiac manifestations, 4789, *4789*
chronic disseminated, 4808–4818, *4810, 4811, 4812, 4813, 4814, 4815, 4816, 4817, 4818*
clinical course, 4787
clinical manifestations, 4786–4787
cutaneous manifestations, 4787, *4788,* 4788–4789, *4789,* 4809–4810, *4810*
diagnosis, 4820, 4822, *4822, 4823, 4824,* 4824–4825, *4825, 4826, 4827,* 4827–4828
early disseminated, 4787–4791, *4789, 4790, 4792, 4793,* 4793–4797, *4794, 4796, 4797, 4798, 4799,* 4799–4803, *4800, 4801, 4802, 4803, 4804,* 4805, *4805, 4806, 4807,* 4807–4808, *4808, 4809*
early localized, 4787
epidemiology, 4783–4786, *4784, 4785*
neurologic manifestations, 4787, 4789–4791, *4790, 4792, 4793,* 4793–4795, *4794, 4796,* 4810–4816, *4811, 4812, 4813, 4814, 4815, 4816*
neuro-ophthalmologic manifestations, 4800–4803, *4802, 4803, 4804,* 4805, *4805, 4806,* 4807–4808, *4808, 4809,* 4816–4818, *4817, 4818*
ocular manifestations, 4787, 4795–4797, *4796, 4798, 4799,* 4799–4800, *4800, 4801, 4816,* 4816–4818, *4817, 4818*
and optic neuritis, 630
pathogen, 4786
pathogenesis, 4818–4820
pathology, 4820, *4820, 4821*
prevention, *4831,* 4831–4832
seronegative, 4828–4829
systemic manifestations, 4787
treatment, 4829–4831
Lymphadenitis, toxoplasmic, 4685
Lymphadenopathy
angioimmunoblastic, 702–703
bilateral hilar, 5480
persistent generalized, 5373
regional, 4200
Lymphadenopathy syndrome, 5363, 5480, *5483*
persistent generalized, 5373
Lymphadenosis benigna cutis, 637
Lymphangioleiomyomatosis, primary, 2692
Lymphedema, cutaneous, 4509
Lymphocyte differentiation, 2330
Lymphocyte-initiated inflammatory reactions, 3726–3727
Lymphocytic adenohypophysitis, *2207,* 2207–2208, *2208*
Lymphocytic choriomeningitis virus, *5154,* 5154–5158, 5155, *5155,* 5155–5158, *5156, 5157, 5158*
Lymphocytic hypophysitis, *2207,* 2207–2208, *2208*
Lymphocytoma, 637, 4788–4789, *4789*
Lymphocytopenia, 3817
Lymphoid stem cells, 2329
Lymphoid system, 2330
Lymphoma, 701–703, *702.* (*See also* Large-cell lymphoma.)
angiocentric T-cell, *3786,* 3786–3788, *3787*
Burkitt's, 2375–2378, *2376, 2377*
cutaneous T-cell, *2386,* 2386–2389, *2387, 2388*
extraorbital, 2378–2379
Hodgkin's disease, 2351, *2351*
general considerations, 2351
neurologic and ocular disorders in, 2352–2353, *2353, 2354, 2355,* 2355–2357, *2356, 2357, 2358,* 2359–2360
prognosis, 2360
systemic symptoms, 2352
treatment, 2360
isolated intraocular large-cell, 2375
mycosis fungoides, *2386,* 2386–2389, *2387, 2388*
non-Hodgkin's, 701–702, 2360–2361, 2364–2366, *2366, 2367, 2368,* 2368–2370, *2369, 2370, 2371, 2372,* 2372–2375, *2373, 2374,* 2378
Burkitt's, 2375–2378, *2376, 2377*
diagnosis, 2385
etiology, 2378
general clinical features, 2378
isolated intraocular large-cell, 2375
neurologic involvement, 2380, *2380, 2381*
orbital involvement, 2378–2380, *2379, 2380*
primary central nervous system large-cell, 2364–2366, *2366, 2367, 2368,* 2368–2370, *2369, 2370, 2371, 2372,* 2372–2375, *2373, 2374*
treatment and prognosis, 2385–2386
visual involvement, *2381,* 2381–2385, *2382, 2383*
primary central nervous system, 5409, 5411–5412, *5412*
systemic diffuse large-cell, 2361–2364, *2362, 2363, 2365*
Lymphomatoid granulomatosis, 703, 3727, *3786,* 3786–3788, *3787*
Lymphomatous meningitis, 5424
Lymphoreticular malignancies, 701
Lyphadenopathy, regional, 4200
Lysosomal storage diseases
mucolipidoses, 2823–2824
mucopolysaccharidoses, 2815, 2816*t*
Hunter syndrome, 2819–2820
Hurler syndrome, *2816,* 2816–2819, *2817, 2818*
Hurler-Scheie compound, 2819
Maroteaux-Lamy, 2821, *2822*
Morquio syndrome, 2820–2821
Sanfilippo syndrome, 2820, *2820, 2821*
Scheie syndrome, 2818–2819, *2819*
Sly syndrome, 2821–2822
sialidoses, 2822
sphingolipidoses
Fabry disease, 2831–2832, *2832, 2833*
Farber disease, 2830–2831, *2831*
gangliosidoses, 2824–2828, *2825, 2826, 2828*
Gaucher disease, 2828–2830, *2829, 2830*
Niemann-Pick disease, 2832–2837, *2834, 2835, 2836, 2837*
Lyssa bodies, 5270, *5270*
Lyssaviruses, 5263–5271, *5264, 5265, 5266, 5267, 5268, 5269, 5270, 5271, 5272, 5273,* 5274–5276
rabies-related, 5276, *5277*
Lytico-Bodig syndrome, 1568

M

Machado-Joseph disease, 763, 1292, 1550, 2791
Macroadenomas, pituitary, 1466
Macrocephaly, 2660
Macroglobulinemia, Waldenström's, 2389, 2399–2400, *2400*, 2565
Macrophages, 2329, 2403
 accumulation of, 3726
 alveolar, 5475–5476
 wandering, 2329, 2404
Macropsia, 468, 947, 1842, 3673
Macrosaccadic oscillations, 1487
Macroscopic appearance
 of hypoxic region of brain, 3324, *3325, 3326*
 of infarct, 3326, *3326*
Macrosquare-wave jerks, 1487
MACULA, sparing of, 354–357, *356, 358*
Macular degeneration, 988
Macular disease, 988
Macular edema, 3462–3463
Maculopapular rash, 4098
Maculopathy, Leber's stellate, 634
Maculoscope ERG, 159
Mad cow disease, 4567
Maddox rod, 1179
Mafucci syndrome, 2735
Magnesium, impact of, on postsynaptic neuromuscular transmission, 1443
Magnetic field-search coil method, 1185
Magnetic resonance angiography (MRA), 1896, *3543*, 3543–3544, *3544*
 in diagnosing aneurysms, 3015, 3109–3110, 3132–3133, *3133, 3134, 3135*, 3135–3137, *3136, 3137*, 3204–3207
 in diagnosing cerebrovascular disease, 3529–3530, *3530*
Magnetic resonance imaging (MRI)
 in diagnosing aneurysms, 3015, 3132–3133, 3204–3207
 in diagnosing cerebrovascular disease, 3527–3529, *3528, 3529*
 in diagnosing intracranial abscess, 3960
 in diagnosing migraines, 3708–3709, *3709*
 in diagnosing optic neuritis, 606, 607, 608, *608*
 in imaging multiple sclerosis, 5617–5619, *5618, 5619, 5620, 5621, 5622, 5623*, 5623–5624, *5624*
Magnocellular cells, 46, 47
Magnocellular layers, 106
Mal mazzuco, 5722
Malaria, cerebral, 4657–4658
Malformations, headaches associated with unruptured vascular, 1711–1712
Malignant atrophic papulosis, 3346, 3859, 3861, 3863–3864, 3888
Malignant histiocytosis, *2413, 2414*, 2414–2415
Malignant melanoma, *2473*, 2473–2474, *2474, 2475, 2476*, 2476–2477, *2477, 2478, 2479*
Malignant meningiomas, 2028
Malignant optic gliomas, 1957, *1958, 1959*
Malignant peripheral nerve sheath tumors, 2316–2318, *2317, 2318*
Malignant phenylalanemia, 2812
Malignant teratoid medulloepithelioma, 691
Malignant tumors of paranasal sinuses, 2450–2453, *2451, 2452, 2453*
Malingering, 1766
Malnutrition and gastrointestinal mucormycosis, 4326–4327
Mamillothalamic tract, 834
Mandibular nerve, 1616, *1617*, 1618, *1618*
Mannan, 4343
Manual pointing, localization using, *393*, 393–394
Maple syrup urine disease, 2813–2814
Marburg virus, 5166
Marchi method, 121
Marcus Gunn phenomenon
 inverse, 1541, *1541*
 paradoxic eyelid retraction evoked by, 1553–1554, *1554*
Marcus Gunn pupil, 939
Marfan's syndrome, *2986*, 2987, *2987*
Marginal corneal ulceration, 3769
Marginal sinus, 848, *848*
Marginal zone, 3
 embryology of, 3–4, *4, 5*
Marie ataxia, 762
Maroteaux-Lamy (MPS VI), 2821, *2822*
Masseter reflex, 1658–1659
Masseter sign, 1681
Mast cells, 855
Mastoiditis, 1722
 as cause of brain abscess, 3945
Maternal insulin-dependent diabetes mellitus, 782
Matrix proteins, 4946
Maxillary nerve, 1616, *1616*
Maxillary sinus mucoceles, 4023, *4023, 4024*
Mean defect on Octopus perimeters, 180
Mean deviation on Humphrey Field Analyzer, 180
Measles, 5200
 clinical manifestations, 5201, *5201*
 complications, 5201, *5202*, 5203–5208, *5204, 5205, 5206, 5208, 5209, 5210*
 and development of viral encephalitis, 3986
 diagnosis, 5209–5210
 epidemiology, 5200
 in immunocompromised patients, 5207–5208, *5209*
 pathogenesis, 5208–5209
 prevention and complications of vaccination, 5210–5213, *5211, 5212, 5213*
 treatment, 5210
Measles inclusion body encephalitis (MIBE), 5213, 5418
Mechanical lid retraction, 1559, *1559*
Mechanical ptosis, 1546–1547
Meckel syndrome, 783
Meckel's cave, 2018
Media, otitis, 4035, 4085
Medial forebrain bundle, 832
Medial geniculate nucleus, 105
Medial inferior pontine syndrome, 3511
Medial longitudinal fasciculus (MLF), 16
Medial medullary syndrome, 3513
Medial midpontine syndrome, 3511
Medial pontine syndrome, 3506, 3509
Medial superior pontine syndrome, 3511
Medial superior temporal area (MST), 1120
Mediterranean Spotted Fever, *4748*, 4748–4751, *4749, 4750, 4751*
Medmont perimeter, 206
Medulla
 lesions of, *1678*, 1678–1680, *1679*
 ocular motor syndromes caused by lesions in, 1283–1285, *1284*
  of anterior inferior cerebellar artery, 1287, *1288*
  skew deviation and ocular tilt reaction, 1287–1289
  Wallenberg's, *1285*, 1285–1287, *1286, 1287*
 tumors of, 1878
Medullary hematopoiesis, 2330
Medullary hemorrhage, 3604
Medullary tractotomy of descending trigeminal root, *1679*, 1679–1680
Medullary veins, 2951
Medulloblastomas, 1293–1294, 1975, 1979–1984, *1981, 1982, 1983*
Medulloepithelioma, 1975, 1984–1985, *1985, 1986*
 malignant teratoid, 691
Megacolon, toxic, 4619
Megakaryocytes, 2329
Megalencephaly, 818
Megalopapilla, 790–791, *791*
Meibomian glands, 1510
Meige syndrome, 1565–1568
 cause of, 1566–1567
Melanin granules, 853, 855
Melanocytes of iris stroma, 853
Melanocytomas, *696*, 696–697, *697, 698*
Melanoma
 malignant, *2473*, 2473–2474, *2474, 2475, 2476*, 2476–2477, *2477, 2478, 2479*
 retinopathy associated with, 39, 219, 2473, 2537–2538, *2539*
Melanosis, neurocutaneous, 2735
MELAS syndrome, 2853–2856, *2854*
Melatonin, 1866–1867
Melphalan, 2564–2565
Membranous nephritis, 3818, *3819*
Memory, 1147
Memory-guided saccades, 1114
Meningeal angiomas, 2712, *2716*, 2716–2718
Meningeal arteries, 2911
Meningeal carcinomatosis, 700–701, 701, 2485–2488, *2486, 2487*, 3351
Meningeal disease, 5407, 5419
Meningeal hemorrhage, 2976
Meningeal leukemia, 2337–2338
Meningeal symptoms, 5495–5496, *5496*
Meningeal veins, 2954
Meninges, anatomy of
 arachnoid, 2018, *2020*, 2020–2021, *2021, 2022, 2023*
 dura mater, *2017*, 2017–2018, *2019*
 pia mater, 2021
Meningioma, 2023, 2660, 2987
 adjuvant therapy, 2031
 angioblastic, 2027–2028, *2028*
 arising from inner sphenoid ridge, 2059–2062, *2060, 2061*
 arising from middle third of sphenoid ridge, 2059, *2059*
 arising from outer sphenoid ridge and pterion, *2057*, 2057–2059, 2057–2062, *2058, 2059, 2061*
 associations, 2030
 cavernous sinus, 2031, *2032, 2033, 2034*, 2034–2036, *2035*
 cerebellopontine angle, 2052–2053
 of clivus, *2053*, 2053–2054
 convexity, *2036*, 2036–2037, *2038, 2039*
 cytogenetics, 2028–2029
 diagnostic neuroimaging, 2030–2031
 diaphragmatic, 2062

ectopic orbital, 2051
en plaque, 2057–2058
endocrinology, 2029–2030
and facial numbness, 1672
falx, 2037, *2039*, 2039–2041, *2040, 2042,* 2043
fibroblastic, 2027, *2028*
in foramen magnum, 2054–2055
of 4th ventricle, 2055
histogenesis, 2024
incidence, 2024–2026
incisural, 2055–2056
in lateral ventricle, 2065, *2065*, 2065–2066, *2066*
malignant, 2028, 2067
local, invasion of brain, 2067–2068
metastasis, 2068
middle cranial fossa, 2043
olfactory groove, 2043–2044, *2045*
optic nerve sheath, 2044–2045, 3424–3425
orbital, 2051
parasagittal, 2037, *2039*, 2039–2041, *2040, 2042,* 2043
pathology, *2025, 2026,* 2026–2028, *2027, 2028*
posterior fossa, 2051–2052
primary optic nerve sheath, 2046–2051, *2047, 2048, 2049,* 2050*t*
psammomatous, 2027
pterional, *2057*, 2057–2059, *2058*
secondary optic nerve sheath, 2051
sphenoid ridge, *2056*, 2056–2057, 2056–2062, *2057, 2058, 2059, 2061*
syncytial, *2026*, 2026–2027
tentorial, 2055–2056
of tentorium cerebelli, 2055–2056
in 3rd ventricle, *51*, 2065, *2065*, 2065–2066, *2066*, 2067, *2067*
transitional, 2027
treatment, 2031
tuberculum sellae, *2062*, 2062–2065, *2064*
Meningitis, 3805, 3821, 3990, 4394, *4395*, 4550. (*See also* Subacute meningitis; Chronic meningitis.)
Acetinobacter, 4104
acute bacterial, 3990, 4028–4029
clinical settings, 3994–3996
diagnosis, 4007–4010, *4008*
etiology, 3990, 3993–3994
meningitis, clinical manifestations, 4001, 4004–4007
pathology, 3998, *3999, 4000,* 4001, *4001, 4002, 4003, 4004, 4005*
pathophysiology, 3996–3998, *3997, 3998*
prognosis, 4011–4012
prophylaxis, 4012–4013
treatment, 4010–4011
acute nonbacterial, 4013–4015, *4014*
aseptic, 2561, 4983, 5053, 5111, 5130–5131, 5146–5147, 5156, 5237–5238, 5241–5242, 5245, 5261
acute, 5387, *5388, 5389*
OKT3 as cause of, 2628–2629
Aspergillus, 4305, 4308–4309, *4313, 4314*
Bacillus, 4108–4109
Bacillus anthracis, 4106
bacterial, 3946, 4069–4070, *4070, 4071, 4076,* 4076–4077, *4077,* 5419–5421, *5420*
acute, 5018–5019
benign recurrent, 5721
blastomycotic, 4337–4338, *4338*
Branhamella catarrhalis, 4103
Brucella species in, 4213–4214
Candida, 4349, 4351
carcinomatous, 701, 2485–2488, *2486, 2487*
caused by *Arcanobacterium haemolyticum,* 4105
caused by *Serratia marcescens,* 4224
chemical, 2339
chronic basal, 3339
of chronic disseminated histoplasmosis, 4397–4398
coccidioidal, 4360, *4361*
Coccidioides immitis (Coccidioidomycosis), 4355, 4364
cryptococcal, 4371, 4374, 4387
enterococcal, 4091
eosinophilic, *4498,* 4498–4499, *4499,* 4503, *4505*
fungal, 5421–5423
gonococcal, 4102–4103
Group A streptococcal, 4086
Group R streptococcal, 4089–4090
group R streptococcal, 4089–4090
Haemophilus influenzae, 4233–4234, *4235*
headaches in, 1716
helminthic, 5423
Kingella kingae, 4103–4104
leptomeningitis, 3990
Listeria, 4131
and Lyme disease, *4790,* 4790–4791
lymphomatous, 5424
meningococcal, 4077, 4094–4100, *4095, 4096, 4097, 4098, 4099, 4100*
Mollaret's, 4982, 5721
mucormycosis in, 4329
neonatal, 4087, 4219
papilledema in, 517–518
carcinomatous lymphomatous, and leukemic, 518
Pasteurella in, 4240
persistent neutrophilic, 4016
plague, 4227–4228
pneumococcal, 4077–4079, *4078, 4079, 4080*
postpartum maternal, 4087
primary anthrax, 4106
Pseudomonas aeruginosa, 4241–4242, *4242*
Salmonella, 4222–4223, *4223*
sarcoid, 5495–5496, *5496*
syphilitic, 636, 5423–5424
tuberculous, 4145, *4148,* 4148–4149, *4149, 4150,* 4151, *4151, 4152, 4153,* 4153–4154, *4154,* 4154–4157, *4155, 4156*
viral, 5424
Meningitis belt, 4094, *4095*
Meningoceles, 3947
Meningococcal disease, 4094
Meningococcal meningitis, 4077, 4094–4100, *4095, 4096, 4097, 4098, 4099, 4100*
Meningococcal meningoencephalitis, 4100
Meningococcemia, 4098
Meningoencephalitis, 1871, 3805, 4087, 4123–4124, 4213, 4369, 4550, 4621, 4686, 4705, 4707, 4891–4892, 5197, 5231, 5248, 5261, 5290, 5416
acute aseptic, 5387, *5388, 5389*
bacterial, 4029
central nervous system (CNS) eosinophilic, 4503, *4505*
chronic, 5240, 5243
cytomegalovirus-associated acute, 5104
eosinophilic, 4503, *4505*
Fusarium oxysporum in, *4389*
Haemophilus influenzae in, 4234
Listeria monocytogenes in, 4132–4133
meningococcal, 4100
primary amoebic, 4623, *4625,* 4625–4626, *4626, 4627, 4628, 4629*
varicella, 5017–5018
Meningohypophyseal trunk, 2873
Meningoradiculitis and peripheral neuropathy, 4794–4795
Meningovascular neurosyphilis, 4883–4884, *4884, 4885,* 4886–4889
Menkes' kinky hair syndrome, 3352
Menstrual cycle, effect of, on corneal sensation, 1664
Mental retardation
in patients with neurofibromatosis type 1, 2661
in patients with Sturge-Weber syndrome, 2717
in patients with tuberous sclerosis, 2684
Mercury intoxication and multiple sclerosis, 5544
MERFF syndrome, 2853
Merlin, 2666
Merozoites, 4644
Mesangial cells, 2403–2404
Mesangial nephritis, 3818
Mesencephalic hemorrhage, *3598,* 3598–3601, *3599, 3600, 3601, 3602*
Mesencephalic lesions, 993–994, *994*
Mesencephalic nucleus of trigeminal nerve, 1628–1629
Mesencephalic parasympathetic outflow pathway, 860
Mesencephalon, 1681–1682, *1683*
neurologic disorders that primarily affect
progressive supranuclear palsy, 1313–1314
Whipple's disease, 1314–1315
ocular motor syndromes caused by lesions of, 1304
interstitial nucleus of Cajal, 1308, 1310
neurologic disorders, 1311, 1313
other sites and manifestations, 1310–1311
periaqueductal gray matter, 1308
posterior commissure, 1304*t*, 1304–1305, *1306,* 1306*t*, 1307, *1307, 1308*
rostral interstitial nucleus of medial longitudinal fasciculus, 1307–1308, *1309, 1310, 1311, 1312, 1313*
tumors of, 1873–1874, *1874*
Mesenchymal chondrosarcomas, 2068
Mesenteric vasculitis, 3819
Mesulergine, 2192
Metabolic acidosis, 671, 673
Metabolic ataxias, 2785–2786, *2786*
Metabolic disorders
amino acid
Lowe syndrome, 2814–2815
maple syrup urine disease, 2813–2814
phenylalaninemia
dihydropteridine reductase defect, 2812
phenylalanine hydroxylase deficiency, 2811–2812
tyrosinemia, 2812–2813, *2813*
coma in, 998
headaches associated with, 1720–1721
lipid
metachromatic leukodystrophy, 2837–2840, *2838, 2839, 2840*

Metabolic disorders—*continued*
Refsum disease, 2840–2841
lysosomal storage diseases
mucolipidoses, 2823–2824
mucopolysaccharidoses, 2815, 2816*t*
Hunter syndrome, 2819–2820
Hurler syndrome, *2816,* 2816–2819, *2817, 2818*
Hurler-Scheie compound, 2819
Maroteaux-Lamy, 2821, *2822*
Morquio syndrome, 2820–2821
Sanfilippo syndrome, 2820, *2820, 2821*
Scheie syndrome, 2818–2819, *2819*
Sly syndrome, 2821–2822
sialidoses, 2822
sphingolipidoses
Fabry disease, 2831–2832, *2832, 2833*
Farber disease, 2830–2831, *2831*
gangliosidoses, 2824–2828, *2825, 2826, 2828*
Gaucher disease, 2828–2830, *2829, 2830*
Niemann-Pick disease, 2832–2837, *2834, 2835, 2836, 2837*
mitochondria, 2853
MELAS syndrome, 2853–2856, *2854*
MERFF syndrome, 2853
neuronal ceroid lipofuscinoses, 2848–2850, *2849, 2850, 2851*
infantile, 2850
juvenile, 2851
late infantile, 2851, *2852*
ocular motor manifestations of, 1330–1331, 1333
peroxisomes, 2841*t,* 2841–2842
hyperoxaluria type 1, 2848
infantile Refsum disease, 2843–2844
neonatal adrenoleukodystrophy, 2843, *2844*
Rhizomelic chondrodysplasia punctata, 2844–2845
X-linked adrenoleukodystrophy, 2845–2847, *2846, 2847, 2848*
Zellweger cerebrohepatorenal syndrome, *2842,* 2842–2843
Zellweger-like disease, 2844
serum lipoproteins, abetalipoproteinemia, 2851–2852
Metabolic encephalopathy, 2631
in Lyme disease, 4814–4816
Metabolism and cerebral blood flow, 2969–2970
Metacercariae, 4479
Metachromatic leukodystrophy (MLD), 765, 2837–2840, *2838, 2839, 2840*
Metacyclic trypomastigotes, 4711
Metamorphopsia, 154, 468–469, 1842, 3673
cerebral, 469
Metaplasia, postpolycythemic myeloid, 2333
Metastatic abscesses, 3948–3950, *3949, 3950, 3951*
Metastatic tumors, 698–700, *699, 700,* 2477
bone, 2477, *2480*
meningeal carcinomatosis, 2485–2488, *2486, 2487*
parenchymal, 2477, 2479, *2479, 2480, 2481, 2482, 2483,* 2483–2484, *2484, 2485, 2486*
Methanol poisoning, 665
Methemoglobinemia and headaches, 1718
Methotrexate, 2554–2558, *2556, 2557, 2558*
neuro-ophthalmologic toxicity, 2557–2558, *2558*
5-fluorouracil, 2558–2560
neurotoxicity, 2554–2555, *2556*
ocular toxicity, 2555–2557, *2557*
systemic toxicity, 2554
Methylprednisolone
for multiple sclerosis, 5629
for optic nerve injury, 729–730
for optic neuritis, 610
Meyer-Archambault loop, 121, *122,* 122–123, 123
Meyer's loop, 121, *122,* 123
Miconazole for coccidioidomycosis, 4365
Microabscesses, 4068
Microaerophilic bacteria, 4066
Microangiopathy
of brain, retina, and inner ear, *3732,* 3732–3734, *3733*
of brain and retina, 3344, *3347*
retinal, 5424–5426, *5426*
Micrococci, 4091–4092, *4092*
Micrococcus kristinae, 4092
Micrococcus luteus, 4092, *4092*
Micrococcus varians, 4092
Microfilaria, 4503
Microglia, 44, 5366
Microglial cells, 2404
Microglial nodule, 5182, *5183*
Microphthalmia, 5292, *5296*
Micropsia, 154, 467–468, 947, 3673
cerebral, 468, *468*67–468
convergence-accomodative, 467–468
Microsaccades, 1105, 1136
Microscopic appearance
of hypoxic brain, 3325, *3326*
of infarcted region, 3327, *3327*
Microscopic polyangiitis, 3750
Microsomia, hemifacial, 1564
Microsporidia, 4646–4647, *4647, 4648, 4649,* 4649–4650
Microtia, 1564
Microtremor, 1136
Microtubule-associated protein (MAPZ), 1920
Microvascular decompression of trigeminal nerve, 1739–1740
Micturition, disturbances of, 5573
Midbrain corectopia, 996
Midbrain disease, poorly reacting pupils from, 990
Middle cerebral artery, 2898–2899, *2900, 2901, 2902, 2903*
aneurysm arising from, 3095, 3097, *3097, 3098, 3099,* 3099–3100, *3100*
Middle cervical ganglion, 838
Middle cranial fossa meningiomas, 2043
Middle ear infection as cause of brain abscess, 3945
Middle meningeal artery, 2945
Middle temporal area, 1120
Migraine aura without headache, 3678–3680, *3679, 3680*
Migraine cervicale, 1723
Migraine headaches, 1693–1695
abortive treatment of, 3710–3711
with aura, 3658, 3664, 3664*t*
aura, 3664
neurologic, 3675–3677
pupillary signs, 3675, *3676*
visual, *3665,* 3665–3675, *3666, 3667, 3668, 3669, 3672, 3673, 3674*
headache, 3677–3678
without aura, 3658, 3662–3664, *3663,* 3663*t*
with aura and permanent visual or neurologic deficit, 3691
permanent diplopia, 3694
permanent neurologic deficits, *3695,* 3695–3696, *3696, 3697*
permanent visual deficits, 3691–3694, *3692, 3693, 3694*
tonic pupil from ischemia of ciliary ganglion or short posterior ciliary nerves, 3694–3695
cardiac, 3699
childhood, 3696–3697
acute confusional, 3698–3699
Alice in Wonderland syndrome, 3697
alternating hemiplegia of, 3699
benign paroxysmal torticollis, 3698
benign paroxysmal vertigo, 3697–3698
cyclic vomiting, 3698
motion sickness in, 3697
somnambulism, 3698
demographics, *3659,* 3659–3660
and disc drusen, 818
effort, 1704
examination of patient, 3707
diagnostic tests, 3707–3709, *3708, 3709*
differential diagnosis, 3707
exertion, 1704
historical review, 3657–3658
innervation of cerebral blood vessels and implications for pathogenesis, 1610, 1613
ophthalmoplegic, 3681–3687, *3682, 3683, 3687*
overlap of icepick headaches and, 1701
pathogenesis, vasogenic theory of, 3701–3703
and photophobia, 3663
predisposing factors, 3660–3662
prodromal symptoms, 3660, 3660*t*
with prolonged aura
basilar artery, 3681
familial hemiplegic, 3678
without headache, 3678–3680, *3679, 3680*
relationship between cluster headache, episodic paroxysmal hemicrania and, 3699–3701
relationship between seizures and, 3701
retinal, 3687–3691, *3688, 3689, 3690*
role of serotonin in, 3705
role of trigeminal nerve in pathogenesis of, 3704–3705, *3705*
in supratentorial arteriovenous malformations, 2257–2258
termination and postdrome, 3660
terminology, 3658*t,* 3658–3659
theory of spreading depression, 3703–3706
transformed, 1752, 3699
treatment
digital temple massage, 3710
management of stress, 3710
medical therapy, 3710–3713
modification of predisposing factors, 3709–3710
unifying theory of, 3705–3706, *3706*
and vasospasm, 3336–3339, *3338*
and vasospastic diseases as causes of decreased cerebral perfusion, 3413
Migrainous hallucinations, 463–464, *464, 465,* 466, *466*
Miliary tuberculosis, 4144, 4145
Millard-Gubler syndrome, 1250, *1251,* 1562, 1874–1875

Miller Fisher syndrome, 5088, 5678, 5695
clinical manifestations, 5696, *5697, 5698,* 5699, *5699, 5700,* 5701
diagnosis, 5702
epidemiology, *5695,* 5695–5696, *5696*
laboratory studies, 5701
neuroimaging studies, 5701–5702
ophthalmoplegia in patients with, 5696
and Q fever, 4769
site of lesion, 5702–5703
treatment and prognosis, 5702
Miller Fisher variant of Guillain-Barré syndrome, 4119
Minimum angle of resolution (MAR), 160
Miosis, 948–949, 964
congenital, 1008–1009
testing, 952
Mirror test, 1768
Misonidazole, 2593
Misplaced pupils, 1008
Mithramycin, 2580
Mitochondria disorders, 2853
MELAS syndrome, 2853–2856, *2854*
MERFF syndrome, 2853
Mitochondrial encephalomyopathies. (*See* Mitochondrial myopathies.)
Mitochondrial encephalopathy, lactic acidosis, and stroke-like episodes (MELAS), 366, 767
Mitochondrial genome, 1388–1389
Mitochondrial myopathies
background of, 1378–1379, *1379*
disorders associated with external ophthalmoplegia
chronic progressive, 1379, 1381, *1381, 1382*
Kearns-Sayre syndrome (KSS), 1381, *1383,* 1383–1385, *1384, 1385, 1386, 1387,* 1387–1388
diagnosis of, in patients with ophthalmoplegia, 1390
genome, 1388–1389
multiple deletions of mtDNA in autosomal-dominant and autosomal-recessive ophthalmoplegia, 1390
point mutations of, tRNAs in maternally inherited ophthalmoplegia, 1389
single deletions of mtDNA in sporadic ophthalmoplegia, 1389–1390
Mitochondrially-inherited optic neuropathies, 666
Mitomycins
ocular toxicity, 2580
systemic toxicity, 2580
Mitotane, 2583–2584
neuro-ophthalmologic toxicity, 2584
neurotoxicity, 2584
ocular toxicity, 2584
systemic toxicity, 2584
Mitral valve annulus, calcification of, 3390
Mitral valve prolapse, 3390–3391
and risk of stroke, 3569
Mitral valve vegetations, 3391–3392
Mixed bulbospinal paralytic poliomyelitis, 5256
Mixed connective tissue disease, 3829–3830, 3835
Mixed cryoglobulinemia, 3783–3786, *3785*
Mixed endophytic-exophytic retinoblastomas, 1994
MNGIE syndrome, 1390
Möbius syndrome, 1238–1240, *1239*
Modified direct agglutination test in diagnosing toxoplasmosis, 4692
Moebius syndrome, 1564
Molds, 4281–4282, *4282*
Aspergillus, 4286–4287, *4287*
clinical manifestations, 4287
allergic, 4287–4290, *4288, 4289, 4290*
aspergillomas, 4290–4294, *4291, 4292, 4293*
invasive aspergillosis, 4294–4299, *4295, 4296, 4297, 4298, 4299, 4300, 4301,* 4301–4306, *4302, 4303, 4304, 4305, 4306, 4307, 4308,* 4308–4310, *4309, 4310, 4311,* 4312, *4312, 4313, 4314, 4315, 4316,* 4316–4317
treatment, 4317
mucorales
appearance, 4318, *4318*
clinical manifestations
central nervous system mucormycosis, *4320,* 4327–4329, *4328, 4329, 4330*
cutaneous mucormycosis, 4325–4326
diagnosis, 4330–4331, *4331*
gastrointestinal mucormycosis, 4326–4327
other forms of mucormycosis of neuro-ophthalmologic interest, 4329
pulmonary mucormycosis, 4319
rhinocerebral mucormycosis, 4319–4322, *4321, 4322, 4323, 4324,* 4324–4325, *4325, 4326, 4327*
epidemiology, 4318–4319
nomenclature, 4317–4318
pathology, 4319, *4320*
pathophysiology, 4319
prognosis, 4332
treatment, 4331–4332
Molecular biology, 1920
Molecular genetic techniques, 5380
Mollaret's meningitis, 4013, 4982, 5721
Molluscum fibrosum pendulum, 2675, *2676*
Mollusks, 4494
Monobasic amino acid antibiotics, 1442
Monocular blindness, 2257
Monocular bobbing movements, 1328–1329
Monocular diplopia, 1169–1170, 1777, 3673, 3694
Monocular downbeat nystagmus, 3501
Monocular paresis of elevation, 3497, 3499, *3499*
Monocular visual loss, 3337–3338
Monomelic motor neuron disease, 2799
Mononuclear phagocytic system, 2329
Mononuclear-phagocytic system. (*See* Histiocytoses.)
Mononucleosis, infectious
complications, 5084–5091, *5085, 5086, 5088, 5089, 5090,* 5091
symptoms and signs of, 5083–5084
Monoplegia, flaccid, 5246
Monosodium glutamate (MSG) and headaches, 1718
Monosporium apiospermum in encephalitis, 3987
Monosymptomatic hereditary optic neuropathies
apparent sex-linked atrophy, 758
congenital recessive, 758
dominant atrophy, 755–758, *757*
Leber's, 744–755
Mooney's Closure Faces Test, 471
Moraxella, 4103
Branhamella catarrhalis, 4103
species, 4103
Morbidity and Mortality Weekly Report, 3988
Morbilliviruses
characteristics of, 5200
clinical manifestations, 5201, *5201*
complications, 5201, *5202,* 5203–5208, *5204, 5205, 5206, 5208, 5209, 5210*
diagnosis, 5209–5210
equine, 5200
measles, 5200
epidemiology, 5200
pathogenesis, 5208–5209
prevention and complication of vaccination, 5210–5213, *5211, 5212, 5213*
treatment, 5210
Morning glory disc anomaly, *785,* 785–788, *786, 787*
Morquio syndrome (MPS IV), 2820–2821
Mortierellaceae, 4318
Morulae, 4765
Mother yaw, 4847
Motion and displacement perimetry, 207–208, *208*
Motion perception, 394–395, *397*
deficits with unilateral cerebral lesions, 438–439, *440, 441, 442*
disorders of. (*See* Akinetopsia.)
Motion processing and area V5, 143–145
Motion sickness in migraine, 3697
Motion-sensitive cells, 130–131
Motor function, tests of, 1652–1653
Motor learning, 1147
Motor neuron disease, 2796, 2796*t*. (*See also* Amyotrophic lateral sclerosis.)
diagnosis, 2800
epidemiology, 2796
etiology, 2796–2797
laboratory and neuroimaging findings, 2800
neurologic manifestations, 2797–2799
neuro-ophthalmologic manifestations, 2799–2800
pathology, 2797, *2797*
prognosis, 2800
treatment, 2800
Motor nucleus of trigeminal nerve, 1618
Motor paralysis, 5245
Motor syndromes, 2627
Mountain ash leaf spots, 2671, *2672, 2673, 2674*
Moyamoya disease, 2609, *2610,* 2978, 3012, *3013,* 3348–3349, *3350*
MPTP-induced parkinsonism, 1568
MTX and radiation therapy, 2596
Mucoceles, 4017
clinical manifestations, 4017, *4019,* 4019–4023, *4020, 4021, 4022, 4023, 4024*
diagnosis, 4024–4025
general features, 4017, *4018*
prognosis, 4025
treatment, 4025
Mucocutaneous candidiasis, 4345–4346, *4347*
Mucocutaneous lesions, 3854–3855
Mucolipidoses, 2823–2824
Mucolipidosis I, 2822–2823

Mucopolysaccharidoses, 764, 2815, 2816*t*
  Hunter syndrome, 2819–2820
  Hurler syndrome, *2816*, 2816–2819, *2817*, *2818*
  Hurler-Scheie compound, 2819
  Maroteaux-Lamy, 2821, *2822*
  Morquio syndrome, 2820–2821
  papilledema in, 519–520
  Sanfilippo syndrome, 2820, *2820*, *2821*
  Scheie syndrome, 2818–2819, *2819*
  Sly syndrome, 2821–2822
Mucor, 4318
Mucoraceae, 4318
Mucorales
  appearance, 4318, *4318*
  clinical manifestations
    central nervous system mucormycosis, *4320*, 4327–4329, *4328*, *4329*, *4330*
    cutaneous mucormycosis, 4325–4326
    diagnosis, 4330–4331, *4331*
    gastrointestinal mucormycosis, 4326–4327
    other forms of mucormycosis of neuro-ophthalmologic interest, 4329
    pulmonary mucormycosis, 4319
    rhinocerebral mucormycosis, 4319–4322, *4321*, *4322*, *4323*, *4324*, 4324–4325, *4325*, *4326*, *4327*
  epidemiology, 4318–4319
  nomenclature, 4317–4318
  pathology, 4319, *4320*
  pathophysiology, 4319
  prognosis, 4332
  treatment, 4331–4332
Mucormycosis, 4281, 4282
  appearance, 4318, *4318*
  clinical manifestations
    central nervous system mucormycosis, *4320*, 4327–4329, *4328*, *4329*, *4330*
    cutaneous mucormycosis, 4325–4326
    diagnosis, 4330–4331, *4331*
    gastrointestinal mucormycosis, 4326–4327
    other forms of mucormycosis of neuro-ophthalmologic interest, 4329
    pulmonary mucormycosis, 4319
    rhinocerebral mucormycosis, 4319–4322, *4321*, *4322*, *4323*, *4324*, 4324–4325, *4325*, *4326*, *4327*
  epidemiology, 4318–4319
  gastrointestinal, 4326–4327
    and malnutrition, 4326–4327
  nomenclature, 4317–4318
  pathology, 4319, *4320*
  pathophysiology, 4319
  prognosis, 4332
  treatment, 4331–4332
Müller cells, *38*, 43–44, *44*
Müller's muscle, 1509, 1512
Multibacillary disease, 4169
Multiceps multiceps, 4440
Multicore disease, 1357, *1358*
Multifocal chorioretinitis, *4866*, 4866–4867, *4867*
Multifocal choroiditis, 4380–4381
Multifocal encephalomyelitis, 5246
Multifocal ERG mapping techniques (topographical ERG), 223, *223*
Multifocal leukoencephalitis, 5064, 5067–5068
Multifocal leukoencephalopathy, 2631
Multilingual Aphasia Examination, 436
Multiple aneurysms, 3016–3018, *3019*
Multiple deletions of mtDNA in autosomal-dominant and autosomal-recessive ophthalmoplegia, 1390
Multiple endocrine adenomatosis syndrome (MEA type I), 2159
Multiple endocrine neoplasia, 2459*t*, 2459–2460, 2989
Multiple myeloma, 703, 2389, *2389*
  etiology, 2389–2390
  familial, 2390
  general considerations, 2389
  general features, 2390
  heavy chain disease, 2401
  macroglobulinemia-associated generalized (systemic) amyloidosis, *2402*, 2403
  neurologic complications, 2390–2392
  ocular involvement in, 2396–2398, *2397*, *2398*
  ocular motor dysfunction, *67*, 2394–2396
  orbital involvement, 2396, *2396*
  papilledema and, 520–521
  plasma-cell granulomas, 2398
  POEMS syndrome (Crow-Fukase syndrome), 2399
  primary generalized (systemic) amyloidosis, 2401–2403, *2402*
  treatment and prognosis, 2398
  visual complications, 2392–2393
  visual sensory dysfunction, *2393*, 2393–2394, *2394*
  Waldenström's macroglobulinemia, 2399–2400, *2400*
Multiple sclerosis, 529, 2664, 5540, *5541*
  associations, 5544
  clinical manifestations, 5567–5568
    asymptomatic involvement of ocular motor system, 5612–5613, *5613*
    combined supranuclear, internuclear, nuclear lesions, and infranuclear lesions, 5609, *5609*, *5610*, 5610–5612, 5611, *5612*, *5613*
    disorders of fixation, 5599, *5602*, 5602–5603
    disorders of ocular motility and alignment, 5603
    infranuclear lesions (ocular motor nerve pareses), 5605–5606, *5607*, *5608*, 5608–5609, *5609*
    internuclear lesions, 5603–5605, *5604*, *5605*, *5606*
    neurologic, 5568–5571, *5569*, *5570*, *5571*, *5572*, *5573*, 5573–5574, *5574*
    neuro-ophthalmologic, 5575
    nuclear lesions, 5603
    psychiatric, 5574–5575
    pupillary disturbances, 5613–5614
    supranuclear lesions, 5603, *5604*
    visual sensory, 5575
  clinically definite, 5627
  clinically probable, 5627
  diagnosis, 5627–5628
  epidemiology, 5540, 5542–5544
  laboratory and neuroimaging findings
    analysis of cerebrospinal fluid, 5614–5616, *5615*
    computer tomography (CT) scanning, *5616*, 5616–5617, *5617*
    magnetic resonance imaging (MRI), 5617–5619, *5618*, *5619*, *5620*, *5621*, *5622*, *5623*, 5623–5624, *5624*
    measurement of evoked potentials, *5625*, 5625–5627
    neuroimaging, 5616
    positron emission tomography, 5616
    proton magnetic resonance spectroscopy, 5624
  laboratory-supported definite, 5627
  laboratory-supported probable, 5627
  and neuroretinitis, 637
  and ocular motor dysfunction, 1330
  and optic neuritis, 615–616
  pathogenesis, 5562–5566, *5564*
  pathology, 5545, *5545*, *5546*, 5547, *5547*, *5548*, *5549*, 5549–5550, *5550*, *5551*, 5552, *5552*, *5553*, *5554*, 5555, *5555*, *5556*, *5557*, *5558*, *5559*, *5560*, *5561*, 5562, *5562*, *5563*
  pathophysiology, 5566–5567, *5567*
  prevention, 5631
  prognosis, 5631–5632
  relationship of optic neuritis to, 617–620
  remyelination in, 3981
  treatment, 5628–5631
Multiple system atrophy (MSA), 2771, 2776, 2776*t*
  epidemiology, 2776
  laboratory and neuroimaging findings, *2778*, 2778–2779
  neurologic manifestations, 2776–2778, 2777*t*
  neuro-ophthalmologic manifestations, 2778
  pathology, 2776, *2777*
  prognosis, 2779
  treatment, 2779
Multiple unilateral and bilateral cranial neuropathies, 3199, 3201
Mumps and development of viral encephalitis, 3986
Mumps encephalitis, 5228–5229
Mumps virus (mumps), 5223
  characteristics of, 5223, *5225*
  clinical manifestations of, 5225, *5226*
  complications of, 5225–5229, *5227*
  diagnosis of, 5229–5230
  epidemiology of, 5223, 5225
  pathogenesis of, 5225
  prevention, 5231
  prognosis of, 5230–5231
  treatment of, 5230
Münchausen syndrome, 1766
Mural thinning, *2979*, 2980
Mural thrombus, 3207
Murray Valley encephalitis, 5175–5176, *5177*, *5178*, 5178–5179, *5179*
  clinical manifestations, 5175–5176
  diagnosis, 5178–5179
  epidemiology, 5175
  pathology, 5176, 5178, *5178*, *5179*, *5180*
  prevention, 5179
  prognosis, 5179
  treatment, 5179
Muscle enlargement, from increased orbital venous pressure, 1398, *1400*, *1401*
Muscle relaxants, 1004–1005
Muscle-eye-brain disease, 1361–1362
Muscular dystrophies, 1360–1361
  congenital, 1361
    Fukuyama, 1361
    muscle-eye-brain disease, 1361–1362
    nosologic relations of, 1362
    Walker-Warburg syndrome, 1362
  myotonic
    clinical manifestations, 1363
      bone involvement, 1364
      cardiac involvement, 1363
      cognition and personality, 1363–1364
      endocrine involvement, 1364
      gastrointestinal tract and smooth muscle involvement, 1364

ocular involvement, *1363,* 1364, *1364, 1365, 1366,* 1366–1367, *1367, 1368,* 1369
respiratory system involvement, 1363
skeletal muscle involvement, 1363, *1363*
diagnosis and treatment, 1370–1371
genetics, 1362
pathology
muscle, *1368,* 1369
ocular, *1369,* 1369–1370, *1370, 1371, 1372*
pathophysiology, 1370
oculopharyngeal dystrophy, 1372–1374, *1373, 1374, 1375,* 1376
proximal myotonic myopathy (PROMM), 1371–1372
Musculoskeletal coccidioidomycosis, 4359, *4359*
Mutation
germinal, 1990
somatic, 1990
Myasthenia
focal, 1424
ocular, 1424
Myasthenia gravis, 999, 1013, 1408, 2629–2630
acquired disorders of neuromuscular transmission other than, 1434–1444, *1435, 1439*
clinical-pathophysiologic correlations, 1408–1409
crisis, 1431
diagnostic testing, *1418,* 1418–1424, *1419, 1421, 1422, 1423*
disorders associated with, 1424
etiology and pathogenesis, 1408, *1409*
natural history, 1410
neonatal, 1431
pediatric, 1431
prognosis, 1430–1431
role of T-lymphocytes and thymus, 1409–1410
symptoms and signs, *1410,* 1410–1418, *1411, 1412, 1413, 1414, 1415, 1416, 1417*
treatment, 1424–1430
Myasthenic crisis, 1431
Myasthenic ptosis, 1546, *1546, 1547, 1548, 1549*
Mycelium, 4281
Mycetoma, 4412
Mycobacteria, 4136
atypical, 4176–4177
Nocardia, 4189, 4189–4192, *4190, 4191*
Tropheryma whippelii, 4180–4189, *4182, 4183, 4184, 4185, 4186, 4187, 4188*
Mycobacterium bovis, 4167–4168
Mycobacterium leprae, 4168–4176, *4169, 4170, 4171, 4172, 4174, 4175*
Mycobacterium tuberculosis, 4136, 4136–4167, *4137, 4138, 4139, 4140, 4141, 4142, 4143, 4144, 4145, 4146, 4147, 4148, 4149, 4150, 4151, 4152, 4153, 4154, 4155, 4156, 4157, 4158, 4159, 4160, 4161, 4162, 4163, 4164, 4165, 4166, 4167, 4168*
Mycobacterium avium, 4176
Mycobacterium avium intracellulare in mycotic aneurysms, 3005
Mycobacterium bovis, 4167–4168
in intracranial brain abscess, 3951–3952
Mycobacterium chelonae, 4176
Mycobacterium fortuitum, 4177, *4177*
Mycobacterium gordonae, 4176
Mycobacterium kansasii, 4177, *4177*
Mycobacterium leprae, 4168–4176, *4169, 4170, 4171, 4172, 4174, 4175*
in granuloma, 3990
in neuritis, 4026
Mycobacterium tuberculosis, 4136, 4136–4167, *4137, 4138, 4139, 4140, 4141, 4142, 4143, 4144, 4145, 4146, 4147, 4148, 4149, 4150, 4151, 4152, 4153, 4154, 4155, 4156, 4157, 4158, 4159, 4160, 4161, 4162, 4163, 4164, 4165, 4166, 4167, 4168*
in chronic basal meningitis, 4030
in granuloma, 3990
in intracranial brain abscess, 3951
pathogenesis, 4137
pathology, 4137–4138
types, 4138–4145, *4143, 4144, 4145, 4146, 4147, 4148,* 4148–4149, *4149, 4150,* 4151, *4151, 4152, 4153,* 4153–4164, *4154, 4155, 4156, 4157, 4158, 4159, 4160, 4161, 4162, 4163, 4164, 4165, 4166,* 4166–4167
Mycoplasma fermentans, 4545
Mycoplasma gallisepticum, 3729
Mycoplasma genitalum, 4545
Mycoplasma hominis, 4554–4555
Mycoplasma penetrans, 4545
Mycoplasma pirum, 4545
Mycoplasma pneumoniae, 4546–4550, *4547, 4548, 4549, 4551,* 4552–4554, 5679
in bacterial encephalitis, 3986
Mycoplasmas, 4545, *4546*
human pathogens
Mycoplasma hominis, 4554–4555
Mycoplasma pneumoniae, 4546–4550, *4547, 4548, 4549, 4551,* 4552–4554
Ureaplasma urealyticum, 4555–4556
properties, 4545–4546
taxonomy, 4545
Mycosis cells, 2386
Mycosis fungoides, *2386,* 2386–2389, *2387, 2388*
Mycotic aneurysms, 2998, 3965, 4070–4071, 4073, *4090,* 4090–4091, 4304–4305, *4306, 4307*
bacterial, 2998–3003, *3000, 3001, 3002,* 3965–3969, *3966, 3968, 3969, 3970*
fungal, *3003,* 3003–3004, *3004,* 3971–3973, *3972, 3973*
miscellaneous, 3005, 3973
spirochetal (syphilitic), 3004–3005, 3973
Mydriasis
congenital, 1009
postoperative, 1011
pupillary, 2183, 3423
Myelin basic protein, 5615–5616
Myelinated (medullated) nerve fibers, 802–804, *803, 804,* 2658
Myelination, *20,* 21–22, *22*
of optic nerve, 76, *77*
Myelinoclastic diffuse sclerosis, 622, 5539
clinical manifestations, 5639
neurologic, 5639
neuro-ophthalmologic, 5639–5641
diagnosis, 5642
laboratory and neuroimaging findings, 5641–5642, *5643, 5644, 5645*
pathogenesis, 5639
pathology, 5639, *5640, 5641, 5642*
treatment and prognosis, 5642
Myelitis, 5019, 5197
herpes zoster, 5056–5057
and Lyme disease, 4791, *4792*
subacute, 2501
transverse, 4113, 5088, 5104, 5195, 5239–5240, 5243
Myeloblastomas, 2338–2339
Myelofibrosis, idiopathic, 2335–2336
Myeloid metaplasia with myelofibrosis, 2335–2336
Myeloid stem cells, 2329
Myeloma, multiple, 703. (*See also* Multiple myeloma.)
familial, 2390
papilledema and, 520–521
Myeloma/macroglobulinemia-associated generalized (systemic) amyloidosis, *2402,* 2403
Myelopathy, 674
early delayed radiation, 2604–2605, *2606*
human immunodeficiency virus-associated vacuolar, 5386
late delayed radiation, 2605–2606, *2607*
necrotizing, 622, *5632,* 5632–5633, *5633, 5634.* (*See also* Necrotizing myelopathy.)
schistosomal, 4488
transverse, 2555
Myelosuppression, 2564–2565
Myoblastoma, granular cell, 2321–2322
Myocardial granulomatous disease and sarcoidosis, 5483
Myocardial infarction, 3395–3396, *3398*
and risk of stroke, 3568–3569
Myocarditis, 3816, 4127, 4705, 5193, 5257
in immunocompetent patients, 5102–5103
Myoclonia, eyelid, 1570
Myoclonic epilepsy with ragged red fibers (MERRF), 767
Myoclonus, 1284, 5239
vertical, 1328
Myoid, 31
Myokymia
facial, 1571, *1572,* 5685
with peripheral neuropathy, 1571–1572
superior oblique, 1259–1261, 1491–1492, 1497
Myopathic complications, 5386–5387
Myopathic disease, insufficiency of eyelid closure caused by, 1565
Myopathic eyelid retraction and lid-lag, 1556–1559, *1557, 1558*
Myopathic origin, excessive eyelid closure of, 1576–1577, *1577*
Myopathic ptosis, *1545,* 1545–1546, *1546*
Myopathies. (*See also* Endocrine myopathies; Inflammatory myopathies; Ischemic myopathy; Mitochondrial myopathies; Ocular myopathy; Traumatic myopathies.)
acute necrotizing, 2530
cachectic, 2530–2531
central core, 1354
centronuclear, 1355, *1356, 1357*
congenital, 1359
cytoplasmic body, 1359
endocrine, 2531
corticosteroids and, 1405
Cushing's syndrome, 1404–1405
Graves' disease, 1399, *1402, 1403,* 1403–1404

Myopathies—*continued*
fingerprint body, 1358
in HIV-seropositive patients, 5387
inflammatory
idiopathic myositis, 1393, 1395, *1395*
infective myositis, 1392–1393, *1394*
ischemic, of extraocular muscles, 1405
myotubular, 1355, *1356, 1357*
necrotizing, ophthalmoplegia with acute, and carcinoma, 1397
nemaline, 1354–1355, *1355*
ocular
associated with celiac disease, 1405
toxic and drug-induced, 1406
proximal myotonic, 1371–1372
reducing body, 1358
resulting from errors in carbohydrate and lipid metabolism, 1405
rod, 1354–1355, *1355*
sarcotubular, 1359
traumatic, 1391–1392, *1392, 1393*
tubular aggregate, 1359
zebra body, 1359
Myopia
empty space, 910
night, 910
Myorhythmia, oculomasticatory, 1314–1315, 4185–4186
Myositis, 5193
amoebic, 4620
idiopathic
dermatomyositis, 1395, 1397
myositis limited to, 1393, 1395, *1395, 1396*
systemic, 1395, 1397
infective, 1392–1393, *1394*
in patients with Legionnaires' disease, 4237
Myotonia, 1362
chondrodystrophic, 1377
congenita, 1376
paramyotonia congenita, 1376
periodic paralysis, 1376–1377, *1377*
Schwartz-Jampel syndrome (chondrodystrophic myotonia), 1377
Myotonia congenita, 1376
Myotonia ion channel disorders, 1376
congenita, 1376
paramyotonia congenita, 1376
periodic paralysis, 1376–1377, *1377*
Schwartz-Jampel syndrome (chondrodystrophic myotonia), 1377
Myotonic cataracts, 1366
Myotonic muscular dystrophies, 1013
clinical manifestations, 1363
bone involvement, 1364
cardiac involvement, 1363
cognition and personality, 1363–1364
endocrine involvement, 1364
gastrointestinal tract and smooth muscle involvement, 1364
ocular involvement, *1363,* 1364, *1364, 1365, 1366,* 1366–1367, *1367, 1368,* 1369
respiratory system involvement, 1363
skeletal involvement, 1363, *1363*
diagnosis and treatment, 1370–1371
genetics, 1362
pathology
diagnosis and treatment, 1370–1371
muscle, *1368,* 1369
ocular, *1369,* 1369–1370, *1370, 1371, 1372*
pathophysiology, 1370
pathophysiology, 1370
Myotubular myopathy, 1355, *1356, 1357*
Myxoma, 3396, 3398, 3400, *3401*

N

N-acetylaspartic aciduria, 766
N-acetyl-*D*-galactosamine (Gal/GalNAc), 4616
Naegleria fowleri, 4623–4626, *4624, 4625, 4626, 4627,* 4628, *4628, 4629*
Naegleria in encephalitis, 3987
Nagel anomaloscope, 212, 407, *407*
Nalorphine, 1005
Naloxone hydrochloride, 1005
Naproxen for cough-induced headache, 1703
Nasociliary nerve, 1613, 1615
Nasopharyngeal carcinomas, 2444–2450, *2446, 2447, 2449, 2450*
Nausea, 3663
Nauta silver-degeneration technique, 133
Near response of pupil, 892–893
Neck, paragangliomas of, 2462–2464, *2463, 2464, 2465*
branchiomeric, 2464–2468, *2466, 2467, 2468, 2469, 2470,* 2470–2471
intravagal, 2471–2472, *2472*
Neck disease, headaches associated with, 1722–1723
Neck manipulation, dissection associated with, 2990, 2991*t*
Necrosis
bilateral retinal, 5091
complete spontaneous, with regression, 1994
progressive outer retinal, 5041, *5042,* 5426
radiation, 2599–2602, *2600, 2601, 2602, 2603,* 2604
treatment of, 52, 2602
Necrotic tissue, debridement of, for mucormycosis, 4331
Necrotizing encephalitis, 4686
Necrotizing microangiopathy and dystrophic calcification, 2611
Necrotizing myelopathy, 622, *5632,* 5632–5633, *5633, 5634*
clinical features, 2514
diagnostic evaluations, 2515
differential diagnosis, 2515
ophthalmoplegia with acute, and carcinoma, 1397
pathogenesis, 2515
pathology, 2514–2515
treatment and prognosis, 2515
Necrotizing pneumonia, 4346
Necrotizing retinitis, 4671, 5023
Nef, 5365
Negative phenomena, 454
Negishi encephalitis, 5189
Neglect dyslexia, 433
Negri bodies, 5269–5270
Neisseria, 4093, 4103
diagnosis, 4100
meningococcal meningitis, 4094–4100, *4095, 4096, 4097, 4098, 4099, 4100*
meningococcal meningoencephalitis, 4100
Neisseria meningitidis, 4093–4094
prophylaxis, 4101
treatment and prognosis, 4100–4101
Neisseria gonorrhoeae, 4101, 4101–4103, *4102*
in bacterial meningitis, 3994
in neuritis, 4026
Neisseria meningitidis, 3943, 4093–4094
in bacterial meningitis, 3993, 3994, 3995
in intracranial abscess, 3950
in septicemia, 4104
Neisseria mucosa in bacterial aneurysms, 2999
Nelson's syndrome, *2162,* 2162–2163
therapy of, 2198
Nemaline myopathy, 1354–1355, *1355*
Nematodes. (*See* Roundworms (nematodes).)
Neocortex and pupillary dilation, 883
Neonatal adrenoleukodystrophy, 2843, *2844*
Neonatal isoimmune thrombocytopenia, 783
Neonatal meningitis, 4087, 4219
Neonatal myasthenia gravis, 1431
Neopallium, 19
Neoplasia, multiple endocrine, 2459*t,* 2459–2460
Neoplasms of neuro-ophthalmologic interest, 2623–2624, *2624, 2625*
Neoplastic aneurysms, 3005–3007, *3006,* 3007, *3008*
Neoplastic angioendotheliosis, 3351
Neoplastic angiopathy, 3351
Neoplastic non-Langerhans cell histiocytoses, *2413, 2414,* 2414–2415
Nephritis
diffuse proliferative, 3817–3818
focal proliferative, 3817, *3817*
immune-mediated poststreptococcal, 4086
membranous, 3818, *3819*
mesangial, 3818
Nephrotic syndrome, 3889–3890
Nerve fiber layer, *50,* 50–51, *51, 52*
Nerve origin, 1571–1572
Nerves of ciliary body, 907
Nervous intermedius neuralgia, 1747
Nervous system toxicity, from radiation therapy, 2596
Nervus intermedius, lesions affecting, 1018–1019
Neural control of ocular motor systems, 1101–1158
abbreviations, 1102*t*
cerebellar control of saccades, 1120, *1121,* 1122–1123
cerebellum and control, 1153
regulation of saccadic amplitude and dysmetria, 1153
regulation of vestibulo-ocular reflex (VOR), 1153
stabilization of images on retina, 1153
fixation, 1156
general principles, 1136–1137
neurophysiology of, 1137
general considerations, 1101–1102
dimensions of eye motion, 1102–1103
phasic velocity and tonic position commands that affect ocular motility, 1103
optokinetic movements, 1157–1158
characteristics of, 1149–1151, *1150*
neurophysiology of, 1151–1153
saccades, 1154, *1155*
saccadic eye movement
basal ganglia, 1120
central midbrain reticular formation, 1120
cerebral control of, 1114
characteristics of, 1103–1107
frontal fields, 1114–1115, *1115, 1116, 1117*
neurophysiology of, 1109–1110
neurotransmitters for premotor neurons, 1114

parietal cortex, 1118–1120
prefrontal cortex, 1118, *1119*
processing of visual information for, 1108–1109, *1109*
quick phases of nystagmus, 1107, *1108*
during sleep, 1107–1108
superior colliculus, 1115–1118
supplementary field, 1118
thalamus, 1120
vision during, 1109
smooth pursuit
characteristics of, 1123–1125, *1124*
neurophysiology of eye movements, 1125–1134, *1126, 1127, 1133*
vergence eye movement, 1134, 1155
characteristics of, 1134
neurophysiology of, 1134–1136, *1135*
vestibulo-ocular reflex, 1156–1157
and eye-head coordination, 1138
cervico-ocular reflex, 1138
combined head and eye pursuit, 1139
reflex, 1139–1149, *1140, 1141, 1143, 1144, 1148*
vestibulo-collic reflex, 1138
Neural crest syndrome, 1027
Neural integration of saccadic pulse, 1113
Neural integrator, 1478
Neural tissue, ectopias of, 2130, *2130*
Neuralgia
atypical facial, *1741,* 1741–1743
facial (geniculate) ganglion, *1742,* 1743–1745, *1745*
glossopharyngeal, 1722, 1745–1747, *1746*
greater auricular, 1749
greater occipital, *1748,* 1748–1749
idiopathic trigeminal, 1750
nervous intermedius, 1747
occipital, 1747–1749, *1748, 1749*
postherpetic, 1729–1730, 5037, 5068, 5072
Raeder's paratrigeminal, 3040
superior laryngeal, 1747
trigeminal, 1735–1741, *1739, 1740,* 1796, 5569–5571, *5570*
vagoglossopharyngeal, 1746
Neuralgic amyotrophy, 5147
Neuritic plaques, 2749, *2749*
Neuritis, 4026, *4027,* 4028, *4028*
acute optic, 5581–5582, *5583, 5584,* 5584–5588, *5585, 5586*
anterior optic, 4872–4873, *4874, 4875,* 5197
asymptomatic optic, *5589,* 5589–5590, *5590*
bilateral optic, 5248
chronic optic, *5588,* 5588–5589
idiopathic perioptic, 709
optic, 264, *4212,* 4212–4213, 4516–4517, *4519,* 4769, 4907, 5229, 5432
acute, 987
asymptomatic demyelinating, 620–622, *621, 622*
autoimmune, 630
bacterial anterior, 4116
bilateral retrobulbar, 4552
chronic demyelinating, 620, *620*
in meningococcal meningitis, 4097
and Q fever, 4769
recurrent, 616, 619
retrobulbar, 599
visual loss from, 4151, 4153
perioptic, 599, 628, *638,* 639, 4872
postinfectious optic, 4967
retrobulbar, 599, 633, 2559–2560, 2576–2577, 4769
retrobulbar optic, 2393
Neuroacanthocytosis, 1319
Neuroblastoma, 1975, 1985–1990, *1987, 1988, 1989, 1991*
olfactory, 1989–1990, *1991*
peripheral, 1985–1988, *1987*
primary cerebral, *1988,* 1988–1989, *1989*
Neurocutaneous melanosis, 2735
Neurocysticercosis, 4462–4463, 5415
asymptomatic, 4463
intravenous, 4466–4467, *4467, 4468*
parenchymal, *4463,* 4463–4465
spinal, 4467, 4476
subarachnoid, *4464, 4465,* 4465–4466, *4466,* 4476
Neurocytomas, 1975
Neuroectodermal tumors, 1999
Neuroeffector junction, 841
Neurofibromas, 2319, *2320,* 2321, *2649,* 2649–2650
within orbit, 2655–2656
plexiform, 2319
visceral, 2661
Neurofibromatosis, 2024, 2300, 2647, 3352
cutaneous, 2664
segmental, 2664
type 1, 3353
association, 2664
cutaneous findings, *2648,* 2648–2650, *2650, 2651,* 2652
genetics, 2647–2648
management, 2665–2666
neuroimaging, *2662, 2663,* 2663–2664, *2664*
neurologic findings, 2659–2661, *2661*
occurrence, 2647, 2648*t*
ocular findings, *2650, 2651, 2652,* 2652–2656, *2653, 2654, 2655, 2656, 2657, 2658, 2659, 2660*
prognosis, 2665, 2665*t*, *2666*
visceral findings, 2661–2663
type 2, 2666
cutaneous findings, 2667
diagnosis and management, *2668,* 2668–2669
genetics, 2666
neurologic findings, *2667,* 2667–2668
ocular findings, 2667
Neurofibromin, 2648
Neurogenic ptosis, *1538,* 1538–1542, *1539, 1540, 1541, 1542, 1543*
Neuroglia
choroid plexus tumors, *1968,* 1968–1970, *1969*
colloid cysts of 3rd ventricle, 1970–1972, *1971*
tumors of, 1920
astrocytic, 1920, *1921*
astrocytomas, 1921–1922
histologic classification, 4–17, *5, 6, 7, 8, 9, 10, 11, 12, 13, 14, 15, 16, 17*
topographic classification, 17–39, *19, 20, 22, 23, 24, 25, 26, 27, 28, 30, 31, 34, 39, 40, 41*
ependymal
ependymomas, *1963,* 1963–1966, *1964, 1965*
subependymomas, 1966–1967, *1967*
oligodendroglia, 1958, *1960,* 1960–1963, *1961*
Neuroglial cells, 1919, 1920
Neurohypophyseal system, 2145–2146
Neurohypophysis, 2141
Neuroimaging
in diagnosing nasopharyngeal carcinoma, 2448
in imaging multiple sclerosis, 5616
Neurologic complications
of HIV-1 infection, 5385, *5386,* 5386*t*
myopathic complications, 5386–5387
peripheral nervous system, 5386–5387
primary intracranial, 5387–5395, *5388, 5389,* 5390*t*, *5391, 5392, 5393, 5394, 5395, 5396, 5397,* 5397–5399, *5398, 5399, 5400, 5401,* 5401–5407, *5402, 5403, 5404, 5405, 5406, 5407, 5408*
primary spinal cord, 5386–5387
of leukemia, 2337–2340, *2338, 2339*
of multiple myeloma, 2390–2392
Neurologic deficit, natural history of arteriovenous malformations presenting with, 2277
Neurologic deterioration syndrome, 2598, *2599*
Neurologic disease, accommodation insufficiency associated with focal or generalized, 1013–1015
Neurologic infections in bone marrow transplantation, 2630
Neurologic involvement in non-Hodgkin's lymphomas, 2380, *2380, 2381*
Neurologic malignancy in bone marrow transplantation, 2630–2631
Neurologic manifestations of ruptured intracranial aneurysms, 3021–3024, *3022, 3023*
Neuroma
acoustic, 1655, 2308
amputation, 1726
Neuromodulation, 841–842
Neuromuscular blockers, impact of, on postsynaptic neuromuscular transmission, 1440
Neuromuscular disorders
accommodation insufficiency associated with, 1013
drugs or toxins as cause of, 1437
insufficiency of eyelid closure caused by, 1564
Neuromuscular eyelid retraction and lid-lag, 1555–1556, *1556*
Neuromuscular junction
congenital and acquired disorders affecting
acetylcholine receptor, 1406, 1408
myasthenia gravis, 1408
clinical-pathophysiologic correlations, 1408–1409
crisis, 1431
diagnostic testing, *1418,* 1418–1424, *1419, 1421, 1422, 1423*
disorders associated with, 1424
etiology and pathogenesis, 1408, *1409*
natural history, 1410
neonatal, 1431
pediatric, 1431
prognosis, 1430–1431
role of T-lymphocytes and thymus, 1409–1410
symptoms and signs, *1410,* 1410–1418, *1411, 1412, 1413, 1414, 1415, 1416, 1417*
treatment, 1424–1430
normal transmission, 1406, *1407*
congenital myasthenic syndromes, 1431–1432
myasthenia gravis, acquired disorders of neuromuscular transmission other than, 1434–1444, *1435, 1439*
disturbances in disorders of, 999

Neuromuscular origin, excessive eyelid closure of, 1576, *1576*
Neuromuscular ptosis, 1546, *1546, 1547, 1548, 1549*
Neuromuscular transmission
  drugs that affect postsynaptic, 1440–1441
  toxins that damage both pre- and postsynaptic, 1443–1444
Neuromyelitis optica, 600, 622, 4164, 4166, 5275, 5539, 5632, *5632, 5635*
  clinical manifestations, 623–625, *624*, 5633
    loss of vision, 5634–5635, *5637*
    miscellaneous, 5637
    paraplegia, 5635, 5637
    prodrome, 5633–5634
  diagnosis, 625, 5637–5638
  epidemiology, 622, 5632
  laboratory studies and neuroimaging, 625, *626*, 5637, *5638*
  pathology, 622–623, *5632*, 5632–5633, *5633, 5634*
  prognosis, 625–626, 5638–5639
  treatment, 625, 5638
Neuromyopathy, carcinomatous, 2524
Neuromyotonia, 2532
  ocular, 1259, *1260*, 1492, 1497, 1554, *2618*, 2618–2619
Neuronal ceroid lipofuscinoses, 2848–2850, *2849, 2850, 2851*
  infantile, 2850
  juvenile, 2851
  late infantile, 2851, *2852*
Neuronolytic demyelination, 3974, 5539
Neurons
  buildup, 1115
  burst, 1109–1110, *1110, 1111, 1112, 1113, 1114*, 1115, *1115, 1116, 1117, 1119, 1121, 1122*, 1122–1123
  fixation, 1115
  omnipause, 1110
Neuro-ophthalmologic complications
  and bone marrow transplantation, 2634–2635, *2636*
  of HIV infection, 5431–5433
Neuro-ophthalmologic manifestations
  of multiple sclerosis, 5575
  of nonorganic disease, 1765
    convergence insufficiency or paralysis, 1780, *1780*
    general considerations, 1765–1766
    monocular diplopia, 1777
    paralysis of horizontal and vertical gaze, 1782
    spasm of near reflex, 1780–1782, *1781*
    specific nonorganic disorders, 1766–1767
      disease affecting afferent visual pathway, *3*, 3–5, *4, 5, 6, 7*, 7–13, *8, 9, 10, 11, 12*
        decreased visual acuity, *3*, 3–5, *4, 5, 6, 7*, 7–10, *8, 9, 10*
    terminology, 1766
    voluntary nystagmus, 1777, 1779, *1779*
    voluntary saccadic oscillations, 1779–1780
  of ruptured intracranial aneurysms, 3021–3024, *3022, 3023*
  of unruptured intracranial saccular aneurysms, 3127
    abducens nerve paresis, 3128
    combined ocular motor nerve pareses, 3128
    miscellaneous, 3130
    oculomotor nerve paresis, 3127–3128
    oculomotor nerve synkinesis, 3128, *3129*
    trochlear nerve paresis, 3128
    visual loss, 3128, 3130
Neuro-ophthalmologic toxicity of chemotherapeutic medications, 5–6, *6*, 7–8, 9–11, 12, 13, 14, 15, 18–21, *20*, 24–26, *25, 26*, 27–28, 29–31, 32, 33–34, *35*, 36–37, *37*, 39–40, 41, 42
Neuroparalytic keratitis, *1676*, 1676–1677
Neuroparalytic keratopathy, 4172
Neuropathic eyelid retraction and lid-lag, 1550–1551, *1551, 1552*
Neuropathic tonic pupils, 978
Neuropathic toxicology of ocular motor system, 1261
  α-2A-interferon, 1263
  antirabies vaccine, 1261
  arsenic, 1261
  arsphenamine, 1261–1262
  aspirin, 1262
  carbon tetrachloride, 1262
  chloroquine, 1262
  colchicine, 1262
  cytosine arabinoside, 1262
  dichloroacetylene, 1262
  diphenylhydantoin (DPH, Dilantin), 1262
  ethylene glycol (antifreeze), 1262
  gelsemium sempervirens (yellow jasmine), 1262
  isoniazid (INH), 1263
  lead, 1263
  nitrofurans, nitrofurantoin (Furadantin) and furaltadone (altafur), 1263
  Orthoclone OKT3, 1263
  pamaquine, 1263
  phenylbutazone, 1263
  piperazine citrate, 1263
  thalidomide, 1263–1264
  thallium, 1264
  trichloroethylene (trichloroethene), 1264
Neuropathies
  acute motor axonal, 5705–5707, *5706*
  acute retrobulbar optic, 4298, *4300*
  acute sensorimotor, 2523–2524
  anterior compressive optic, 649–653, *650, 651, 652*
  anterior ischemic optic, 58, 259–260, *263, 264*
  anterior optic, 717, *5501*, 5503–5504
  arteritic anterior ischemic optic, 571–572
  arteritic ischemic optic, 5047–5048
  arteritic optic, 583–585, *585*
  arteritic posterior ischemic optic, 583–585, *585*
  bilateral optic, 2582, 5184
  bilateral subacute progressive optic, 2561
  bilateral trigeminal, 5248
  chronic progressive sensorimotor, 2522–2523
  compressive optic, 264
    with optic disc swelling, 649–653, *650, 651, 652*
    without optic disc swelling, *653, 654, 656*, 657
  cranial, 1835, 2269, 2362–2363, *2363*, 2391, 2612, 4889, *5032*, 5032–5033, *5033, 5034*, 5035, *5035, 5036, 5037*, 5037–5041, *5038, 5040, 5041*, 5042, *5043*, 5043–5047, *5044, 5045, 5046, 5047, 5048, 5049*, 5049–5051, *5050, 5051*, 5238–5239, 5242, 5492, 5699–5700
    radiation therapy in, 2612
    as sign of tumors, 1794–1797
  cryptococcal optic, 710
  cyanide optic, 675
  cytomegalovirus-multifocal, 5112–5113
  distal optic, 294, *297, 298*
  dominantly-inherited, 666
  epidemic nutritional optic, 667–668
  ethambutol optic, 674
  facial, 2612, 4373
  glaucomatous optic, 253, *255*, 255–256, *256, 257*
  HIV-associated peripheral, 5386–5387
  infiltrative optic, 266, *269*
  ischemic optic, 259–260, *263, 264*
  Kjer's, 666
  Leber's optic, 666, 744–755
    ancillary testing, 749–750
    associated findings, 746, 749
    clinical features, 744–746, *747, 748*
    determinants of expression, 753–755
    hereditary, 987
    inheritance and genetics, 750–751, *752*, 753
    treatment, 755
  mitochondrially-inherited optic, 666
  nonarteritic optic, 585, *586, 587, 588, 589*, 592
  nonarteritic posterior ischemic optic, 585, *586, 587, 588, 589*, 592
  nutritional optic, 663–664
  olfactory, 2612
  optic, 4373, 5046–5047
    bilateral toxic, 4142
  paraneoplastic optic, 2541–2543, *2542*
  peripheral, 674, 2353, 2561, 2573–2574
    facial myokymia with, 1571–1572
  posterior ischemic optic, 583, 2619
  posterior optic, 717
  probable ischemic optic, 5051–5052
  progressive visual dysfunction in optic, *8*, 653–656, *654*
  radiation optic, 2619–2622, *2620, 2621*
  retrobulbar compressive optic, *653, 654, 656*, 657
  retrobulbar ischemic optic, 5052
  retrobulbar optic, 5197, *5500*, 5503
  role of radiation therapy in facial, 2612
  subacute motor, 2522
  subacute sensorimotor, 2523–2524
  subacute sensory, 2521–2522
  toxic and deficiency optic, 663
    clinical characteristics of, 664–666
    differential diagnosis, 666–667
    etiologic criteria, 663–664
    evaluation, 667
    specific nutritional amblyopias, 667–671
  toxic and drug-induced optic, 1406
  toxic and metabolic optic, 264–265
  toxic optic, 664, 2560
  trigeminal, 2619, 4373
  trigeminal sensory, 1675
  tropical optic, 670–671
  unilateral optic, 4487
  vestibulocochlear, 2612–2613
  vestibulocochlear, role of radiation therapy in, 2612–2613
Neuropathy, ischemic optic, 3447–3448
Neurophysiologic tests, 1652–1653
Neurophysiology
  of fixation, 1137
  of optokinetic movements, 1151–1153

of pursuit eye movements, 1125–1134, *1126, 1127, 1133*
of saccadic eye movements, 1109
Neuropsychiatric manifestations of multiple sclerosis, 5574–5575
Neuropsychology, of face perception, 415–416
Neuroretinitis, 599, 602, 628, 634–639, *635,* 4202–4207, *4204, 4205, 4206,* 4671, 4873–4874, *4875, 4876,* 4967–4968, 5195–5196, 5237, 5275, 5501
arcuate, 636
diffuse unilateral subacute, 636–637
Leber's idiopathic stellate, 634
optic, 4518
treatment of, 637–638
Neurosarcoidosis, 706, 5491–5493, *5495, 5496, 5497,* 5498, 5514
Neurosyphilis, 4882*t*, 4882–4884, 4883*t*
asymptomatic, 4882–4883
meningovascular, 4883–4884, *4884, 4885,* 4886–4889
parenchymatous, 4883, 4886–4887
symptomatic, 4883
syphilitic, 5423–5424
tests for, 4928–4929
Neurotoxicity
and bone marrow transplantation, 2627–2630, *2628, 2629, 2630*
of chemotherapeutic medications, 2554–2555, *2556,* 2558–2559, 2560–2561, *2561,* 2562, 2563–2564, *2564,* 2565, 2566, 2567, 2568, *2569,* 2573–2574, 2578–2579, 2581, 2583, 2584, 2587–2588, 2590, *2590,* 2593–2594, *2594*
from radiation therapy, *50,* 2598–2602, *2600, 2601, 2603,* 2604–2609, *2605, 2606, 2607, 2608, 2609, 2610, 2611,* 2611–2613
Neurotransmitters
for saccadic premotor neurons, 1114
and vestibulo-ocular reflex (VOR), 1148–1149
Neurotrophic keratitis, *1676,* 1676–1677, 5040
Neutrophils, 2329
Nevi of uveal tract, 2658
Nevus flammeus, 2709
Niacin deficiency
as cause of optic neuropathy, 670
and headaches, 1718
Nicaraven for aneurysms, 3175
Nicardipine for delayed cerebral ischemia, 3172
Niemann-Pick disease, 1326, 2832–2837, *2834, 2835, 2836, 2837*
type 2, 1319, 1326
Night myopia, 910
Night presbyopia, 910
Nimidipine for delayed cerebral ischemia, 3171
Nissl-Alzheimer arteritis, 4912
Nitrofurans, 1263
Nitrofurantoin, 1263
Nitrogen mustards, 2563–2564, *2564*
neuro-ophthalmologic toxicity, 2564
neurotoxicity, 2563–2564, *2564*
ocular toxicity, 2564
systemic toxicity, 2563
Nitroglycerin (NTG) and headaches, 1717–1718
Nitroglycerine for delayed cerebral ischemia, 3172
Nitrosoureas
neuro-ophthalmologic toxicity, 2570–2573, *2572*
neurotoxicity, 2568, *2569*
ocular toxicity, 2568–2570, *2569, 2570, 2571*
systemic toxicity, 2568
Nocardia, 4189, 4189–4192, *4190, 4191*
in intracranial abscess, 3950
Nocardia asteroides, 4189, 5421
in intracranial brain abscess, 3952
Nocardia brasiliensis, 4190
Nocardiosis, *4189,* 4189–4192, *4190, 4191*
Nodes of Ranvier, 3974
Nodulus, experimental lesions of, 1290
Nona, 5722
Nonanthrax *Bacillus* species, 4107–4109, *4109*
Nonarteritic anterior ischemic optic neuropathy (NAION)
bilateral, 565–566, *566*
clinical characteristics, 557–559, *558, 559, 560, 572,* 572–573, *573*
appearance of disc, 559, *559, 560*
color vision, 557
fluorescein angiography, 559
initial symptoms, 557
initial visual acuity, 557
pain, 557
pupils, 559
visual field, 557–559, *558*
course, 559–560, *561, 562,* 563, 573, *574*
demographics, 550
diabetic papillopathy, *16,* 564–565
diagnosis and ancillary tests, 576–578
disc swelling preceding visual loss, 564
pathogenesis, 566–568, 573, *574*
pathology, 568–570, *569, 570,* 573, *575,* 576, *576, 577*
prevention, 571
arteritic anterior, 571–572
recurrent, 562–563
risk factors and associated conditions, 550–557
acute blood loss, anemia, and hypotension, 553–555
cardiac disease, 551–552
carotid artery disease, 552
cataract surgery, 556
cerebrovascular disease, 551
coagulopathies, 551
diabetes mellitus, 551
elevated intraocular pressure, 555–556
embolism, 552–553
favism, 555
hypertension, 551
migraine, 556
miscellaneous associations, 556–557
nocturnal hypotension, 555
treatment
medical, 570
surgical, 570–571
vasculitides other than giant cell arteritis, 578, *579,* 580, *580, 581, 582*
visual outcome, 560
Nonarteritic posterior ischemic optic neuropathy, 585, *586, 587, 588, 589,* 592
Nonatheromatous emboli, 3424
Nonbacterial thrombotic (Marantic) endocarditis, 2520–2521
Noncalcifying diffuse corticomeningeal angiomatosis, 2275
Noncaseating granulomatous infiltration of meninges, 5532
Nonclonal erythrocytosis, 2332
Non-communicating (obstructive) hydrocephalus, 3035
Nondural arteriovenous malformations (AVMs), natural history of, 2277
Nonhemolytic streptococci, 4074, 4075
Non-Hodgkin's lymphoma, 701–702, 2360–2361, 2364–2366, *2366, 2367, 2368,* 2368–2370, *2369, 2370, 2371, 2372,* 2372–2375, *2373, 2374,* 2378
Burkitt's, 2375–2378, *2376, 2377*
diagnosis, 2385
etiology, 2378
general clinical features, 2378
isolated intraocular large-cell, 2375
neurologic involvement, 2380, *2380, 2381*
orbital involvement, 2378–2380, *2379, 2380*
primary central nervous system large-cell, 2364–2366, *2366, 2367, 2368,* 2368–2370, *2369, 2370, 2371, 2372,* 2372–2375, *2373, 2374*
treatment and prognosis, 2385–2386
visual involvement, *2381,* 2381–2385, *2382, 2383*
Nonhuman primates
blindsight in, 400–402, *402*
face perception in, 421–423
physiology of motion perception in, 439, 441–443
Noninfected prosthetic valves, 3392–3393
Noninfectious arteritis, 3340, 3342
Noninfectious inflammatory disorders, headaches associated with, 1716
Noninfective valvular disease, 3389–3392
Noninvasive luminal infection, 4619
Nonischemic dilated cardiomyopathies, 3569
Non-Langerhans cell histiocytoses, 2413, *2415,* 2415–2416, *2416, 2417,* 2418, *2418, 2419,* 2420, *2420*
Non-nucleoside reverse transcriptase inhibitors, 5383
Nonorganic blepharospasm, 1570
Nonorganic disease, neuro-ophthalmologic manifestations of, 1765
convergence insufficiency or paralysis, 1780, *1780*
general considerations, 1765–1766
monocular diplopia, 1777
paralysis of horizontal and vertical gaze, 1782
spasm of near reflex, 1780–1782, *1781*
specific nonorganic disorders, 1766–1767
disease affecting afferent visual pathway, *3,* 3–5, *4, 5, 6, 7,* 7–13, *8, 9, 10, 11, 12*
decreased visual acuity, *3,* 3–5, *4, 5, 6, 7,* 7–10, *8, 9, 10*
terminology, 1766
voluntary nystagmus, 1777, 1779, *1779*
voluntary saccadic oscillations, 1779–1780
Nonorganic disturbances
of accommodation, 1784
of eyelid function, 1784
of lacrimination, 1784–1785
of ocular and facial sensation, 1784
Nonparalytic poliomyelitis, 5254
Nonreactive tuberculosis, 4138
Nonspecific corneal changes, 1366–1367
Nonspecific nontreponemal reaginic antibody tests, 4925–4927

Nonsteroidal anti-inflammatory drugs (NSAIDs) for Kawasaki disease, 5740
Nonstreptococcal pharyngitis, 4105
Nonstriate visual areas, relation of blindsight to, 147–148
Nonsystemic vasculitic neuropathy, 3727
Nonvascular intracranial disorders, headache associated with, 1714–1717
Nonvisual manifestations in papilledema, 509–510
Norepinephrine, 841
Normal tear film, 926
Normochromic normocytic anemia, 3772–3775, *3774*
Normokalemic periodic paralysis, 1377
North Asian Tick Typhus, 4751
Nosologic relations of congenital muscular dystrophies, 1362
Nothnagel's syndrome, 1199, 1873
Notochord, 2437–2438, *2438*
  compression of, 2438
NPC, 952
Nuclear and infranuclear ocular motility disorders, 1189–1190
  abducens nerve palsy and nuclear horizontal gaze paralysis, 1237
    acquired, 1244–1245, *1248*, 1248–1256, *1249, 1250, 1251, 1252, 1253, 1254, 1255*
    congenital, 1237–1242, *1238, 1239, 1240, 1241, 1242, 1243*, 1244, *1244, 1245, 1246, 1247*
    cyclic esotropia and its relationship to, 1258
    divergence weakness and its relationship to, 1257
    evaluation and management of, 1256–1257
  diagnosis of infranuclear ophthalmoplegia, 1258–1259
  evaluation and management of patients with, acquired oculomotor nerve palsy, 1225–1227
  hyperactivity of ocular motor nerve
    neuromyotonia, 1259, *1260*
    superior oblique myokymia, 1259–1261
  neuropathic toxicology of ocular motor system, 1261
    α-2A-interferon, 1263
    antirabies vaccine, 1261
    arsenic, 1261
    arsphenamine, 1261–1262
    aspirin, 1262
    carbon tetrachloride, 1262
    chloroquine, 1262
    colchicine, 1262
    cytosine arabinoside, 1262
    dichloroacetylene, 1262
    diphenylhydantoin (DPH, Dilantin), 1262
    ethylene glycol (antifreeze), 1262
    furaltadone (altafur), 1263
    gelsemium sempervirens (yellow jasmine), 1262
    isoniazid (INH), 1263
    lead, 1263
    nitrofurans, 1263
    nitrofurantoin (Furadantin), 1263
    Orthoclone OKT3, 1263
    pamaquine, 1263
    phenylbutazone, 1263
    piperazine citrate, 1263
    thalidomide, 1263–1264
    thallium, 1264
    trichloroethylene (trichloroethene), 1264
  oculomotor nerve palsies
    acquired, 1194–1200, *1197, 1198, 1199, 1200, 1201, 1202*, 1202–1209, *1203, 1204, 1205, 1206, 1207, 1208, 1209, 1210, 1211*, 1211–1216, *1212, 1213, 1214, 1216, 1217, 1218, 1219*, 1220–1225, *1221, 1222, 1223, 1224, 1225*
    congenital, *1190*, 1190–1194, *1191, 1192, 1193, 1194, 1195, 1196*
  synkinesis involving ocular motor and other cranial nerves, 1261
  trochlear nerve palsies, 1227, *1228, 1229, 1230*
    acquired, 1227, 1229, *1230, 1231*, 1231–1232, *1232, 1233*, 1234–1236, *1235*
    congenital, 1227
    differential diagnosis of acquired, 1236
    evaluation and management of, 1236–1237
Nuclear lesions, 5603
Nucleocapsid, 4946
Nucleoside reverse transcriptase inhibitors, 5383
Nucleus
  dorsal, 105, 106
  droplet, 4136–4137
  paraventricular, 830
  supraoptic, 830
  ventral, 105
Nucleus (pars) caudalis, 1631
Nucleus (pars) interpolaris, 1631
Nucleus (pars) oralis, 1631
Nucleus ventralis posterior, 1634, 1636
Nucleus ventralis posterolateralis, 1636
Nucleus ventralis posteromedialis, 1629–1630
Null point, 1465
Numb cheek syndrome, 1669, *1669*
Numb chin syndrome, 1669
Nutritional optic neuropathy, 663–664
  epidemic, 667–668
Nystagmus, 1416, 1462, 1723, 1824, 1848, 1869, 1893, 3826, 4889, 4908, 5256, 5433, 5599, 5728, 5729
  on abduction in contralateral eye, 1295
  acquired pendular, 1466–1468, *1467*, 1467*t*, 1496
    relationship to disease of visual pathways, 1466–1468, *1467*, 1467*t*
  arthrokinetic, 1462, 1471
  association with cerebellar abscesses, 3959
  audiokinetic, 1462, 1471
  bilateral conjugate downbeat, 3501
  botulinum toxin as treatment of, 1498
  Bruns', 1294, 1480, 2311
  caused by central vestibular imbalance, 1472*t*, 1472–1475, 1473*t*
  caused by peripheral vestibular imbalance, 1470–1472
  central vestibular, 1473–1475, *1474, 1475*
  central vestibular, pathogenesis of, 1473–1475, *1474, 1475*
  classification of, based on pathogenesis, 1464
  clinical features of, with lesions affecting visual pathway, 1464–1466
  congenital, 1482
    clinical features, *1482*, 1482–1483
    pathogenesis of, 1483–1484
  convergence, 1781–1782
  convergence-retraction, 1304–1305, 1480–1481, *1481*, 1794, 3501–3502
  cyclovergence, 1469
  definition of, 1462
  difference between physiologic and pathologic, 1462
  dissociated, 1479, *1480*
  dissociated vertical, 1296
  downbeat, 1472, 1472*t*, 1495–1496, 2702
  elliptical, 1326
  epileptic, 1485–1486
  eyelid, 1486, 1550–1551
  familial episodic ataxia with, 1496
  in familial paroxysmal ataxia, 1479–1480
  gaze-evoked, *1478*, 1478–1480, 1479–1480
  hemi-seesaw, 1477, *1477*, 1477*t*
  horizontal, 1473
  induced by auditory stimuli, 1471
  induced by change of head position, 1470–1471
  induced by proprioceptive and auditory stimuli, 1471
  jerk, 1107, 1462, *1462*
  jerk seesaw, 1477
  jerk-waveform divergence, 1481
  latent, 1484
  lid, 1873
  in meningococcal meningitis, 4096
  methods of observing and recording, *1463*, 1463–1464
  monocular downbeat, 3501
  and *Mycoplasma pneumoniae* infection, 4552
  occlusion, 1484
  optokinetic, 370, 1462, 1848
  origin and nature of, associated with disease of visual pathways, 1464
  patients with tuberculous meningitis, 4151
  pendular, 1462
  pendular seesaw, 1478
  periodic alternating, 1475–1476, *1476*, 1476*t*, 1496
  periodic alternating windmill, 1476
  peripheral vestibular
    clinical features of, 1470
    induced by caloric or galvanic stimulation, 1471–1472
  physiologic, 1462
  pseudocaloric, 1176
  pursuit paretic, 1128
  quick phases of, 1107, *1108*
  rebound, *1481*, 1481–1482
  recovery, 1470
  seesaw, 1477, *1477*, 1477*t*, 1496, 2180, 3501
  as sign of tumor, 1797
  surgical procedures for, 1498
  torsional, 1473, 1473*t*
  treatments for, 1494–1499, 1495*t*
  upbeat, 1326, 1472–1473, 1473*t*, 1495–1496
  vestibular, 1462
  from vestibular imbalance, 1495–1496
  voluntary, 1490, 1777, 1779, *1779*
  in Wallenberg's syndrome, 1286

O

Obesity and incidence of atherosclerosis, 3330
Object recognition, disturbances of. (*See* Prosopagnosia.)
Obligate anaerobes, 4066

Obligate intracellular parasites, 3989–3990, *3992*
Occipital artery, 2871, 2941
Occipital lobe
abscesses of, 3957, 3958–3959
anatomy and functions of, 1844, *1845*
hemorrhage of, 3597
lesions of, 1322, 3671–3672, *3672*
bilateral, 357, *359, 360,* 360–361, *362, 363, 364*
bilateral effects of unilateral, 352, 354
unilateral anterior, 347–348, 349–350, 352, *353, 354, 355*
unilateral posterior, 349, *350, 351, 352, 353*
nonvisual symptoms and signs of disease in, 374–375
tumors involving, 1844–1848, *1845, 1846,* 1847, *1847*
visual features of damage to, 370–371
Occipital neuralgia, 1747–1749, *1748, 1749*
Occipital sinus, 2961
Occipitomesencephalic excitation, 877–878, *878*
Occlusion
of anterior choroidal artery, 3434–3436, *3435, 3436, 3437, 3438*
of anterior parietal artery, 3440
of branch retinal artery, *3446, 3447,* 3447–3450, *3448*
of cerebral artery, 3432–3434, *3433*
of cortical branches, 3440, *3441*
of internal carotid artery, 3010–3011, *3011,* 3428–3432, *3429, 3430*
of middle cerebral artery, 3436–3438, *3439*
of ophthalmic artery, 3432
of posterior branches of middle cerebral artery, 3440–3441
of Rolandic artery, 3440
of superior vena cava, 3929
Occlusion nystagmus, 1484
Occult giant cell arteritis, 3775
Ochroconis gallopavum, 4353
Octopus perimeter, 177
Octreotide for pituitary adenomas, 2192
Ocular abnormalities, 4621
Ocular alignment, 1176–1183
disorders of, *1780,* 1780–1782, *1781,* 2617–2619, *2618,* 5603
Ocular apraxia, 445
Ocular blastomycosis, 4338, *4339–4340, 4341,* 4341–4342, *4342*
Ocular blepharospasm, 1569
Ocular bobbing, 1328, 1492–1493, *1493,* 3023, 3511
Ocular candidiasis, 4348, *4348, 4349*
Ocular complications
of bone marrow transplantation, 2632, *2633,* 2634, *2634, 2635, 2636*
of HIV infection, 5424, *5425*
anterior segment disease, 5429–5430
retinal microangiopathy, 5424–5426, *5426*
retinitis and chorioretinitis, *5426,* 5426–5429, *5427, 5428, 5429*
Ocular cryptococcosis, 4378–4381, *4379, 4380, 4381*
Ocular cysticercosis, 4468–4469, *4469, 4470,* 4471, *4471, 4472, 4473*
Ocular dipping, 3512
Ocular disease, headache associated with, 1723–1726, 1726*t*
Ocular dominance columns, *132,* 133, *133, 134, 135*
and amblyopia, 133–134
Ocular fixation, abnormalities of, 433
Ocular flutter, 1487, 1491, 1497, 1987, 5433, 5509
Ocular histoplasmosis, 4397
Ocular hypotony, 1369, 3768–3769
Ocular involvement
in multiple myeloma, 2396–2398, *2397, 2398*
in tertiary syphilis, 4900–4902
Ocular ischemic syndrome, 3457–3458, *3458, 3459, 3460,* 3460–3462, *3461, 3462, 3463,* 3767, *3771*
Ocular loiasis, 4505, *4506, 4507*
Ocular media, 154
Ocular migraine, 3687
Ocular misalignment, 941
Ocular motility, 1169
disorders of, *1780,* 1780–1782, *1781,* 2617–2619, *2618,* 5603
examination, 1171
alignment, 1176–1183
fixation and gaze-holding ability, 1171
performance of versions, 1183
quantitative analysis of eye movements, 1185
range of eye movements, *1171,* 1171–1176, *1173, 1174*
history, 1169
blurred vision, 1170
diplopia, 1169–1170
vestibular symptoms, 1170
visual confusion, 1170
Ocular motor abnormalities, 1824, 1843–1844
and disease of basal ganglia, 1316
Huntington's disease, 1318–1319
Parkinson's disease, 1316–1318, *1318*
Ocular motor apraxia, *1325,* 1325–1326, 2661
Ocular motor disorders in sarcoidosis, 5509
Ocular motor disturbances, 3214–3215
Ocular motor dysfunction, 2177–2180, *2179,* 2179*t*, *2180,* 2394–2396, *2395*
from brainstem damage, 2619
and multiple sclerosis, 1330
Ocular motor manifestations of some metabolic disorders, 1330–1331, 1333
Ocular motor nerve palsies, 1738–1739, 1865, 2177–2178
Ocular motor nerve paresis, 1848, 2617–2618, 3466, 3826, 4077–4078, 4127, 4151, *4153,* 5043, 5433, 5508–5509, 5605–5606, *5607, 5608,* 5608–5609, *5609,* 5729
in pituitary adenomas, 2179*t*
Ocular motor nerves, 1075, 1077–1079, *1078, 1079*
schwannomas of, 2302, *2303*
Ocular motor nuclei, 1075, 1077–1079, *1078, 1079*
Ocular motor syndromes
and disease of the cerebellum, 1290, 1290*t*
degenerative, 1292–1293
developmental anomalies of hindbrain, 1291–1292, 1292*t*
location of lesions and their manifestations, 1290–1291
mass lesions, 1293–1294
vascular, *1292,* 1293, *1293*
and lesions in cerebral hemispheres, 1319
abnormal eye movements and dementia, 1326–1327
acute, 1319–1320, *1320, 1321*
apraxia, *1325,* 1325–1326
eye movements in stupor and coma
gaze deviations, 1327–1328
reflex, 1329–1330
spontaneous, 1328–1329
focal, 1322
frontal lobe, 1324–1325
occipital lobe, 1322
parietal lobe, 1322–1323
temporal lobe, 1323–1324
manifestations of seizures, 1327
persistent deficits caused by large unilateral, 1320–1322, 1321*t*, *1322*
and lesions in medulla, 1283–1285, *1284*
of anterior inferior cerebellar artery, 1287, *1288*
Wallenberg's, *1285,* 1285–1287, *1286, 1287*
and lesions of mesencephalon
neurologic disorders that primarily affect, 1311, 1313
progressive supranuclear palsy, 1313–1314
Whipple's disease, 1314–1315
sites and manifestations of
interstitial nucleus of Cajal, 1308, 1310
other, 1310–1311
periaqueductal gray matter, 1308
posterior commissure, 1304*t*, 1304–1305, *1305, 1306,* 1306*t*, 1307, *1307, 1308*
rostral interstitial nucleus of medial longitudinal fasciculus, 25–26, *27, 28, 29, 30, 31*
and lesions of pons
of abducens nucleus, 1298–1299
combined unilateral conjugate gaze palsy and internuclear ophthalmoplegia, *1301,* 1301–1303, *1302*
of internuclear system, internuclear ophthalmoplegia
etiologies, 1297, 1298*t*, *1299, 1300*
manifestations, *1294,* 1294–1297, *1295, 1296, 1297*
posterior, of Lutz, 1297–1298
of paramedian pontine reticular formation, 1299–1301
saccadic oscillations from pontine, 1303
slow saccades from pontine, 1303, 1303*t*
and lesions of superior colliculus, 1315
and lesions of thalamus, *1315,* 1315–1316, *1317*
Ocular motor system, 1041
abnormalities in, 3805
anatomy and embryology of, 1043, *1044, 1045,* 1045–1052, *1046, 1047, 1048,* 1049*t*, *1050, 1052*
abducens nerve, 1067, 1070, *1070, 1071, 1072, 1073*
abducens nucleus, 1066–1067, *1068, 1069, 1070*
fascicular portion of oculomotor nerve, 1055, *1055, 1056,* 1057, *1057*
fascicular portion of trochlear nerve, 1064, *1065*
levator palpebrae superioris, 1052, *1053*
oculomotor nerve, 1057, *1058,* 1059, *1059, 1060,* 1061, *1061, 1062, 1063*

Ocular motor system—*continued*
oculomotor nucleus, 1053–1055, *1054, 1055*
trochlear nerve, 1066, *1066, 1067*
trochlear nucleus, 1064, *1064*
embryology of
extraocular muscles, 1072–1075, *1074, 1075, 1076, 1077*
levator palpebrae superioris, 1075, *1078*
nuclei and nerves, 1075, 1077–1079, *1078, 1079*
supranuclear components of, 1079
cerebellum, 1092, *1093,* 1094, *1094*
cerebral cortex, 1082–1087, *1084, 1085, 1086*
immediate premotor structures of brainstem, 1080–1082, *1081*
internuclear system, 1080, *1080*
vestibular system, 1087–1092, *1088, 1089, 1090, 1091*
Ocular movement, limitation of, 1804
Ocular myasthenia, 1424
Ocular myoclonus, 3603
Ocular myopathy
associated with celiac disease, 1405
toxic and drug-induced, 1406
Ocular neuromyotonia, 1259, *1260,* 1492, 1497, 1554, *2618,* 2618–2619
Ocular orbital coccidioidomycosis, 4361–4362, *4364, 4365, 4366*
Ocular pain, 1726–1727, 3467
in optic neuritis, 601
Ocular pneumoplethysmography (OPPG), 3538–3539
Ocular pulsation, 3275, *3277, 3278*
Ocular sensation, nonorganic disturbances of, 1784
Ocular sensitivity, 1606
Ocular signs of bilateral carotid artery occlusive disease, 3467, 3469
Ocular symptoms and signs, 1860–1861
of ophthalmic artery occlusion, 3469–3471, *3471*
Ocular tilt reaction, 1141, 1286, 1288, 1477, 3501, *3502,* 3513–3514, 5602, *5602*
Ocular torsion, 1172
Ocular toxicity of chemotherapeutic medications, 2555–2557, *2557,* 2559, 2561, 2562, 2563, 2564, 2565, 2566, 2567–2570, *2569, 2570, 2571, 2574,* 2574–2576, 2579, 2580, 2581, 2584–2585, *2585, 2586,* 2588, 2590–2591, *2591,* 2593
Ocular toxocariasis, 4516
Ocular toxoplasmosis, *4681,* 4681–4683, *4682, 4683*
diagnosis of, 4698–4699
pathology of, 4687, *4690,* 4691, *4691, 4692*
treatment of, 4700–4701
Ocular tuberculosis, 4144–4145
Oculocardiac reflex, 1656–1657
Oculocephalic testing, 1174–1175
Oculocerebrorenal syndrome, 2814–2815
Oculocerebrovasculometry (OCVM), 3539
Oculoglandular tularemia, 4229
Oculogyric crisis, *5731,* 5731–5732, *5732*
Oculomasticatory myorhythmia, 1314–1315, 4185–4186
Oculomotor apraxia, 2722
Oculomotor nerve, 1053, 1057, *1058,* 1059, *1059, 1060,* 1061, *1061, 1062, 1063,* 1520–1522, *1521*
aberrant regeneration of, 3128, *3129*
aberrant reinnervation of, 1014
damage to cavernous portion of, 977
damage to pupillomotor fibers in, 975, *975*
subarachnoid portion of, 975–977, *976*
dysfunction, 2976
and aneurysmal rupture, 3022
dysfunction of, 1795
fascicular palsies of, 1014
fascicular portion of, 1055, *1055, 1056,* 1057, *1057*
involvement in cavernous sinus, 1215, *1216, 1217*
lesions of
in cavernous sinus and superior orbital fissure, 1212–1216, *1214*
within orbit, 1215–1216, *1218, 1219*
in subarachnoid space, 1202–1203
of uncertain or variable locations, 1218, *1219, 1220*
palsies
acquired, 1194–1200, *1197, 1198, 1199, 1200, 1201, 1202,* 1202–1209, *1203, 1204, 1205, 1206, 1207, 1208, 1209, 1210, 1211,* 1211–1216, *1212, 1213, 1214, 1216, 1217, 1218, 1219,* 1220–1225, *1221, 1222, 1223, 1224, 1225*
congenital, *1190,* 1190–1194, *1191, 1192, 1193, 1194, 1195, 1196*
eyelid retraction associated, 1554
paresis, 3046–3047, 3075, 3127–3128, 4373, 5023, 5087
paresis associated with small pupil, 1805, *1808*
peripheral palsies of, 1014
primary synkinesis of, 3081
pupillary fibers in, 861–862, *863*
synkinesis, 3128, *3129*
primary, 1225, *1225*
secondary, 1224–1225
Oculomotor nerve fascicle, lesions of, 1198–1200, *1201, 1202, 1203, 1204*
Oculomotor nucleus, 1053–1055, *1054, 1055,* 1520–1522, *1521*
lesions of, 1194–1198, *1197, 1198, 1199, 1200, 1201*
Oculomotor nucleus fascicle, ptosis from lesions of, 1540–1542, *1541, 1542, 1543*
Oculomotor palsy with cyclic spasms, 1554
Oculomotor paresis with cyclic spasms, 1192–1194, *1196*
Oculopalatal myoclonus syndrome, 1284, 1468–1469, *1469*
Oculopharyngeal dystrophy, 1372–1374, *1373, 1374, 1375,* 1376
Oculoplethysmography, 3538
Oculosympathetic dysfunction, 3896
Oculosympathetic paresis, 964
Oculosympathetic pathways, ptosis from lesions of, 1542, *1544*
OFF-center bipolar cell, 40
OKT3 as cause of aseptic meningitis, 2628–2629
Olfactory groove
meningiomas of, 2043–2044, *2045,* 2987
tumors of, *1825,* 1825–1827
Olfactory nerve dysfunction, 1794–1795
Olfactory neuroblastoma, 1989–1990, *1991*
Olfactory neuroepithelium, 5182
Olfactory neuropathy, role of radiation therapy in, 2612
Oligodendrocytes, 44, 65–66
interfascicular, 21, 3974
Oligodendroglia tumors, 1958, *1960,* 1960–1963, *1961*
Oligodendrogliomas, 1919, 1958, *1960,* 1960–1963, *1961*
Oligomenorrhea and Cushing's syndrome, 2160
Olivopontocerebellar atrophy, 762, 1568
Omnipause neurons, 1110, 1535
ON-center bipolar cell, 40
Onchocerca volvulus, 4507–4511, *4509, 4510*
diagnosis of, 4510–4511
treatment of, 4511
Onchocerciasis, 4507–4511, *4509, 4510*
diagnosis of, 4510–4511
treatment of, 4511
Oncospheres, 4439
Oncoviruses, 5433–5434
human T-cell leukemia virus type I, 5434
diagnosis, 5435
diseases associated with HTLV-I infection, *5433,* 5435–5438, *5436, 5437, 5438, 5439, 5440,* 5440–5442, *5441*
epidemiology, 5434
transmission, 5434
human T-cell leukemia virus type II, 5441–5442
counseling, 5442
Ondine's curse, 3515, 4132
One-and-a-half syndrome, *1301,* 1301–1303, *1302,* 1331, 3023, 3509–3510, *3510,* 5612
On-off channels, 118
Oocysts, 4667
Oophoritis, 5226
Open-angle glaucoma, 2350
Ophthalmic artery, 7, 61
aneurysms arising from, 3066–3067, *3067, 3068, 3069, 3070*
occlusion of, 3432
Ophthalmic collateral circuit, 3415–3416
Ophthalmic division pain
associated with occlusion of internal carotid artery, 1707
associated with occlusion of posterior cerebral artery, 1707–1708
Ophthalmic migraine, 3687
Ophthalmic nerve, 1606–1607, *1607, 1608, 1609,* 1610, *1610, 1611, 1612, 1613*
Ophthalmic segment of internal carotid artery, 2877, *2878, 2879, 2880,* 2880–2881, *2881, 2882, 2883,* 2884, *2884, 2885, 2886, 2887, 2888*
Ophthalmic vein
inferior, 2966
superior, 2965–2966
thrombosis of, 3915–3918, *3916, 3917*
Ophthalmicus, herpes zoster, 3973, 5033–5035
Ophthalmodynamometry (ODM), 3536–3541, *3537, 3538, 3539, 3540*
compression, 3537, 3538, *3538*
suction, 3537–3538, *3538*
Ophthalmodynia periodica, 1727
Ophthalmologic examination, 3525
Ophthalmoparesis, 1411–1416, *1413, 1414, 1415,* 2179, 2995, 3896, 4036, 5256, 5685, 5705, 5726, *5727*
diabetic, 3685

Ophthalmoplegia, 1029, 2183–2184, 2333, 2976, 4113
with acute necrotizing myopathy and carcinoma, 1397
ataxia, and areflexia, 1029
bilateral internal, 5023
bilateral internuclear, 4375
chronic progressive external, 1545
complete, 2722
internal and external, 4113
diagnosis of mitochondrial myopathy in patients with, 1390
encephalomyopathy with, from vitamin E deficiency, 1391
external, 3837
infranuclear, 1258–1259
internal, 974, 5248
internuclear, 1289, 1294, *1301,* 1301–1303, *1302,* 4375, 5256, 5433, 5603, 5703
multiple deletion of mtDNA in autosomal-dominant and autosomal-recessive, 1390
from orbital and muscle tumors, 1397, *1398*
in patients with Miller Fisher syndrome, 5696
point mutations of mitochondrial tRNAs in maternally inherited, 1389
posterior internuclear, 1294
of Lutz, 1297–1298
single deletion of mtDNA in sporadic, 1389–1390
unilateral internal, 5022–5023
wall-eyed bilateral internuclear, 5605
Ophthalmoplegia syndrome, 1727
Ophthalmoplegic migraine, 3681–3687, *3682, 3683, 3687*
Ophthalmoscopic appearance in optic neuritis, *604,* 604–605, *605*
Ophthalmoscopy in diagnosing traumatic optic neuropathy, 720
Opsoclonus, 1487, 1491, 1497, 1987, 5239, 5254
biotin-responsive, 1497
Opsoclonus-myoclonus syndrome, 5087, 5248
Ophthalmic artery, carotid-ophthalmic aneurysms arising from junction with, *3059,* 3059–3060, *3060, 3061, 3062,* 3062–3063, *3063, 3064, 3065,* 3065–3066, *3066, 3067*
Ophthalmicus, herpes zoster, trigeminal pain during and after, 1729
Optic aphasia, 3484–3485
Optic ataxia, 445, 448, 451, *451, 452*
Optic atrophy, 274, 276, 1835, 1844, 1848, 2044, 3805, 4887–4889
differential diagnosis of, *289,* 291–292, *292, 293, 294*
nerve injury in, 743
ophthalmoscopic features of, 285–288, *286, 287, 288, 289,* 290, *290, 291*
pathology of, 278, 280–281, *283,* 283–284
Optic canal
decompression, 735
relationship between paranasal sinuses and, 71
Optic chiasm, 3828
critique of nerve fiber schemata of, 99
disease affecting, 1466, *1466*
embryology of, *14,* 14–15
gross anatomy of, and its relationship to surrounding structures, 85, *86, 87*
inferior, 85–87, *88, 89,* 90, *90*
lateral, 92–93
posterior, *86, 92,* 93
superior, 90–92, *91*
nonvisual fibers in, 99
syndrome of, 1811, *1812*
type, number, and organization of nerve fibers within, *93,* 93–97, *94, 95, 96, 97, 98*
visual symptoms originating in, 3674
Optic chiasm and intracranial optic nerves and sarcoidosis, 5505–5507, *5506*
Optic chiasmal apoplexy, 2258
Optic chiasmal gliomas, 1945, 1951–1956, *1952, 1954*
Optic chiasmal ischemia, permanent bitemporal hemianopia from, 3692–3693
Optic chiasmal lesions
chiasmal syndrome of Cushing, 321–323
etiologies of optic chiasmal syndrome, 313, 318–319
neuro-ophthalmologic signs associated with optic chiasmal syndromes, 320–321, *321, 322*
neuro-ophthalmologic symptoms associated with optic chiasmal syndromes, *319,* 319–320, *320*
visual field defects, 307, *308, 309,* 309–311, *310, 312–313,* 313, *314–315, 316, 317, 318*
Optic chiasmal neuritis of multiple sclerosis, 5590, *5591, 5592, 5593, 5594,* 5595, *5595*
Optic chiasmal syndrome, 5087
etiologies of, 313, 318–319
neuro-ophthalmologic symptoms associated with, *319,* 319–320, *320,* 320–321
Optic disc, 58, 547
anomalous elevation of, 266, 269, *269, 270,* 271, *272, 273,* 274, *274, 275, 276, 277, 278, 279*
appearance of, 559, *559, 560*
in optic neuritis, *605,* 612, 613, *614*
in retinal disease, 252–253, *253, 254*
congenital anomalies of, 777–778
doubling of, *800,* 800–801
hyperemia of, 487
nonpathologic pallor of, 276, 278
swelling of, 488
tilted, 274, *278, 279*
Optic disc atrophy, 274, 276
differential diagnosis of, *289,* 291–292, *292, 293, 294*
nonpathologic pallor of disc, 276, 278
ophthalmoscopic features of, 285–288, *286, 287, 288, 289,* 290, *290, 291*
pathogenesis of acquired pallor, *284,* 284–285
pathology of, 278, 280–281, *283,* 283–284
Optic disc coloboma, *12,* 785, 788–789, 789*t,* 790*t*
Optic disc drusen, 988
pseudopapilledema associated with, 805
ancillary studies, 808–810, *809, 810, 811*
anomalous disc elevation without visible or buried, *817,* 818
complication, 810
central visual loss, 812
ischemic optic neuropathy, 813
peripapillary central serous choroidopathy, 814
peripapillary subretinal neurovascularization, 814
prepapillary or peripapillary hemorrhages, 812–813
retinal vascular occlusions, 813
transient visual loss, 813–814
visual field defects, 810–812, *812*
distinguishing buried, from papilledema, 807–808, *808,* 808*t*
epidemiology, 805
histology of, 814, *815*
natural history, 805
ophthalmoscopic appearance
of buried, 806–807, *807*
of visible drusen, 805–806, *806*
pathogenesis of, 814, 816
systemic
angioid streaks with and without pseudoxanthoma elasticum, 817–818
megalencephaly, 818
migraine headaches, 818
retinitis pigmentosa, *816,* 816–817
Optic disc dysplasia, 182*1,* 796, *796*
Optic disc gliomas, *1956,* 1956–1957
Optic disc margins, blurring of, 488
Optic disc neovascularization, 3462
Optic disc pallor, pathogenesis of acquired, 284–285
Optic disc swelling, 259, *260,* 1801–1802, *1802*
anomalous elevation of, 266, 269, *269, 270,* 271, *272, 273,* 274, *274, 275, 276, 277, 278, 279*
compressive optic neuropathies without, *653, 654, 656,* 657
infiltrative neuropathy, 266, *269*
true, 259, 260, *261, 262, 263,* 264–265
Optic disc trauma, 717
Optic foramen, 66, *68,* 71
Optic nerve, 57, *58, 59,* 4469, *4471*
aplasia in, *801,* 801–802
apoplexy in, 2258
bilateral lesions of, 298, *299,* 300, *300*
centrifugal fibers in, 78
compression of, 988
damage in scleroderma, 3838
demyelinated, 5547
disease of, 1465–1466, 4872
dysfunction of, 1795
and sarcoidosis, *5498, 5499,* 5499–5501, *5500, 5501, 5502, 5503, 5504,* 5505
embryology of, 4, *6,* 6–8, *7, 8, 9, 10, 11*
gliomas of, 681–689, *682, 683, 684, 685, 686, 687, 688, 689, 1945,* 1945–1951, *1946, 1948, 1949,* 2652–2654, *2653, 2654, 2655*
hemangioblastoma in, 694, *695,* 696, *696*
hemorrhage within, 3032, *3033*
hypoplasia in, 778
associated central nervous system malformations, 780, *781,* 782, *782*
associated endocrinologic deficiencies, 779–780
association between albinism and, 783
electrophysiological studies, 779
histopathology, 778, *779*
ophthalmoscopic appearance, 778, *778*
pathogenesis, 784
quantitative analysis, 778–779
segmental hypoplasia, *783,* 783–784, *784*
systemic and teratogenic associations, 782–783
visual function, 778

Optic nerve—*continued*
injury to. (*See also* Traumatic optic neuropathy.)
primary mechanisms of, 725
prognosis of, 715
secondary mechanisms of, 725–729, *726*, *727*
intracanalicular, 7, 66, *68*, 69, *69*, *70*, 70*t*, *71*, 71–72, *72*
intracranial, 7–8, 16, 72, *73*, *74*, *75*, *76*, 717
intraocular, 57–58, *59–60*
astrocytes, 58–59, *62*
axons, 58, *61*, *62*
blood vessels, 59, 61–62, *63*, *64*
extracellular space, 62–64
lesions of
appearance of disc in patients with congenital and acquired disease, 259
atrophy, 274, 276
differential diagnosis of, *289*, 291–292, *292*, *293*, *294*
nonpathologic pallor of disc, 276, 278
ophthalmoscopic features of, 285–288, *286*, *287*, *288*, *289*, 290, *290*, *291*
pathogenesis of acquired pallor, *284*, 284–285
pathology of, 278, 280–281, *283*, 283–284
swelling, 259, *260*
anomalous elevation of, 266, 269, *269*, *270*, 271, *272*, *273*, 274, *274*, *275*, *276*, *277*, *278*, *279*
infiltrative neuropathy, 266, *269*
true, 259, 260, *261*, *262*, *263*, 264–265
bilateral, 298, *299*, 300, *300*
superior or inferior (altitudinal) hemianopia, *299*, 300, *300*, *301*
bilateral ''checkerboard'' altitudinal hemianopia and vertical hemifield slide phenomenon, 300, 302, *302*
syndromes of unilateral dysfunction, 292, 294
anterior optic chiasm syndrome, 294, *297*, *298*
distal optic neuropathy, 294, *297*, *298*
distal syndrome, 294, *297*, *298*
Foster Kennedy syndrome, 296, 298
optociliary shunts and syndrome of chronic optic nerve compression, 294
prechiasmal compression syndrome, 294
unilateral and bilateral nasal hemianopia, 302–304, *303*, *304*, *305*, *306*, *307*
leukemic involvement of, 2341–2343, *2343*, *2344*
monitoring function of, during decompression, 657
myelination of, 76, *77*
and optic chiasmal hemorrhage, *3607*, 3607–3608, *3608*
orbital, *64*, 64–66, *65*, *66*, *67*, *68*
quantitative histology of, 76–78
topographic anatomy of, 78–79, *79*, *80*, 81
visual symptoms originating in, 3674–3675
Optic nerve sheath, 73
decompression surgery, 562
Optic nerve sheath hemorrhage, 3029, *3029*, *3030*, *3031*, *3032*
Optic nerve sheath meningioma, 2044–2045, 3424–3425
Optic neuritis, 264, 599, 1725, 3855, *4212*, 4212–4213, 4516–4517, *4519*, 4907, 4956, 4967, 5087, 5229, 5237, 5289, 5432, 5640, 5687, *5691*, 5699, 5728
acute, 5581–5582, *5583*, *5584*, 5584–5588, *5585*, *5586*
asymptomatic (subclinical), *5589*, 5589–5590, *5590*
autoimmune, 630
bacterial anterior, 4116
bilateral retrobulbar, 4552
causes of, *631*, 631–632, *632*
in children, *36*, 632–634
chronic, *5588*, 5588–5589
definition of, 599
historical perspective of, 600
acute idiopathic demyelinating, 600
demographics, 600–601
diagnostic, etiologic, and prognostic studies, 605–608, *606*, *608*
management recommendations for patients with presumed acute, 616
neurologic prognosis, 615–616
pathogenesis of visual loss in, 617
pathology, 616–617
recurrent, 616
relationship of, to multiple sclerosis, 617–620
residual visual deficits after resolution of, *605*, 612–615, *614*
signs of, 601–602, *603*, *604*, 604–605, *605*
symptoms of, 601
treatment of, *609*, 609–610, *610*
visual function in fellow eye, 605
visual prognosis, 610–612, *611*
asymptomatic demyelinating, 620–622, *621*, *622*
chronic demyelinating, 620, *620*
encephalitis periaxialis concentrica (concentric sclerosis of Baló), 628
in myelinoclastic diffuse sclerosis (encephalitis periaxialis diffusa, Schilder's disease), 626–628
neuromyelitis optica (Devic's disease), 622
clinical manifestations, 623–625, *624*
diagnosis, 625
epidemiology, 622
laboratory studies and neuroimaging, 625, *626*
pathology, 622–623
prognosis, 625–626
treatment, 625
in HIV-positive patients and patients with AIDS, 630
in meningococcal meningitis, 4097
of multiple sclerosis, 5581–5582, *5583*, *5584*, 5584–5590, *5585*, *5586*, *5588*, *5589*, *5590*
in myelinoclastic diffuse sclerosis (encephalitis periaxialis diffusa, Schilder's disease), 626–628
optic neuropathies that mimic acute, 639
parainfectious, 628–629
in patients with Lyme borreliosis, 630
and Q fever, 4769
recurrent, 616, 619
retrobulbar, 2393
in sarcoidosis, 629
and sinus disease, 630–631
from syphilis, 629–630
in systemic lupus erythematosus and other vasculitides, 630
after vaccination, 629
from viral and bacterial diseases, 628
visual loss from, 4151, 4153
Optic neuropathy, 987, 4373, 5046–5047
bilateral, 2582
subacute progressive, 2561
toxic, 4142
cyanide, 675
and cyclosporine, 2634
epidemic nutritional, 667–668
ethambutol, 674
hereditary. (*See* Hereditary optic neuropathies.)
as manifestation of hereditary degenerative or developmental diseases
ataxias, 762–763
polyneuropathies, 763–764
storage, and cerebral degenerations of childhood, 764–767
nutritional, 663–664
syndrome of, 674
in systemic lupus erythematosus, 3826–3827
that mimic acute optic neuritis, 639
toxic, 664, *671*, 671–675
tropical, 670–671
Optic neuroretinitis, 4518
Optic perineuritis, 599, 628, *638*, 639, 4097, 4872, 5432
Optic pit, 791–793, *792*, *793*
Optic pit-associated macular detachment, risk of, 792–793
Optic radiation lesions
internal capsule, 337, *337*, *338*, *339*
parietal lobe, *343*, *344*, *345*, 347, *347*, *348*, 349
temporal lobe, 339–340, *340*, *341*, *342*, 344, 347
Optic radiations, anatomy and physiology of, 121–126, *122*, *123*, *124*, *125*, 126
Optic strut, 71
Optic tract, 101
anatomy of, 101, *102*, *103*, 104, *104*
embryology of, 15, *16*
fiber organization in, 104
lesions of, 325–326, *326*, *327*, *328*, *329*, *330*, 330–331, *331*, *332–333*
syndrome of, 1811–1812, *1813*, *1814*
Optica, neuromyelitis, 4164, 4166
Opticoacoustic nerve atrophy with dementia, 760
Optico-cerebral syndrome, 586, 3449
Optochiasmatic arachnoiditis, 4153, 4373–4374, 4876, 4878–4880
Optociliary shunt vessels, 1802, *1803*
Optociliary shunts and syndrome of chronic optic nerve compression, 294
Optokinetic after-nystagmus, 1149
Optokinetic drum, use of, to detect nonorganic unilateral blindness, 1767–1768, *1768*
Optokinetic movements, 1157–1158
Optokinetic nystagmus, 1462, 1848
in cortical and cerebral blindness, 370
Optokinetic system, 1185
characteristics of movements, 1149–1151, *1150*
clinical examination of, 1185
neurophysiology of movements, 1151–1153

Oral contraceptives
as risk factor for stroke, 3567
and risk of thrombotic cerebrovascular and ocular disease, 3359, 3361
Orbicularis oculi involvement, 1416, *1416*, *1417*
Orbicularis oculi muscle, 1509, 1510–1511, *1511*
innervation of, 1513–1514, *1514*, *1515*, *1516*, *1517*, 1517–1520, *1518*, *1519*, 1520*t*
Orbit
abscess of, 4298, *4298*
aspergillomas of, 4290–4291
echinococcal cyst of, 4452
effect of radiation therapy on, 2615, 2617
inflammation and infection, 1725
leukemic involvement of, *2340*, 2340–2341, *2341*, *2342*
paragangliomas of, 2471
postoperative pain, 1726
sensory nerve endings in, 1602
syndrome of floor of, 1804
trauma, 1725–1726
tumors in, 1725, *1726*, *1798*, 1798–1804, *1800*, *1801*, *1802*, *1803*, *1804*
ophthalmoplegia from, 1397, *1398*
Orbit tumors in, ophthalmoplegia from, 1397, *1398*
Orbital angiomas, *2243*, *2244*, 2244–2245
Orbital apex, syndrome of, 1668
Orbital apex syndrome, 4291, 4299
Orbital arteriovenous malformations (AVMs), 2266
natural history of, 2279
Orbital artery, 2897
Orbital aspergillosis, *4296*, *4297*, 4298–4299
Orbital blastomycosis, 4338, *4339–4340*, *4341*, 4341–4342, *4342*
Orbital cellulitis, 1725, 4035
as cause of brain abscess, 3945–3946, *3947*
as cause of septic cavernous sinus thrombosis, 3894–3895
Orbital complications of HIV infection, *5430*, 5430*t*, 5430–5431, *5431*
Orbital cryptococcosis, 4378–4381, *4379*, *4380*, *4381*
Orbital cysticercosis, 4468–4469, *4470*
Orbital disease
headache associated with, 1723–1726, 1726*t*
signs of, 1804
Orbital echinococcosis, 4447, *4449*
Orbital emphysema, 716–717
Orbital granulomas, 3796
Orbital hemorrhage, 3024, *3025*
management of, 732–733
after retrobulbar block, 716
Orbital involvement
in multiple myeloma, 2396, *2396*
in non-Hodgkin's lymphomas, 2378–2380, *2379*, *2380*
Orbital meningiomas, 2051
Orbital pain in optic neuritis, 601
Orbital sarcoidosis, 5470, 5486–5487
Orbital septum, 1510
Orbital tumors, imaging of, 1897–1898, *1898*
Orbital veins, *2964*, *2965*, 2965–2966, *2966*
Orbital venous pressure, muscle enlargement from, 1398, *1400*, *1401*
Orbitofrontal artery, 2897
Orbitopathy, thyroid, 1556–1557
Orbiviruses, *5259*, 5259–5261, *5260*
Organic brain syndrome, 4814, *4816*
Organic disease
accommodation spasm associated with, 1016
accommodation spasm unassociated with, 1016–1018, *1017*
Organism emboli, 3379, *3382*
Orgasmic headache, 1704
Oriental Spotted Fever, 4751
Orientation-selective, 130, 141
Oropharyngeal tularemia, 4229
Orthoclone OKT3, 1263
Orthomyxoviridae
characteristics of, 5190, *5191*
influenza viruses, 5190–5198, *5191*, *5194*, *5195*, *5197*
Orthoreoviruses, 5261
Orungo virus, 5261
Oscillations
macrosaccadic, 1487
voluntary saccadic, 1490
Oscillopsia, 1170, 1462, 2223, 3474
Oscilloscope screen projections, 622
Osler-Weber-Rendu syndrome, 2735
Osteal granulomas, 5482, *5484*
Osteitis, 1722
Osteochondromas, 2443, *2443*
Osteoclast activating factor (OAF), 2390
Osteoclastomas, 2443–2444
Osteoclasts, 2404
Osteogenesis imperfecta, 783, 3012
Osteogenic sarcoma, 2069–2070
Osteoma, 2442–2443
within optic chiasm, 4153–4154
Osteomyelitis, 4088
Osteoporosis and Cushing's syndrome, 2160
Osteoporosis-pseudoglioma syndrome, 767
Oticus, herpes zoster, 1744–1745, *5033*, 5033–5035, *5034*, *5035*, *5036*, 5037–5038
Otis media as cause of septic cavernous sinus thrombosis, 3894
Otitic hydrocephalus, 3900, 4040
Otitis media, 4035, 4085, 5201, 5203
Otolaryngologic symptoms and signs, 3038
Otolithic inputs, imbalance of, 1288
Otolith-ocular reflexes, 1140–1142, *1141*, 1175
Otologic complications, radiation therapy in, 2597
Otorrhagia, 3038
Otorrhea, 3038
Outer plexiform layer, 35–36, *38*
Outer protein shell, 4946
Oxidative stress hypothesis, 2796
Oxygen, hyperbaric, 3175
for mucormycosis, 4331–4332
for radionecrosis, 591–592
for radionecrosis of bone, 2622
Oxytocin, 835, 2146

P

Pacchionian bodies, 2020
Pachymeningitis, 4308
cranial hypertrophic, 4136
idiopathic hypertrophic cranial, 5529–5533, *5530*, *5531*, *5532*
Padilledema, chronic, 494, *494*
Paget's disease, skull as frequent site of, 1722
Pain
associated with iris, 1724–1725
congenital universal absence of, 1686–1687
corneal, 1606–1607, 1724
facial, with sixth nerve palsy, *1730*, 1730–1731
in ischemic optic neuropathies, 557
in nonarteritic anterior ischemic optic neuropathy (NAION), 557
ocular, 601, 1726–1727, 3467
after instillation of pilocarpine, 1724
in optic neuritis, 601
ophthalmic division
associated with occlusion of internal carotid artery, 1707
associated with occlusion of posterior cerebral artery, 1707–1708
orbital, 601
postoperative orbit, 1726
related to teeth, 1733
retroauricular, 1702
retrobulbar, 1726–1727
skin, 1606
thalamic, 1750
trigeminal, during and after herpes zoster oph, 1729
Pain sensation, 1650
Pain syndromes, 5569
Palate, paralysis of, 4127
Palato-ocular myoclonus, 5602
Paleopallium, 19
Palinopsia, 454, 1842
anatomic correlations, 456, *456*, *457*
associated findings, 454–455
etiology, 456
features, 454
pathophysiology, 455–456
prognosis, 455
psychogenic, 456
Palpebral fissure, 1510, *1510*
Palpebromandibular reflex, 1571, 1658
Palsy
abducens nerve
chronic, isolated paralysis, 1255–1256
cyclic esotropia and its relationship to, 1258
evaluation and management of, 1256–1257
lesions of
in cavernous sinus and superior orbital fissure, 1253–1254, *1254*, *1255*
extradural portion of, at petrous apex, 1253
within orbit, 1254–1255
in subarachnoid space, 1250–1253, *1252*
in uncertain or variable location, 1255
and nuclear horizontal gaze paralysis, 1237
acquired, 1244–1245, *1248*, 1248–1256, *1249*, *1250*, *1251*, *1252*, *1253*, *1254*, *1255*
congenital, 1237–1242, *1238*, *1239*, *1240*, *1241*, *1242*, *1243*, 1244, *1244*, *1245*, *1246*, *1247*
cyclic esotropia and its relationship to, 1258
divergence weakness and its relationship to, 1257
evaluation and management of, 1256–1257
acquired oculomotor nerve
evaluation and management of patients with, 1225–1227
recovery from, 1220
acquired trochlear nerve
differential diagnosis of, 1236

Palsy—*continued*
evaluation and management of, 1236–1237
Bell's, 1562, 1563, 4982
diagnosis of, 1563
treatment of, 1563–1564
congenital adduction, with synergistic divergence, 1191–1192, *1192, 1193*
conjugate gaze, 1848
contralateral trochlear nerve, 968
double elevator, 1311
facial nerve, insufficiency of eyelid closure from, *1558,* 1560–1564, *1562*
facial pain with sixth nerve, *1730,* 1730–1731
isolated oculomotor nerve, 3118
ocular motor nerve, 1865, 2177–2178
oculomotor, with cyclic spasms, 1554
progressive bulbar, 2799
progressive supranuclear, 2771
pseudo-6th nerve, 1781
pseudo-abducens, 1304
subarachnoid oculomotor nerve
from involvement at or near its entrance to cavernous sinus, 1209, *1211,* 1211–1212, *1212, 1213*
isolated fixed, dilated pupil as sole manifestation of, 1203–1204
supranuclear gaze, 5509
Pamaquine, 1263
Pancreatic cysts, 2705
Pancreatitis, 3819, 5105, 5226
Pandysautonomia, acute, 1028–1029
Panencephalic Creutzfeldt-Jakob disease, 4584, *4586*
Panencephalitis
progressive rubella, 5290–5291
subacute sclerosing, 5213
clinical manifestations, *5214,* 5214–5216, *5215, 5216, 5217*
diagnosis, 5217, 5220, *5223, 5224*
epidemiology, 5213–5214
pathogenesis, 5217
pathology, 5216–5217, *5218, 5219*
treatment and prognosis, 5220, *5224*
Panhypopituitarism, 2159, 2165, 4159
Panophthalmitis of meningococcal meningitis, 4096–4097
Panuveitis, 5236
Papaverine for delayed cerebral ischemia, 3172
Papaverine hydrochloride, 1004–1005
Papilledema, 259, *261, 262, 263,* 485, 1795, 1824, 1835, 1844, 1848, 1860, 1865, 2044, 2338, 2577, 3032–3033, 3797, 3805, 3958, 4160–4161, 4184, 4373, 4876, 5088, 5256, 5431–5432, *5498,* 5500, 5641, 5687, *5690,* 5709, 5728
from acute and chronic subdural hematoma, 516
and age, 504
and aqueductal stenosis, 515
and arteriovenous malformations (AVMS), 516
asymmetric, *498,* 498–499, *499, 500*
from brain abscesses, 516
in carcinomatous lymphomatous, and leukemic meningitis, 518
in cerebral and leptomeningeal gliomatosis, 518
in chronic inflammatory demyelinating polyneuropathy (CIDP), 518–519, *519*
and craniosynostosis, 520
development, 503
diagnosis, 501–502, *502*
differential diagnosis, 503, 503*t*
from epidural hematoma, 516
etiology, 514–533
and hyperthyroidism, 521
from intracranial masses, 515
in Landry-Guillain-Barré syndrome (GBS), 518–519, *519*
and late-onset citrullinemia, 521
measurements of intracranial pressure, 486–487, *487*
in meningococcal meningitis, 4097
monitoring, 533–534
in mucopolysaccharidoses, 519–520
and multiple myeloma, 520–521
nonvisual manifestations, 509–510
ophthalmoscopic appearance
chronic, 494, *494*
early, 487–489, *488, 489, 490, 491*
fully developed, *491, 492,* 492–494, *493*
postpapilledema atrophy, 494, *495, 496,* 496–497, *497, 498*
unilateral or asymmetric, *498,* 498–499, *499, 500*
pathogenesis, 507–509, *509*
pathology, 504, *506,* 506–507, *507, 508*
in Poems syndrome (Crow-Fukase syndrome), 520
resolution, 504, *505*
in septic and aseptic meningitis and encephalitis, 517–518
as sign of tumors, 1791
and spinal cord lesions, 518
from subarachnoid hemorrhage, 516–517
in systemic lupus erythematosus, 3829
terminology, 485–486
after trauma, 517
treatment, 534–536
true, 673
in tuberculous meningitis, 4154–4155
unilateral, *498,* 498–499, *499, 500*
visual manifestations, 510, *511,* 512, *512, 513,* 514
visual prognosis, 504
Papillomacular bundle, 50
Papillomacular fibers, 50
Papillopathy, diabetic, *564,* 564–565
Papillophlebitis, 583, *584,* 3919–3920
Papovaviridae, 5131, *5131*
papillomaviruses, 5132
polyomaviruses, 5132
BK virus, *5132,* 5132–5133
JC virus, *5133,* 5133–5139, *5134, 5135, 5136, 5137, 5138, 5139, 5140, 5141,* 5141–5142, *5142*
Pappataci fever, 5163
Paracentral artery, 2897
Paracentral scotomas, 602
Paraclinoid aneurysms, *3055, 3056,* 3056–3059, *3057, 3058*
Paracoccidioides brasiliensis, 4282, 4406–4407, *4408*
clinical manifestations, 4408–4410, *4409, 4410*
demographics, 4407–4408
diagnosis, 4410–4411
pathology, 4410, *4411*
pathophysiology, 4408
treatment, 4411–4412
Paracoccidioidomycosis, 4407, 5422
Paracusia, 1831
Paradoxic gustolacrimal reflexes, crocodile tears, 1022–1025, *1023*
Paradoxic levator excitation
eyelid retraction and ptosis from combined, 1554, *1555*
eyelid retraction from, 1551, *1553,* 1553–1555, *1554, 1555*
Paradoxic levator inhibition, eyelid retraction and ptosis from combined, 1554, *1555*
Paradoxical reaction of pupils to light and darkness, 990
Paraflocculus, experimental lesions of, 1290
Paraganglia, 2462
Paragangliomas, 2321
branchiomeric, 2464–2468, *2466, 2467, 2468, 2469, 2470,* 2470–2471
carotid body, 2465–2468, *2468*
of glomus jugulare, 2468, *2469,* 2470–2471
of head and neck, 2462–2464, *2463, 2464, 2465*
branchiomeric, 2464–2468, *2466, 2467, 2468, 2469, 2470,* 2470–2471
intravagal, 2471–2472, *2472*
intravagal, 2471–2472, *2472*
of orbit, 2471
Paragonimiasis, 4479, *4481,* 4481–4483, *4482, 4483, 4484,* 4485
Paragonimus species in intracranial brain abscess, 3952
Paragonium, 4479, *4481,* 4481–4483, *4482, 4483, 4484,* 4485
Paragonium heterotremus, 4479
Paragonium mexicanus, 4479
Paragonium miyazaki, 4479
Paragonium westermani, 4479
Parainfectious optic neuritis, 628–629
Parainfluenza viruses, 5231
characteristics of, 5231, *5231*
clinical manifestations, 5232
Paralysis
accommodation for distance, 1016
bulbar, 5245
of divergence, 5727
flaccid motor, 5239, 5242
Paralytic poliomyelitis, 5254–5255
Paralytic pontine exotropia, 1302, 3510, 5612, *5612*
Paralytic rabies, 5273
Paramedian infarction, 3483
Paramedian mesencephalic syndrome, 3506
Paramedian pontine reticular formation, 1080–1081, 1299–1301
Paramyotonia congenita, 1376
Paramyxoviridae, 5198, *5199,* 5200
measles, 5200
clinical manifestations, 5201, *5201*
complications, 5201, *5202,* 5203–5208, *5204, 5205, 5206, 5208, 5209, 5210*
diagnosis, 5209–5210
epidemiology, 5200
pathogenesis, 5208–5209
prevention and complications of vaccination, 5210–5213, *5211, 5212, 5213*
treatment, 5210
morbilliviruses, 5200–5201, *5201, 5202,* 5203–5217, *5204, 5205, 5206, 5208, 5209, 5210, 5211, 5212, 5213, 5214, 5215, 5216, 5217, 5218, 5219,* 5220, *5220*
characteristics of, 5200
measles, 5200

clinical manifestations, 5201, *5201*
complications, 5201, *5202,* 5203–5208, *5204, 5205, 5206, 5208, 5209, 5210*
diagnosis, 5209–5210
epidemiology, 5200
pathogenesis, 5208–5209
prevention and complication of vaccination, 5210–5213, *5211, 5212, 5213*
treatment, 5210
parainfluenza viruses, 5231
characteristics of, 5231, *5231*
clinical manifestations, 5232
paramyxoviruses, 5220
mumps virus, 5223
characteristics of, 5223, *5225*
clinical manifestations of, 5225, *5226*
complications of, 5225–5229, *5227*
diagnosis of, 5229–5230
epidemiology of, 5223, 5225
pathogenesis of, 5225
prognosis of, 5230–5231
treatment of, 5230
prevention, 5231
pneumoviruses (respiratory syncytial virus), *5232,* 5232–5233, *5233*
subacute sclerosing panencephalitis, 5213
clinical manifestations, *5214,* 5214–5216, *5215, 5216, 5217*
diagnosis, 5217, 5220, *5223, 5224*
epidemiology, 5213–5214
pathogenesis, 5217
pathology, 5216–5217, *5218, 5219*
treatment and prognosis, 5220, *5224*
Paramyxoviruses, 5220
mumps virus, 5223
characteristics of, 5223, *5225*
clinical manifestations of, 5225, *5226*
complications of, 5225–5229, *5227*
diagnosis of, 5229–5230
epidemiology of, 5223, 5225
pathogenesis of, 5225
prognosis of, 5230–5231
treatment of, 5230
prevention, 5231
Paranasal sinus blastomycosis, 4338
Paranasal sinuses, 72, 5470
aspergillomas in, 4291
malignant tumors of, 2450–2453, *2451, 2452, 2453*
relationship between optic canal and, 71
Paranasal sinusitis as cause of brain abscess, 3945
Paraneoplastic cerebellar degeneration, 1293
Paraneoplastic disorders, 2360
of voluntary muscle
acute necrotizing myopathy, 2530
cachectic myopathy, 2530–2531
dermatomyositis, 2527–2530, *2528*
endocrine myopathies, 2531
polymyositis, *2527,* 2527–2530, *2529*
Paraneoplastic encephalomyelitis, 2498
brainstem (bulbar), 2498–2500, *2500*
cerebellar, 2500–2501
cerebral (limbic), 2498, *2499*
diagnostic evaluations, *2502,* 2502–2503, 2503*t*
differential diagnosis, 2503–2504
pathogenesis, anti-Hu syndrome, *2504,* 2504–2505, *2505*
pathology, 2501–2502
prognosis, 2505
subacute myelitis, 2501
treatment, 2505
Paraneoplastic optic neuropathy, 2541–2543, *2542*
Paraneoplastic peripheral neuropathies, 2521
acute sensorimotor, 2523–2524
carcinomatous neuromyopathy, 2524
chronic progressive sensorimotor, 2522–2523
subacute motor, 2522
subacute sensorimotor, 2523–2524
subacute sensory, 2521–2522
Paraneoplastic retinopathies, 2532, 2533*t*
cancer-associated, 2533, *2534, 2535,* 2535–2537, *2536, 2537*
cancer-associated cone dysfunction, 2537
diffuse uveal melanocytic proliferation, 2538–2541, *2540*
melanoma-associated, 2537–2538, *2539*
uveomeningitis, 2541
Paraneoplastic rigidity, 2531–2532
Paraneoplastic syndromes, 2497–2498
affecting central nervous system (CNS)
encephalomyelitis, 2498
brainstem (bulbar), 2498–2500, *2500*
cerebellar, 2500–2501
cerebral (limbic), 2498, *2499*
diagnostic evaluations, *2502,* 2502–2503, 2503*t*
differential diagnosis, 2503–2504
pathogenesis, anti-Hu syndrome, *2504,* 2504–2505, *2505*
pathology, 2501–2502
prognosis, 2505
subacute myelitis, 2501
treatment, 2505
necrotizing myelopathy
clinical features, 2514
diagnostic evaluations, 2515
differential diagnosis, 2515
pathogenesis, 2515
pathology, 2514–2515
treatment and prognosis, 2515
of opsoclonus, myoclonus, and ataxia, 2510
clinical features, 2510–2511
diagnostic evaluations, 2511–2513, *2512*
differential diagnosis, 2513
pathogenesis, 2513
pathology, 2511, *2511*
prognosis, 2514
treatment, 2513–2514
subacute cerebellar degeneration, 2505
clinical features, 2505–2507
diagnostic evaluations, 2507, *2509*
differential diagnosis, 2507
pathogenesis, 2507–2509, *2510*
pathology, 2507, *2508*
prognosis, 2509–2510
treatment, 2509
involving eyes and optic nerves
optic neuropathy, 2541–2543, *2542*
retinopathies, 2532, 2533*t*
cancer-associated, 2533, *2534, 2535,* 2535–2537, *2536, 2537*
cancer-associated cone dysfunction, 2537
diffuse uveal melanocytic proliferation, 2538–2541, *2540*
melanoma-associated, 2537–2538, *2539*
uveomeningitis, 2541
tonic pupils, 2543–2544, *2544*
of opsoclonus, myoclonus, and ataxia, 2510
clinical features, 2510–2511
diagnostic evaluations, 2511–2513, *2512*
differential diagnosis, 2513
pathogenesis, 2513
pathology, 2511, *2511*
prognosis, 2514
treatment, 2513–2514
Paranodal region, 3974
Paraplegia, 5635, 5637
hereditary spastic, 2794, 2795*t*
complicated forms of, 2795
pure, 2794–2795
in neuromyelitis optica, 624–625
Paraproteinemias, 3359
Parasagittal meningiomas, 2037, *2039,* 2039–2041, *2040, 2042,* 2043
Parasol cells, 46, 47
Parasympathetic nervous system, in lacrimal secretion, 925
Parasympathetic pathway to lacrimal gland, 2–3, *3, 4,* 5, *5, 6,* 7–8, 228, *1175*
Parasympatholytic agents, *1000, 1001,* 1001–1003, *1002, 1003*
pharmacologic blockade with, 984, *985*
Parasympathomimetic drugs, 1005, *1006*
Paratrigeminal neuralgia, 1700–1701
Paratrigeminal syndrome, 1701
Paratyphoid fever, 4221
Paraventricular nucleus, 830
Parenchyma, leukemic involvement of brain, 2338, *2338*
Parenchymal central nervous system (CNS) disease, 5409–5424, *5410, 5412, 5413, 5414, 5418, 5420*
Parenchymal damage, 3805–3806
Parenchymal disease, 5407
Parenchymal metastatic tumors, 2477, 2479, *2479, 2480, 2481, 2482, 2483,* 2483–2484, *2484, 2485, 2486*
Parenchymal neurocysticercosis, *4463,* 4463–4465
Parenchymatous neurosyphilis, 4883, 4886–4887
Parent vessel ligation, 3152
Paresis
abducens nerve, 3128, 3214, 5606, 5608, 5709
bilateral abducens, 5087
bilateral horizontal gaze, 5603
combined ocular motor nerve, 3128
cranial nerve, 5087, 5245
general, 4889–4891
horizontal gaze, 5433, 5603, 5727
isolated abducens, 3118
isolated facial nerve, 5023
ocular motor nerve, 1848, 2617–2618, 5043, 5433, 5508–5509, 5605–5606, *5607, 5608,* 5608–5609, *5609,* 5729
in pituitary adenomas, 2179*t*
oculomotor nerve, 3046–3047, 3075, 3127–3128, 5023, 5087
oculosympathetic, 964
of one or more ocular motor nerves, 3043
trochlear nerve, 3043, 3046, 3128, 5087
unilateral abducens, 5248
unilateral facial nerve, 5248
vertical gaze, 5433, 5727
Parietal arteries, superior, 2897
Parietal cortex in saccadic eye movements, 1118–1120

Parietal lobes
  abscesses of, 3957, 3958
  anatomy and functions of, 1837–1838, *1838*
  hemorrhage in, 3597
  lesions of, *343, 344, 345,* 347, *347, 348,* 349, 1322–1323
  tumors involving, 1837–1844, *1838, 1839, 1843*
    symptoms and signs produced by, 1838–1844, *1839, 1843*
  visual attention and, 1129–1130
Parieto-occipital artery, 2931
Parinaud's syndrome, 1853–1854, 1868, 1873, 3497
Parkinsonism, 1316–1318, *1318,* 1550, 1568, 2039
  drug-induced, 2771
  MPTP-induced, 1568
Parkinson's disease, 4605
  and other basal ganglia disorders
    corticobasal ganglionic degeneration
      laboratory studies, 2780, *2781*
      neurologic manifestations, 2779–2780
      neuro-ophthalmologic manifestations, 2780
      pathology, 2779, *2779*
      pathophysiology, 2780
      treatment, 2780
    Huntington's
      diagnosis, 2783–2784
      epidemiology, 2780–2781
      etiology, 2781–2782
      genetic testing, 2784
      laboratory and neuroimaging studies, 2783
      neurologic manifestations, 2782–2783
      ocular motor manifestations, 2783
      pathology, 2781, *2782*
      pathophysiology, 2782
      prognosis, 2784
      treatment, 2784
      visual sensory manifestations, 2783
    idiopathic, 2764
      differential diagnosis, 2770–2771
      epidemiology, 2764
      etiology, 2767–2768
      laboratory and neuroimaging findings, 2770
      neurologic manifestations, 2768–2769
      ocular motor manifestations, 2770
      pathology and neurochemistry, *2764,* 2764–2767, *2765, 2766, 2767*
      pathophysiology, 2768, *2769*
      prognosis, 2772
      treatment, 2771–2772
      visual sensory manifestations, 2770
    multiple system atrophy, 2776, 2776*t*
      epidemiology, 2776
      laboratory and neuroimaging findings, *2778,* 2778–2779
      neurologic manifestations, 2776–2778, 2777*t*
      neuro-ophthalmologic manifestations, 2778
      pathology, 2776, *2777*
      prognosis, 2779
      treatment, 2779
    Steele-Richardson-Olszewski syndrome
      epidemiology, 2772
      etiology, 2773
      eyelid manifestations, 2775
      laboratory and neuroimaging findings, 2775–2776
      neurologic manifestations, 2773
      neuro-ophthalmologic manifestations, 2773–2775, *2775*
      pathology, *27,* 2772–2773, *2774*
      prognosis, 2776
      treatment, 2776
Parotitis of mumps, 5225
Paroxysmal nocturnal hemoglobinuria, 523–524
Parry-Romberg syndrome, 1801
Pars distalis, 2141
Pars intermedia, 2141
Pars nervosa, 2141
Pars planitis, 5581
Partial nonprogressing stroke (PNS), 3324
Parvocellular cells, 46
Parvocellular layers, 106
Parvoviridae, 5142–5143, *5143, 5144, 5145,* 5145–5147, *5146*
  vaccinia virus, 5149–5154, *5151, 5152, 5153*
  variola, 5148–5149, *5150*
Parvovirus B19, 5146
Passive immunization. (*See* Vaccines.)
Pasteurella, 4240
Pasteurella haemolytica, 4193
Pasteurella multocida, 4240
Past-pointing, 1177, *1178*
Patau's syndrome, 2336
Pathergy phenomenon, 3805
Pattern Deviation Plot, 182
Pattern electroretinogram (PERG), 159, *221,* 222–223
Pattern Standard Deviation (PSD) on Humphrey Field Analyzer, 180
Paucibacillary disease, 4169
Pautruer's microabscesses, 2386, *2387, 2388*
Pearly tumors, 2108–2110, *2109*
Pediatric myasthenia, 1431
Peduncular hallucinations, 463–464
Peduncular hallucinosis, 1873
Peek phenomenon, 1564
Pelizaeus-Merzbacher disease, 766, 798, 1326, 1331, 1468, 2856–2857
Pelli-Robson chart, 168–169, 622
Pelopsia, 1842
Pendular nystagmus, 1462
Pendular seesaw nystagmus, 1478
Penicillium in fungal aneurysms, 3004
Peninsula pupils, 1008
Pentoxifylline for cerebral malaria, 4662
Peptic disc, angiomas of, 2707
Peptostreptococci, 4092
Peptostreptococcus
  in empyema, 3983
  in intracranial brain abscess, 3947, 3950, 3952
Peptostreptococcus anaerobius, 4092
  in intracranial brain abscess, 3952
Peptostreptococcus micros, 4092
  in intracranial brain abscess, 3952
Perceptual deficit in prosopagnosia, 416–417
Percutaneous radiofrequency trigeminal rhizotomy, 1739, 1741
  for trigeminal neuralgia, 1738
Percutaneous retrogasserian glycerol rhizotomy for trigeminal neuralgia, 1738
Percutaneous transluminal angioplasty, 3566, 3576
Percutaneously placed vascular stents, *3164,* 3164–3165, *3165, 3166, 3167*
Perfusion, agents to increase, 3562
Pergolide mesylate for pituitary adenomas, 2192
Perianal amoebiasis, 4619
Periaqueductal gray matter, 1308
Periarteritis nodosa. (*See* Polyarteritis nodosa.)
Periaxial demyelination, 3974, 5539
Pericallosal artery, 2891
  aneurysms, 3093
Pericardial amoebiasis, 4620
Pericarditis, 4347, 5103, 5193
  acute, 3816
Perifascicular myofiber necrosis or atrophy, 1395
Perimesencephalic hemorrhage, 3131
Perimetry, 204
  Amsler grid, *157,* 174–175
  ancillary information, 178, *181*
  confrontation, 172–174, *173, 174*
  five-step approach to interpretation, 185–186, *186, 187, 188, 189, 190, 191, 192, 193,* 194, 194*t*, *195, 196, 197, 198, 199, 200, 201, 202, 203*
  flicker, 207
  frequency doubling, 208–209, *209*
  general principles, 169–171
  Goldmann manual projection perimeter, 176–177, *177*
  graphic representation of data, 178, *180*
  high-pass resolution perimetry (HRP), 205–207, *207*
  indices, 180, 182
  interpretation of information, 178
  motion and displacement, 207–208, *208*
  new, *204,* 204–209, *205, 206, 207, 208, 209*
  probability plots, 182, *182, 183*
  progression of loss, 182, *184,* 184–185, *185*
  psychophysical basis for, *171,* 171–172, *172*
  reliability indices, 178–180
  Short Wavelength Automated Perimetry, *204,* 204–205, *205, 206*
  static, 177, *177*
  in studying anterior limit of Meyer-Archambault loop, 122–123
  suprathreshold static, 177–178, *179*
  tangent (Bjerrum) screen, *175,* 175–176, *176*
  techniques for, 172
Perineural invasion in cylindroma, 2454
Perineuritis, optic, 599, 628, *638,* 639, 4097, 4872, 5432
Perinodal region, 3974
Periodic alternating gaze deviation, 1494
Periodic alternating nystagmus, 1475–1476, *1476,* 1476*t*, 1496
Periodic alternating windmill nystagmus, 1476
Periodic paralysis, 1376–1377, *1377*
  hyperkalemic, 1377, *1378*
  hypokalemic, 1377, *1377*
Perioptic neuritis, 599, 628, *638,* 639, 4872
Periorbital directional Doppler ultrasonography, 3540–3541
Periorbital skin, effects of radiation therapy on, 2613
Periostitis, syphilitic, 1722
Peripapillary central serous choroidopathy, 814
Peripapillary retinal nerve fiber layer
  evaluation of, in diagnosis of optic atrophy, 287–288, *288, 289,* 290, *290*
  hemorrhage of, 488–489, *490*
Peripapillary staphyloma, *780,* 785, 789–790
Peripapillary subretinal neurovascularization, 814

Peripheral autonomic nervous system, 837–838
parasympathetic (craniosacral), 839–840, *840*
sympathetic (thoracolumbar), 838–839
Peripheral eosinophilia, 4287, 4452
Peripheral nerves
damage to, 5497–5498
malignant sheath tumors of, 2316–2318, *2317, 2318*
miscellaneous tumors of, 2321–2322
schwannomas of, 2316
Peripheral nervous system, 5386–5387
gonococcal infection of, 4102
Peripheral neuroblastoma, 1985–1988, *1987*
Peripheral neuropathy, 674, 2353, 2561, 2573–2574, 3744, 3757–3758, 3837, 4141–4142, 5539
in Lyme disease, 4814
Peripheral parasympathetic (craniosacral) nervous system, 839–840, *840*
Peripheral polyneuritis, 4127
Peripheral sympathetic (thoracolumbar) nervous system, 838–839
Peripheral vestibular nystagmus
clinical features of, 1470
induced by caloric or galvanic stimulation, 1471–1472
Peripheral visual field defects, 810–812, *812*
Peripheral wedge-shaped cataracts, 2667
Periphlebitis, retinal, 5491, *5491, 5492*
Peritonsillar abscess, 4085
Peritonsillar cellulitis, 4085
Periungual fibromas, 2675, *2675*
Perivascular pseudorosettes, *1964,* 1964–1965
Permanent diplopia, 3694
Permanent neurologic deficits, *3695,* 3695–3696, *3696, 3697*
Pernicious anemia, 668, 669, 675
Peroxisomes disorders, 2841*t*, 2841–2842
hyperoxaluria type 1, 2848
infantile Refsum disease, 2843–2844
neonatal adrenoleukodystrophy, 2843, *2844*
Rhizomelic chondrodysplasia punctata, 2844–2845
X-linked adrenoleukodystrophy, 2845–2847, *2846, 2847, 2848*
Zellweger cerebrohepatorenal syndrome, *2842,* 2842–2843
Zellweger-like disease, 2844
Persistent generalized lymphadenopathy, 5373
Persistent hepatitis B virus infection, 4965–4966
Persistent neutrophilic meningitis, 4016
Persistent primitive acoustic (otic) artery, 2936, *2940*
Persistent primitive hypoglossal artery, 2936, *2939, 2941, 2942*
Persistent primitive trigeminal artery, 2935, *2939*
Persistent pupillary membrane remnants, 1008
Pertussis, *4209,* 4209–4210
Pertussis encephalopathy, 4210
Petechial lesions, 4098
Petrosal nerve, lesions affecting greater superficial, 1019, *1020, 1021*
Petrosal sinuses, 2964, *2965*
Petrous segment, 2871, *2871, 2872*
Peutz-Jeghers syndrome, 2735
Phacomatoses, 2647. (*See also* Ataxia telangiectasia; Encephalotrigeminal angiomatosis; Klippel-Trénaunay-Weber syndrome; Neurofibromatosis; Tuberous sclerosis; von Hippel-Lindau (VHL) disease; Wyburn-Mason syndrome.)
Phagocytic activity, 3328
Phakomatoses, 2083
Pharmacologic agents
accommodation insufficiency and paralysis from, 1016
accommodation spasm from, 1018
Pharmacologic stimulation
of iris dilator, 974
of iris sphincter, 974
Pharmacologic tests, 1419–1420
Pharmacologically dilated pupils, *1783,* 1783–1784
Pharyngitis, 4981
nonstreptococcal, 4105
Pharyngoconjunctival fever (PCF), 4956
Phase, acquisition, 450
Phenacetin, for headaches, 1718
Phencyclidine, 3586
Phenelzine, for cough-induced headache, 1703
Pheneramine maleate, 1004
Phenothiazine toxicity, 5731
Phenothiazines
impact of, on postsynaptic neuromuscular transmission, 1441
for pituitary adenomas, 2196
Phenylalanemia, malignant, 2812
Phenylalanine hydroxylase deficiency (phenylketonuria), 2811–2812
Phenylalaninemia
dihydropteridine reductase defect, 2812
phenylalanine hydroxylase deficiency, 2811–2812
Phenylbutazone, 1263
Phenylephrine, 1003
Phenylketonuria, and dietary management, 2811–2812
Phenylpropanolamine, 3586
Phenytoin for neuromyotonia, 2532
Pheochromocytoma, *2458,* 2458–2460, 2459*t*, *2460, 2461,* 2462, 2661, 2705, 3012
headaches associated with, 1713
Phialophora verrucosa, 4353
Philophthalmus, 4494
Phlebovirus, *5163,* 5163–5165, *5164*
Phonologic dyslexia, 435
Phosphenes, 5582
Photo stress recovery time (PSRT), 157–158
Photo stress test, 157–158
Photo-oculodynia syndrome, 1726
Photophobia, 930, 1731, 2176–2177, 3675
and migraines, 3663
Photopsias, 154, 601, 2257
Photoreceptors, 30–35, *32, 34*
degeneration of, 2535
Photosensitivity, 3813
Phthisis bulbi, 1997
Phycomycetes
in fungal aneurysms, 3971
in intracranial brain abscess, 3952
Physiologic anisocoria, 936
Physiologic nystagmus, 1462
Physiologic pupillary unrest, 885–887
Physostigmine, 1005
Pia mater, 73, 2021
external cellular layer of, as barrier to infection, 3941
Pickford-Nicholson anomaloscope, 212
Pick's disease and other lobar degenerations, 2759–2764, *2761, 2762, 2763*
Pickwickian syndrome, 528
Picornaviridae, 5233–5234, *5234*
coxsackieviruses, 5235–5241
echoviruses, 5241–5243
enteroviruses, 5234–5235, 5243–5250, *5244, 5246*
polioviruses, 5250–5258, *5251, 5252, 5253, 5254*
rhinovirus, 5258
Picotamide, 3561
Pigmentary retinopathy, 1383, 5292
Pigmented ciliary epithelium, 900
Pigmented lesions, 2649
Pigmentosa, retinitis, 4907
Pilocarpine, ocular pain after instillation of, 1724
Pilocytic astrocytes, 1921, *1922*
Pilocytic astrocytomas, *1930,* 1930–1931, *1931*
Pineal artery, 1865
Pineal body, 17
Pineal gland
astrocytomas of, 1936–1937, *1937*
tumors involving, *1851, 1865,* 1865–1871, *1866, 1868, 1869*
Pineal parenchymal cells
embryonal tumors
ependymoblastoma, 1979
medulloblastoma, 1979–1984, *1981, 1982, 1983*
medulloepithelioma, 1984–1985, *1985, 1986*
neuroblastoma, 1985–1990, *1987, 1988, 1989, 1991*
primitive neuroectodermal, *1999,* 1999–2000, *2000*
retinoblastoma, 1990–1999, *1992, 1993, 1994, 1995, 1996*
tumors of, 1972–1973, *1974,* 1975
neurons, 1975
ganglion cell
central neurocytoma, 1977–1978, *1978*
disembryoplastic infantile gangliogliomas, 1977
dysembryoplastic neuroepithelial, 1978–1979, *1979*
dysplastic cerebellar gangliocytoma, 1977, *1978*
gangliocytomas, 1975–1977, *1976*
gangliogliomas, 1975–1977, *1976*
pinealomas, 1972–1973, *1974,* 1975
Pinealocytes, 1865
Pinealomas, 1972–1973, *1974,* 1975
ectopic, 2085
Pineoblastomas, 1972, 2085
Pineocytomas, 1972
Ping-pong gaze, 1329
Pinta, 4844, *4845, 4846*
Pintids, 4844, *4846*
Piperazine citrate, 1263
Pituitary adenomas, 2987
associated with intracranial lesions, 2203
classification of, 2152–2154
clinical manifestations, 2155
of apoplexy, 2180
endocrine, 2155–2165, *2157, 2159, 2160, 2161, 2162*
other, caused by, 2185–2186
visual, 2165, *2166, 2167,* 2168, *2169, 2170,* 2170–2171, *2171, 2172, 2173,* 2174, *2174, 2175,* 2176–2180, *2177, 2178, 2179,* 2179*t*, *2180*
diagnosis of, *2152, 2153, 2154, 2161, 2179, 2181, 2184,* 2186–2187, *2188, 2189*

Pituitary adenomas—*continued*
  general considerations, 2149, *2150, 2151,* 2152, *2152, 2153, 2154, 2155*
  invasive (malignant), 2203–2204
  and pregnancy, 2201–2203
  prognosis in patients with, 2199
    endocrine, 2199–2200
    systemic, 2201
    visual, *2200,* 2200–2201
  therapy for, 2187–2188
    ACTH-secreting, 2197–2198
    associated with dysthyroidism, 2199
    gonadotropin-secreting, 2198–2199
    medicine, 2191–2192
    nonsecreting, 2193–2194
    PRL-secreting, 2194–2196, *2195, 2197*
    radiation, 2192–2193
    surgery, 2188–2191
    therapeutic options, 2188
Pituitary apoplexy, 2180–2185, *2181, 2182, 2183, 2184*
  manifestations of, 2180–2185, *2181, 2182, 2183, 2184*
  in patients with adenomas, *2181,* 2181–2185, *2182, 2183, 2184*
  syndrome of, 1815, 1816, *1816*
Pituitary carcinoma, *2205,* 2205–2206
Pituitary dysfunction, 5495
  syndromes of, 1815
Pituitary fossa, lesion of, 2206
Pituitary gland, 87
  anatomy of, 2141–2142, *2143, 2144,* 2144–2145, *2145*
  endocrine functions of anterior, 2146–2148
    adrenocorticotropic hormone (ACTH), 2147
    gonadotropins, luteinizing hormone (LH) and follicle-stimulating hormone (FSH), 2148
    growth hormone (GH), 2148–2149
    β-lipotropin hormone (β-LPH), 2147–2148
    prolactin (PRL), *2148,* 2149
    thyrotropin (thyroid-stimulating hormone, TSH), 2146–2147
  metastases to, 2206
  shape of, 87–88
Pituitary hyperthyroidism, 2163–2164
Pituitary macroadenomas, 1466
Plague
  bubonic, *4226,* 4226–4227, *4227*
  primary pneumonic, 4226–4227
  septicemic, 4227
Plague meningitis, 4227–4228
Plaque, 5547
  chronic active, 5552, 5555
  chronic inactive, 5552, *5553, 5554, 5555*
  demyelinating, 5549–5550
  shadow, 5555, 5558, *5559*
Plasma cells, 2329, 2330
Plasma exchange, beneficial effect of, 5692
Plasma-cell granulomas, 2398
Plasmacytomas, 2389
  intracranial, 2391
Plasmapheresis, 3811
  for Kawasaki disease, 5740
  for Lambert-Eaton myasthenic syndrome, 1437
  for myasthenia gravis, 1429–1430
  for neuromyotonia, 2532
Plasmodium species
  cerebral, 4657–4658
    clinical manifestations, *4658,* 4658–4659
    diagnosis, 4662
    pathogenesis, *4659,* 4659–4661, *4660*
    pathology, *4661,* 4661–4662, *4662, 4663, 4664, 4665*
    prognosis, 4664, 4666–4667
    treatment, 4662, *4664*
  clinical manifestations, 4654–4655, *4655*
  diagnosis, 4656
  epidemiology, 4651, 4653
  life cycle of, *4650,* 4650–4651, *4651, 4652, 4653*
  pathogenesis, 4653, *4654*
  prevention, 4667
  treatment, *4656,* 4656–4657, *4657*
Plasmotomy, 4613
Platelet activating factor (PAF), 3561
Platelet aggregation in migraines, 1695
Platelet-derived growth factor (PDGF), 3334
Platelet-fibrin emboli, 3367, *3370,* 3370–3371, *3371, 3372*
Pleomorphic xanthoastrocytomas, 1934, *1934*
Plerocercoids, 4443
Plesiomonas shigelloides, 4245
Pleurodynia, epidemic, 5235
Pleuropulmonary amoebiasis, 4620
Plexiform neurofibromas, 2319
Plexopathy
  brachial, 2607–2609
  lumbosacral, 2607–2609
Pluripotential stem cells, 2329
Plus-minus syndrome, 1549, *1552*
Pneumococcal meningitis, 4077–4079, *4078, 4079, 4080*
Pneumococcus, *4075,* 4075–4080, *4076, 4077, 4078, 4079, 4080*
Pneumoencephalogram, 2101
Pneumolysin, 4075
Pneumonia
  Mycoplasma pneumoniae in, 4546–4550, *4547, 4548, 4549, 4551,* 4552–4554
  necrotizing, 4346
  primary viral, 5192–5193
  Q fever presentation as, 4767
  secondary bacterial, 5193
Pneumonitis, 5104
  interstitial, in immunocompetent patients, 5102
  varicella, 5016
Pneumosinus dilatans, 72, 2048
Pneumoviruses, *5232,* 5232–5233, *5233*
POEMS syndrome, 2399
  papilledema in, 520
Point mutations of mitochondrial tRNAs in maternally inherited ophthalmoplegia, 1389
Pol gene, 5364–5365, 5365, 5434
Polar spongioblastomas, 1934, *1935*
Polioencephalitis, 5257
Poliomyelitis
  abortive, 5254
  bulbar paralytic, 5255–5256
  mixed bulbospinal paralytic, 5256
  nonparalytic, 5254
  paralytic, 5254–5255
  spinal paralytic, 5255
Polioviruses (polio), 5250–5258, *5251, 5252, 5253, 5254,* 5258
  clinical manifestations, 5253–5257
  diagnosis, 5257
  epidemiology, 5250–5251
  pathogenesis, 5251–5252, *5252*
  pathology, 5252–5253, *5253*
  prevention, 5258
  prognosis, 5257–5258
  treatment, 5257
Polyangiitis overlap syndrome, 529
Polyarteritis nodosa, *3743, 3744,* 3744–3751, *3745, 3746, 3747, 3748, 3750, 3751*
  central nervous system manifestations, 3745
  demographics, 3744
  diagnosis, 3749–3750, *3751*
  ocular and neuro-ophthalmologic manifestations, *3746,* 3746–3749, *3747, 3748*
  pathology, 3749, *3750*
  prognosis and treatment, 3751
  systemic manifestations, *3744,* 3744–3745
Polyarthritis, 3744
Polychondritis, relapsing, 3842–3845, *3844, 3845*
Polycoria, 1008
Polycystic kidney disease and development of aneurysms, 3010, *3011*
Polycythemia, 2705, 3357, *3358*
Polycythemia vera
  diagnosis, 2333
  general clinical manifestations, 2332
  neurologic manifestations, 2332
  ocular manifestations, 2332–2333, *2333, 2334*
  prognosis and treatment, 2333–2334
Polymerase chain reaction, 4100
  in diagnosing bacterial meningitis, 4010
  in diagnosing *E. histolytica,* 4622
Polymorphic cell sarcoma, 2071
Polymorphonuclear leukocytes, 2329
Polymorphonuclear neutrophils, 4001
  in host defense, 3996–3998
Polymyositis, 1397, *2527,* 2527–2530, *2529,* 2629, 3838–3841, *3839, 3840, 3841, 3842*
Polyneuritiformis, heredopathia atactica, 2840–2841
Polyneuritis, peripheral, 4127
Polyneuropathy
  acute inflammatory demyelinating, 5539
  chronic inflammatory demyelinating, 5539, 5707
    clinical manifestations, 5709–5710, *5710, 5712, 5713*
    diagnosis, 5711–5712
    epidemiology, 5707
    laboratory findings, 5710–5711
    natural history, 5712
    pathogenesis, 5708–5709
    pathology, 5707–5708, *5708*
    prognosis, 5712
    treatment, 5712
  chronic inflammatory demyelinating, papilledema in, 518–519, *519*
  demyelinating, 2561
  hereditary, 763–764
Polyneuropathy, organomegaly, endocrinopathy, monoclonal gammopathy, and skin changes (POEMS), 703
Polyomaviruses, 5132

BK virus, *5132,* 5132–5133
JC virus (progressive multifocal leukoencephalopathy), *5133,* 5133–5139, *5134, 5135, 5136, 5137, 5138, 5139, 5140, 5141,* 5141–5142, *5142*
Polyopia, 454, 3673
cerebral, 456–457, 1170
Polypoid tarsitis, 4901
Polyradiculitis, 5261
Polyradiculomyelopathy, subacute ascending, 5111–5112
Polyvalent ABE antitoxin, 4120
Polyvalent pneumococcal polysaccharide vaccine, 4079–4080
Pons
lesions of, 1680–1681, *1681*
ocular motor syndromes caused by lesions of
abducens nucleus, 1298–1299
combined unilateral conjugate gaze palsy and internuclear ophthalmoplegia, *1301,* 1301–1303, *1302*
internuclearophthalmoplegia, *1294,* 1294–1298, *1295, 1296, 1297,* 1298*t*, *1299, 1300*
paramedian pontine reticular formation, 1299–1301
saccadic oscillations from pontine, 1303
slow saccades from pontine, 1303, 1303*t*
tumors of, 1874–1875, *1876, 1877,* 1877–1878
Pontiac fever, 4237, 4239
Pontine hemorrhage, 3023, 3601–3604, *3603, 3604*
Pontine lesions, slow saccades from, 1303, 1303*t*
Port-wine stain, 2709
Positional exophthalmos, 2655
Positive phenomena, 454
Positive scotoma, 154
Positive sputum smear, 4140
Positive visual phenomena, 454
hallucinations, 457–464, *458, 459, 460, 461, 464, 465, 466,* 466–467
in optic neuritis, 601
perseveration, 454–457
Positron emission tomographic scanning, 3530, *3531,* 3532
in imaging multiple sclerosis, 5616
Postcentral gyrus, involvement of, 1685
Postchiasmal demyelinating neuritis of multiple sclerosis, *5595,* 5595–5596, *5597, 5598*
Postchiasmal visual pathway, sarcoidosis in, *5507,* 5507–5508, *5508*
Post-chiasmal visual system, disease affecting, 1466
Postconcussive syndrome, 1706
Posterior cerebral arteries, 3440–3441. (*See also* Cerebral arteries.)
aneurysms arising from, 3123, *3125,* 3125–3127, *3126*
and its branches, 2921–2922, *2922, 2923, 2924, 2925,* 2928–2929, *2929, 2930, 2931,* 2931–2932, *2932, 2933, 2934, 2935*
occlusion of, 3440–3441
ophthalmic division pain associated with occlusion of, 1707–1708
Posterior choroidal arteries, infarction, 3483
Posterior commissure, nucleus of, 1082
Posterior communicating arteries, 2884, 2886
aneurysms arising from, 3083, *3089*
internal carotid artery, aneurysms arising from junction with, *3075,* 3075–3083, *3076, 3077, 3078, 3079, 3081, 3082, 3083*
Posterior cortical atrophy, 469
Posterior fossa arteriovenous malformations (AVMs), 2261, 2263
dural, 2274, 2278
Posterior fossa hemangioblastomas, 2223, 2225, *2225*
Posterior fossa meningiomas, 2051–2052
Posterior fossa microvascular decompression, 1574
of trigeminal nerve for trigeminal neuralgia, 1738
Posterior fossa veins, 2952–2953
Posterior inferior cerebellar artery, *2904, 2905, 2906, 2908,* 2908–2910, *2909, 2910, 3207*
aneurysms arising from, 3108–3109, *3112, 3113*
Posterior inferior cerebellar artery syndrome, 3513
Posterior internuclear ophthalmoplegia, 1294
of Lutz, 4375
Posterior ischemic optic neuropathy (PION), 583, 2619, 3339, 3763–3764, *3765, 3766*
arteritic, 583–585, *585*
nonarteritic, 585, *586, 587, 588, 589,* 592
Posterior optic neuropathy, 717
Posterior pituitary ectopia, 782
Posterior scleritis, 1724
Posterior spinal artery, 2907–2908
Posterior subcapsular cataracts, 2667
Posterior superior alveolar artery, 2945
Posterior uveitis, 5581
Posterolateralis, nuclear ventralis, 1636
Posteromedialis, nuclear ventralis, 1629–1630
Postganglionic Horner's syndrome, 2447–2448, 3043
Postganglionic neuron, 969
Postganglionic sympathetic pathway, *881, 882,* 882–883
Postgeniculate congenital homonymous hemianopia, 989
Postgeniculate visual sensory pathway, embryology of, 16–17, *17, 18, 19,* 29
Postherpetic neuralgia, 1729–1730, 5037, 5068, 5072
Postictal cerebral blindness, 369
Postinfectious encephalomyelitis, 3989
Postinfectious optic neuritis, 4967
Postmicturition dysuria, 4488
Postmicturition hematuria, 4488
Postnatally acquired rubella, 5287–5289, *5288, 5289*
Postoperative mydriasis, 1011
Postpapilledema atrophy, 494, *495, 496,* 496–497, *497, 498*
Postpapilledema optic atrophy, 4153, 4184
Postpartum maternal meningitis, 4087
Postpoliomyelitis paralytic syndrome, 5258
Postpolycythemic myeloid metaplasia, 2333
Postprandial transient visual loss, 3422
Poststreptococcal acute glomerulonephritis, 4085
Poststreptococcal vasculitis, 4086
Postsynaptic congenital myasthenic syndromes, 1432, *1433,* 1434
Postsynaptic neuromuscular transmission, drugs that affect both, 1441–1443
Post-transplant lymphoproliferative disorder (PTLD), 2630–2631
Posttraumatic syndrome, 1706
Post-treatment reactive encephalopathy (PTRE), 4719
Postural suboccipital headache, 1704
Potential Acuity Meter, 154, 1769, 1771
Potter syndrome, 783
Pott's disease, 4163–4164, *4166*
Powassan encephalitis, 5189–5190
Power Doppler imaging, 3535–3536
Poxviridae, 5147–5148, *5148, 5149*
Praziquantel for neurocysticercosis, 4477
Prechiasmal optic nerve compression syndrome, 294
Predictive saccades, 1114
Prednisone for optic neuritis, 609–610
Pre-eclampsia, association with central retinal vein occlusion, 3918–3919
Preexcitation syndromes, 746
Prefrontal cortex in saccadic eye movements, 1118, *1119*
Preganglionic Horner's syndrome, 969
Preganglionic neuron, 968
Preganglionic sympathetic fibers, *880,* 880–881
Pregnancy
association with central retinal vein occlusion, 3918–3919
and development of multiple sclerosis, 5543
and pituitary adenomas, 2201–2203
as risk factor in aneurysms, 3012
thrombotic strokes during, 3362
Premammillary thalamoperforating artery, 2886
Preretinal hemorrhages, 3025
Presbyopia, 913–914
night, 910
Preseptal orbicularis oculi subdivision, 1510
Presumed ocular histoplasmosis syndrome, 4404–4406, *4405, 4406, 4407*
Presynaptic congenital myasthenic syndromes, 1432
Presynaptic neuromuscular transmission
drugs that affect both, 1441–1443
toxins that damage, 1437–1440
Pretectal syndrome, 1868
Primary acetylcholine receptor deficiency, 1432, 1434
Primary acquired autonomic dysfunction, 1028
Primary amoebic meningoencephalitis, 4623, *4625,* 4625–4626, *4626, 4627, 4628, 4629*
Primary anthrax meningitis, 4106
Primary axonal degeneration syndromes, 5703
acute motor neuropathy, 5705–5707, *5706*
Guillain-Barré, 5703–5705, *5704*
Primary axonal Guillain-Barré syndrome (GBS), 5703–5705, *5704*
Primary central nervous system (CNS) large-cell lymphoma, 2364–2366, *2366, 2367, 2368,* 2368–2370, *2369, 2370, 2371, 2372,* 2372–2375, *2373, 2374*
Primary central nervous system lymphoma, 5409, 5411–5412, *5412*
Primary central nervous system vasculitides, 3727–3729, *3728, 3729, 3730,* 3731–3732
Primary cerebral neuroblastoma, *1988,* 1988–1989, *1989*

Primary degenerative dementia, 2747–2748, 2748*t*
  Alzheimer's disease
    biochemical pathology, 2750
    clinical features, 2751–2755, 2752*t*
    diagnosis, 2755
    epidemiology, 2748–2749
    laboratory investigations, 2755
    neurologic manifestations, 2751–2753
    ocular motor manifestations, 2754–2755
    pathogenesis, 2751
    pathology, *2749,* 2749–2750, *2750, 2751*
    prognosis, 2756
    pupillary disturbances, 2755
    treatment, 2755–2756
    visual sensory manifestations, 2753–2754, *2754, 2755*
  frontotemporal
    behavioral and psychiatric manifestations, 2760–2762
    epidemiology, 2759
    laboratory and neuroimaging findings, 2762, *2762*
    neurologic manifestations, 2759–2760
    pathology, 2759, *2760, 2761*
    prognosis, 2762
  with Lewy bodies
    diagnosis, 2758, 2758*t*
    epidemiology, 2756
    laboratory and neuroimaging findings, 2758
    neurologic and psychiatric manifestations, 2757–2758
    neuro-ophthalmologic manifestations, 2758
    pathology, 2756–2757, *2757*
    pathophysiology, 2757
    prognosis, 2759
    treatment, 2758–2759
  Pick's disease and other lobar degenerations, 2759–2764, *2761, 2762, 2763*
  primary progressive aphasia, 2762–2763
    clinical manifestations, 2763
    epidemiology, 2763
    laboratory and neuroimaging findings, *2763,* 2764
    pathology, 2763
Primary deviation, 1176
Primary exoerythrocytic forms, 4650
Primary generalized (systemic) amyloidosis, 2401–2403, *2402*
Primary intracranial complications, 5387–5395, *5388, 5389,* 5390*t, 5391, 5392, 5393, 5394, 5395, 5396, 5397,* 5397–5399, *5398, 5399, 5400, 5401,* 5401–5407, *5402, 5403, 5404, 5405, 5406, 5407, 5408*
Primary intracranial sarcomas, 2071–2072
Primary intraventricular hemorrhage, 3597
Primary lateral sclerosis, 2799
Primary leptomeningeal gliomatosis, 1941, *1941*
Primary lymphangioleiomyomatosis, 2692
Primary neurologic complications, 5385
Primary ocular motor nerve synkinesis, 1805, 1807, *1809*
Primary oculomotor nerve synkinesis, 1225, *1225,* 3047, *3050*
Primary optic nerve sheath meningiomas, 2046–2051, *2047, 2048, 2049,* 2050*t*
Primary pneumonic plague, 4226–4227
Primary progressive aphasia, 2762–2763
  clinical manifestations, 2763
  epidemiology, 2763
  laboratory and neuroimaging findings, *2763,* 2764
  pathology, 2763
Primary sarcoma of meninges and brain, *2070,* 2070–2072, *2071, 2072*
Primary somatic sensory cortex, 1637, *1638, 1639,* 1640, *1640*
Primary spinal cord, 5386–5387
Primary synkinesis of oculomotor nerve, 3081
Primary syphilis, 4857, *4857, 4858*
Primary viral pneumonia, 5192–5193
Primary visual cortex, 126
  anatomy and histology of, 126, *127,* 128, *128, 129*
    layer 1, 128
    layer 2, 128
    layer 3, 128
    layer 4, 128
    layer 5, 128–129
    layer 6, 129
  physiology, 129–132, *130,* 131
    binocularity and ocular dominance columns, *132,* 132–133, *133, 134, 135*
    ocular dominance columns and amblyopia, 133–134
    organization and modularity, 134–135, *135, 136*
Primitive hypoglossal artery, 2870–2871
Primitive neuroectodermal tumors (PNETS), *1999,* 1999–2000, *2000*
Primitive or nuclear zone, 3
Prince Rule, 949
Prions, 4561–4562, 4562*t*
  animal diseases, 4567
    bovine spongiform encephalopathy, 4567
    scrapie, 4567
  future, 4605
  human diseases
    Creutzfeldt-Jakob disease, 4568–4569
      diagnosis, 4584, *4587,* 4587–4591, *4588, 4589, 4590, 4591*
      epidemiology, 4569, 4571
      familial, 4576–4577
      Iatrogenic, *4578,* 4578–4579
      pathology, 4580–4581, *4581, 4582, 4583,* 4584, *4584, 4585, 4586*
      prevention of Iatrogenic, 4592
      sporadic, 4571–4574, *4572, 4574, 4575,* 4576, *4576*
      treatment, 4592
    fatal familial insomnia, 4595, 4598
      cerebral metabolism, 4601–4602
      clinical characteristics, 4598–4599
      genetics, 4599–4600, *4601*
      pathology, 4600–4601, *4601, 4602*
    Gerstmann-Sträussler-Scheinker disease, 4592, 4594
      clinical characteristics, *4593,* 4594
      pathology and genetics, *4594,* 4594–4595, *4595, 4596, 4597, 4598, 4599, 4600*
    kuru, 4567, *4568*
      clinical characteristics, 4568
      diagnosis, 4568
      neuro-ophthalmologic features, 4568
      pathology, 4568, *4569, 4570, 4571*
      treatment, 4568
    other inherited diseases, 4602–4604
  myopathy and neuropathy, 4605
  protein gene, 4564
    function of normal, 4564–4565
    propagation and pathophysiology of, 4565–4566, *4566*
  proteins, 4562–4564, *4563, 4564*
Prism dissociation tests, 1772
PRNP gene, 4576–4577, 4602–4604
Probability plots, 182, *182, 183*
Probable ischemic optic neuropathy, 5051–5052
Procarbazine, 2565
  neuro-ophthalmologic toxicity, 2565
  neurotoxicity, 2565
  ocular toxicity, 2565
  systemic toxicity, 2565
Procercoids, 4443
Procerus, 1513, *1513*
Prodromal symptoms and signs, before rupture of intracranial aneurysm, 3021
Progestins for pituitary adenomas, 2196
Proglottids, 4439, *4440*
Progressing stroke, 3324
Progression of visual field loss, 182, *184,* 184–185, *185*
Progressive bulbar palsies, 2799
Progressive encephalopathy with edema, hypsarrhythmia, and optic atrophy (Peho syndrome), 760
Progressive multifocal leukoencephalopathy (PML), 2339–2340, 3978, *5133,* 5133–5139, *5134, 5135, 5136, 5137, 5138, 5139, 5140, 5141,* 5141–5142, *5142,* 5409, 5412–5413, *5413*
Progressive muscular atrophy, 2798–2799
Progressive optic atrophy with juvenile diabetes mellitus, diabetes insipidus, and hearing loss, 760–761
Progressive outer retinal necrosis (PORN), 5041, *5042,* 5426
Progressive rubella panencephalitis, 5290–5291
Progressive supranuclear palsy, 1313–1314, 1568, 2771. (*See also* Steele-Richardson-Olszewski syndrome.)
Progressive thrombosis, 3209
Progressive visual dysfunction in retrobulbar compressive optic neuropathies, *8,* 653–656, *654*
Progressive visual loss, 1824
Prolactin (PRL), *2148,* 2149
Prolactin secreting pituitary adenomas, treatment of, 2195–2196
Prolactin-inhibiting factor (PIF), 2146
Prolactinomas, 2155–2156
Prolactin-releasing factor (PRF), 2146
Prophylactics
  in preventing Lyme disease, 4831–4832
  in treating migraines, 3711–3713
Prophylaxis against influenza, 5198
Propionibacteria, 4135–4136
Propionibacterium acnes, 4135–4136
  in empyema, 3983
Propionibacterium in intracranial brain abscess, 3952
Propranolol for coital headaches, 1705
Proprioceptive stimuli, nystagmus induced by, 1471
Proptosis, 1799–1800, *1800, 1801,* 1825, 1835, 3050, 3130, 3269, 5729
  axial, 1799
  intermittent, 2252
  recurrent, 2252
  unilateral, 2260–2261
Prosencephalon, 16

Prosopagnosia, 142, 391, 1840, 3485
  anatomy, 417–419, *418, 419, 420*
  anterograde, 423–424
  apperceptive, 416
  associated deficits, 414–415
  associative, 416
  covert facial recognition, 414, *415*
  developmental, 420
  face perception in nonhuman primates, 421–423
  forms of, 416
  functional imaging, 423, *423*
  neuropsychology of face perception, 415–416
  other disorders of face perception, 424
  pathology, 419–420
  perceptual deficit in, 416–417
  recognition deficit in, 417, *417*
  specificity of impairment for faces in, 413–414
  symptoms, 413
Prostacyclin, 3557
Prostigmin test, *1417,* 1421–1422, *1422*
Protease, 5363, 5365
Protease inhibitors, 5383
Protein C, deficiency of, 3889
Protein gene, 4564
  function of normal, 4564–4565
  propagation and pathophysiology of, 4565–4566, *4566*
Protein S clotting assays, 3889
Proteinuria, Bence Jones, 2390
Proteus, 4220–4221
  in empyema, 3983
  in intracranial abscess, 3950
Proteus mirabilis, 4104, 4220
  in bacterial meningitis, 3994
  in sinusitis, 4025
Proteus myxofaciens, 4220
Proteus vulgaris, 4220
Proton magnetic resonance spectroscopy in imaging multiple sclerosis, 5624
Protoplasmic astrocytes, 1920
Protoplasmic astrocytomas, 1934–1935, *1935*
Protosis as sign of tumor, *1797,* 1798
Prototheca wickerhamii, 4419
Protozoa
  amoebae (amoebiasis), 4614, *4614*
    free-living, 4623
      Acanthamoeba species, 4628–4630, *4630, 4631,* 4632, *4632, 4633, 4634,* 4635, *4635, 4636, 4637,* 4638, *4638*
      Balammuthia mandrillaris (Leptomyxida), 4638, *4639, 4640,* 4640–4641, *4641*
      Naegleria fowleri, 4623–4626, *4624, 4625, 4626, 4627,* 4628, *4628, 4629*
    life cycle, *4614,* 4614–4615, *4615, 4616*
      clinical manifestations, 4619
      diagnosis, 4621–4623
      epidemiology, 4615
      extraintestinal disease, 4619–4621
      intestinal disease, 4619
      pathogenesis, 4615–4617
      pathology, 4617, *4617, 4618,* 4619
      prognosis, 4623
      treatment, 4623
  Babesia species
    clinical manifestations, 4644–4645
      neurologic, 4645
      systemic, 4645
    diagnosis, 4645–4646
    laboratory findings, 4645
    life cycle, *4642,* 4642–4644, *4643, 4644*
    pathology, 4644
    treatment and prognosis, 4646
  microsporidia, 4646–4647, *4647, 4648, 4649,* 4649–4650
  Plasmodium species
    cerebral malaria, 4657–4658
      clinical manifestations, *4658,* 4658–4659
      diagnosis, 4662
      pathogenesis, *4659,* 4659–4661, *4660*
      pathology, *4661,* 4661–4662, *4662, 4663, 4664, 4665*
      prognosis, 4664, 4666–4667
      treatment, 4662, *4664*
    clinical manifestations, 4654–4655, *4655*
    diagnosis, 4656
    epidemiology, 4651, 4653
    life cycle, *4650,* 4650–4651, *4651, 4652, 4653*
    pathogenesis, 4653, *4654*
    prevention, 4667
    treatment, *4656,* 4656–4657, *4657*
  Toxoplasma gondii
    clinical manifestations, 4670–4671
      acute acquired toxoplasmosis in immunocompetent patient, *4671,* 4671–4672, *4672*
      acute toxoplasmosis in immunodeficient patient, 4672–4673, *4674,* 4675, *4675, 4676,* 4677–4678, *4678, 4679*
      congenital toxoplasmosis, 4678, *4680,* 4681
      ocular toxoplasmosis, *4681,* 4681–4683, *4682, 4683*
    diagnosis, 4691–4694, *4694, 4695, 4696,* 4696–4699
    epidemiology, 4668–4670
    life cycle, *4666,* 4667–4668, *4668, 4669, 4670*
    pathogenesis, 4670, *4671*
    pathology, 4683, 4685
      of acquired central nervous system toxoplasmosis, *4686,* 4686–4687, *4687, 4688*
      of central nervous system toxoplasmosis, 4685
      neuro, of congenital toxoplasmosis, 4687, *4690*
      of ocular toxoplasmosis, 4687, *4690,* 4691, *4691, 4692*
      of toxoplasmic lymphadenitis, 4685
    prevention, 4701
    treatment and prognosis, *4699,* 4699–4701
  Trypanosoma species, 4701
    Trypanosoma brucei, 4710, *4710*
      clinical manifestations, *4714,* 4714–4715
      diagnosis, 4717–4719
      epidemiology, 4711, 4713–4714
      life cycle, *4710,* 4710–4711, *4711, 4712*
      pathology and pathogenesis, 4715–4717
      prognosis, 4719
      treatment, 4719
    Trypanosoma cruzi, 4701–4702, *4702*
      clinical manifestations, 4705–4706
      diagnosis, 4708–4709
      epidemiology, 4703–4705
      life cycle, *4702,* 4702–4703, *4703*
      pathogenesis, 4708
      pathology, 4706–4708, *4709*
      prevention, 4710
      treatment, 4709–4710
Protozoal disease, 5415–5416
Proximal myotonic myopathy (PROMM), 1371–1372
Pruritus, 2650, 2652
Psammoma bodies, 2027
Psammomatous meningiomas, 2027
Pseudallescheria boydii, 4282, *4412,* 4412–4415, *4413, 4414*
  in encephalitis, 3987
  in intracranial brain abscess, 3952
  in sinusitis, 4026
Pseudo-6th nerve palsy, 1781
Pseudo-abducens palsy, 1304
Pseudo-abducens paresis, 1781
Pseudoallescheriasis, 4412, 5422
Pseudoaneurysm, 3016
Pseudocaloric nystagmus, 1176
Pseudo-Hurler syndrome, 2823, 2827
Pseudohyphae, 4282
Pseudoisochromatic plates, 211
  in color vision testing, 156
Pseudomonas, 4240, 4243–4244
Pseudomonas aeruginosa, 4124, 4240–4243
  in bacterial meningitis, 3995
  in empyema, 3983
  in meningitis, 4241–4242, *4242*
  in sinusitis, 4025
Pseudomonas mallei, 4240
Pseudopapilledema, 805
  associated with optic disc drusen, 805
    ancillary studies, 808–810, *809, 810, 811*
    anomalous disc elevation without visible or buried or, *817,* 818
    complications with
      central visual loss, 812
      ischemic neuropathy, 813
      peripapillary central serous choroidopathy, 814
      peripapillary subretinal neurovascularization, 814
      prepapillary or peripapillary hemorrhages, 812–813
      retinal vascular occlusions, 813
      transient visual loss, 813–814
      visual field defects, 810–812, *812*
    distinguishing pseudopapilledema associated with buried drusen from papilledema, 807–808, *808,* 808*t*
    epidemiology, 805
    histology of, 814, *815*
    natural history, 805
    ophthalmoscopic appearance
      of buried disc drusen, 806–807, *807*
      of visible drusen, 805–806, *806*
    pathogenesis of, 814, 816
    systemic associations with
      angioid streaks with and without pseudoxanthoma elasticum pseudoxanthoma elasticum, 817–818
      megalencephaly, 818
      migraine headaches, 818
      retinitis pigmentosa, *816,* 816–817
Pseudopodia, 4614, *4614*
Pseudopolycoria, 1006, 1008

Pseudoptosis, 1547, *1549, 1550, 1551,* 1784
Pseudotumor cerebri, 486, 3829, 3927, 4040
associated findings in idiopathic, 530
clinical manifestations, 522
complications of, 530–532
definition of, 521
diagnosis of, 532–533
endocrine and metabolic dysfunctions, *524t,* 524–525
epidemiology, 521–522
etiology, 522
exogenous substances, *525t,* 525–527
familial, 530, *531*
obstruction or impairment of intracranial venous drainage, 522–524, *523t*
pathophysiology of idiopathic, 532
systemic illnesses, 527–530
Pseudotumor syndrome, 527
Pseudoxanthoma elasticum, 2987, *2988, 2989,* 3352
Psittacosis, 529
Psoriatic arthritis, 3857, *3857, 3858*
Psychiatric disease, disturbances in, 998–999
Psychogenic disturbance, 1766
Psychogenic headaches, 1698
Psychogenic palinopsia, 456
Psychogenic tears, 926
Psychomotor epilepsy, 1834
Psychophysical basis for perimetry and visual field testing, *171,* 171–172, *172*
Psychophysical tests, 159–160
PTC syndrome, 2588–2589, 2593
Pterional meningiomas, *2057,* 2057–2059, *2058*
Pterygoid portion of internal maxillary artery, 2945
Ptosis, 964, 1537–1538, 1784, 3826, 4887, 5685, 5726, *5727*
acquired myopathic, 1545–1546
associated with eye movements, *1540,* 1540–1541, *1541*
associated with mouth opening, 1541, *1541*
bilateral, 4117
bilateral cortical, *1538,* 1539
congenital, 1545, *1545, 1546*
developmental myopathic, 1545, *1545, 1546*
eyelid retraction associated with contralateral, 1555, *1556*
levator aponeurotic, 1542–1543, *1544,* 1545
mechanical, 1546–1547
myasthenic, 1546, *1546, 1547, 1548, 1549*
myopathic, *1545,* 1545–1546, *1546*
neurogenic, *1538,* 1538–1542, *1539, 1540, 1541, 1542, 1543*
neuromuscular, 1546, *1546, 1547, 1548, 1549*
from paradoxic supranuclear inhibition of levator, 1540
signs of levator palpebrae superioris, *1410,* 1410–1411, *1411*
treatment of, 1547
unassociated with either oculomotor nerve paresis, 3466, *3466, 3467*
unilateral, 2260, *2263*
unilateral cortical, *1538,* 1538–1539
Pubertas praecox, 1869–1870
Pulfrich phenomenon, 158, 622, 5590
testing for, 330, 612, 945
Pulmonary coccidioidomycosis, 4357–4358, *4358*
Pulmonary cryptococcosis, 4370, *4373*
Pulmonary embolism as causes of decreased cerebral perfusion, 3407, 3409
Pulmonary fibrosis, 5514
Pulmonary granulomas, 5467–5468
Pulmonary infiltrates without lymphadenopathy, 5514
Pulmonary schistosomiasis, 4488
Pulmonary tuberculosis, clinical manifestations, 4138–4139, *4164, 4165, 4166,* 4166–4167
Pulmonary veno-occlusive disease, 3929
Pulsatile tinnitus, 3217
Pulsating exophthalmos, 3275, 3277, *3279*
Pulsation phenomena, 3674
Pulse of innervation, 1103
Pulsed Doppler, 3533
Pulsed transcranial Doppler, 3541–3543
Pulseless disease, 3788. (*See also* Takayasu's arteritis.)
Punctata profunda, 4901
Punctate inner retinal lesions, 4682
Punctate keratitis, 4509
Punctate outer lesions, 4682
Pupil cycle induction test, 946
Pupillary capture, 936
Pupillary constriction
brainstem and spinal cord inhibition of, 879
relation between accommodation and, 912
Pupillary dilation, 1844
assessment of, 937–938, *938*
bilateral, 4373
limbic cortex and, 883
neocortex and, 883
unilateral, 3675
Pupillary disturbances, 5613–5614, 5729–5730
Pupillary disturbances in patients with giant cell arteritis, 3767
Pupillary examination, 158
Pupillary fibers in oculomotor nerve, 861–862, *863*
Pupillary function, abnormalities of, 5052
Pupillary function and accommodation, 1416–1417
Pupillary involvement, subarachnoid oculomotor nerve palsy with, 1204–1208, *1205, 1206, 1207, 1208, 1209*
Pupillary light reaction
effect of age on, 888
effect of stimulus intensity on, 889, *889*
latent period of, 889
role of, 888–889
spectral sensitivity of, 889–890, *890*
Pupillary light reflex
integration of, at pretectum, 871–875, *872, 873, 874, 875, 876, 877*
retinal ganglion cell contribution to, 868–869, *869, 870*
rod and cone contribution to, 868
Pupillary light response, 1865
conditioning of, 891
interocular modification of, 890–891
modification of, by emotion and fatigue, 890, *892*
as servomechanism, 891–892
Pupillary miosis, 947
Pupillary mydriasis, 2183
Pupillary near response, testing, 937, *937*
Pupillary reaction, 602, 604
in assessing traumatic optic neuropathy, 719
in optic neuritis, 613
testing to light, *936,* 936–937
Pupillary ruff, 850
Pupillary signs, 3675, *3676*
Pupillary size and reactivity, abnormalities of, 5728
Pupillary size and reactivity, nonorganic disorders of, 1782–1784, *1783*
Pupillary sparing, subarachnoid oculomotor nerve palsy with, 1208–1209, *1210*
Pupillary zone, 850
Pupillography, use of, 936–937
Pupillometry, infrared video, 934
Pupillomotor sensitivity of retina, 890, *891*
Pupils
anatomy and physiology, 847–894
embryology of iris, *848,* 848–850, *849, 850*
gross and microscopic anatomy of iris, 850, *851*
anterior border layer, 852, *852*
anterior epithelium-dilator muscle layer, *851, 854,* 855–857, *856*
blood vessels of, 858, *858*
nerves of, 858–860
posterior pigmented epithelium, *857,* 857–858
sphincter muscle, *851, 854,* 855, *855*
stroma, 853, *853*
influence of pupil size on iris structure, 860
normal pupillary reflexes
dilation, 893–894
after eyelid closure, 893
reaction to darkness, 892
reaction to light, *887,* 887–892, *889, 890, 891, 892*
reaction to near, 892–893
physiology of iris, 860
motor control of sphincter muscle, 860–879, *861, 862, 863, 864, 865, 866, 867, 869, 870, 871, 872, 873, 874, 875, 876, 877, 878*
Argyll Robertson, *991,* 991–993, 4887, 4889–4890, 5510, *5511,* 5614
inverse, 993
assessment of accommodation, convergence, and near response, 947
examination, 948–952, *949, 950, 951*
history, 947–948
assessment of lacrimation, 953
examination, 953–956, *954t, 955*
history, 953
assessment of size, shape, and function, 933
examination, 934–935
assessing size, 935–936
consensual response to light, 937
edge-light pupil cycle time, *945,* 945–946
for light-near dissociation, 938
for Pulfrich phenomenon, 945
pupil cycle induction test, 946
of pupillary dilation, 937–938, *938*
pupillary near response, 937, *937*
pupillary reaction to light, *936,* 936–937
for relative afferent pupillary defect, 938–941, *939, 940, 941, 942, 943t,* 943–944
for subjective relative afferent defect, brightness comparison test, 944–945
history, 933–934
pharmacologic testing, *946t,* 946–947, *947t*

bilateral tonic, 5145
cat-like, 1006
disorders of, 961–962
disturbances during seizures, 994–995
disturbances in, of neuromuscular junction
botulism, 999
myasthenia gravis, 999
disturbances in coma, 995–998
central syndrome of rostral-caudal deterioration, 996–997
syndrome of uncal herniation, 997–998
disturbances in psychiatric disease, 998–999
drug effects, 999–1001
muscle relaxants, 1004–1005
others that affect, 1005–1006
parasympatholytic (anticholinergic), *1000, 1001,* 1001–1003, *1002, 1003*
parasympathomimetic (cholinergic), 1005, *1006*
sympatholytic (antiadrenergic), 1005
sympathomimetic (adrenergic), 1003–1004, *1004*
efferent abnormalities, anisocoria, 962, *962,* 962*t*
acquired Horner's syndrome in children, 971
Adie's tonic syndrome, 978–983, *979, 980, 981, 983, 984*
congenital Horner's syndrome, 971–973, *972, 973*
damage to cavernous portion of oculomotor nerve, 977
damage to ciliary ganglion and its roots in orbit, *977,* 977–998
damage to iris sphincter, 983–984, *985*
damage to pupillomotor fibers in oculomotor nerve, 975, *975*
damage to pupillomotor fibers in subarachnoid portion of oculomotor nerve, 975–977, *976*
differentiation of, 986–987, *988*
Horner's syndrome, 963–971, *964, 965, 967, 971*
local tonic, 977–978
more, in light, 974–975
neuropathic tonic, 978
paradoxical reaction of, to light and darkness, 990
pharmacologic blockade with parasympatholytic agents, 984, *985*
pharmacologic stimulation of iris dilator, 974
pharmacologic stimulation of iris sphincter, 974
poorly reacting, from midbrain disease, 990
relative afferent pupillary defect, 987–990
simple, 962–963, *963*
sympathetic hyperactivity, *973,* 973–974
Tournay's phenomenon, 984–986
transient unilateral dilation of, in young, 986, *986, 987*
Wernicke's, 990
light-near dissociation, 990
Argyll Robertson, *991,* 991–993
inverse Argyll Robertson, 993
lesions of afferent pathway, 994
mesencephalic lesions, 993–994, *994*
drugs that affect, 1005–1006
drugs that constrict, *1004,* 1005
drugs that dilate, *1000, 1001,* 1001–1003, *1002, 1003*
ectopic, 1008
hypersensitivity of, 974
inverse Argyll Robertson, 993
isolated fixed, dilated, as sole manifestation of subarachnoid oculomotor nerve palsy, 1203
local tonic, 977–978
Marcus Gunn, 939
misplaced, 1008
neuropathic tonic, 978
paradoxical reaction of, to light and darkness, 990
peninsula, 1008
pharmacologically dilated, *1783,* 1783–1784
scalloped, 1008
size of
and intraocular pressure, 884
and pupillary movements, 883–884
square, 1006
tadpole, *973,* 973–974
tonic, 2543–2544, *2544,* 3767, 5052–5053, 5433, 5509–5510, *5510*
from ischemia of ciliary ganglion or short posterior ciliary nerves, 3694–3695
transient unilateral dilation of, in young, 986, *986, 987*
Wernicke's, 990
Pure alexia, 424–428
anatomy, pathology, and mechanisms of, *426, 427,* 427–428, *428, 429, 430, 431*
associated signs of, 425
covert reading in, 425–427
Pure hereditary spastic paraplegia, 2794–2795
Pure motor hemiplegia, 3517
Pure sensory stroke, 3517
Purine analogs
neuro-ophthalmologic toxicity, 2562–2563
pyrimidine analogs, 2563
neurotoxicity, 2562
ocular toxicity, 2562
systemic toxicity, 2562
Purpura, thrombocytopenic, 530
Pursuit, clinical examination of, 1184–1185
Pursuit initiation, 1123–1124, *1124*
Pursuit maintenance, 1124
Pursuit paretic nystagmus, 1128
Push-up method, 949
Putamen, 1862–1863
Putaminal hemorrhages, 3022, 3593, 3594, 3611
Pyoceles, 4017
clinical manifestations, 4017, *4019,* 4019–4023, *4020, 4021, 4022, 4023, 4024*
diagnosis, 4024–4025
general features, 4017, *4018*
prognosis, 4025
treatment, 4025
Pyogranulomas, 4332, 4337, 4394, *4397*
Pyramidal signs as sign of tumor, 1797
Pyramidalis, lamina, 128
Pyrazinamide for tuberculosis, 4143–4144
Pyribenzamine, 3586
Pyridoxine deficiency as cause of optic neuropathy, 670
Pyrimethamine, 4699, *4699*
Pyrimidine analogs
ocular toxicity, 2563
hydroxyurea, 2563
systemic toxicity, 2563
Pyuria, 4139

Q

Q fever, 4737, 4738, 4766
clinical manifestations, *4767,* 4767–4770, *4768, 4769*
diagnosis, 4770–4771
epidemiology, 4766–4767
pathogen, 4766, *4766*
pathology, 4770
prevention, 4771
treatment and prognosis, 4771
Quadrantanopsia, homonymous, 3691–3692
Quadrantic scotoma, 3691–3692
Queensland Tick Typhus, 4751
Quick phases, 1107
Quinagolide, 2192
Quivering eye motions in botulism, 4119

R

Rabies
hysteric, 5273
paralytic, 5273
Rabies virus, 5263
clinical manifestations, *5266,* 5266–5268, *5267*
diagnosis, 5274
differential diagnosis, 5273–5274
in endemic encephalitis, 3985
epidemiology, 5264, *5264*
hysteric, 5273
paralytic, 5273
pathogenesis, 5264–5266, *5265, 5266*
pathology, *5269,* 5269–5271, *5270, 5271,* 5273
prevention, 5274–5276
prognosis, 5274
treatment, 5274
Rabies-related lyssaviruses, 5276, *5277*
Race as factor in optic neuritis and multiple sclerosis, 618
Racemose angioma, 2725
Racemose cyst, 4473
Radiation, 1902
for arteriovenous malformations (AVMs), 2282
for Cushing's disease, 2198
general considerations, 2595
nervous system toxicity, 2596
risk factors of damage, 2596
strategies to improve outcome, 2595–2596
interstitial, 2595
for nasopharyngeal carcinoma, 2448–2449
for pituitary adenomas, 2192–2193, 2196
toxicity
bony abnormalities, 2597
endocrine abnormalities, 2597–2598
neurotoxicity, 2598–2602, *2600, 2601, 2602, 2603,* 2604–2609, *2605, 2606, 2607, 2608, 2609, 2610, 2611,* 2611–2613
otologic complications, 2597
systemic, 2596–2598
Radiation angiopathy, 3350–3351, *3352*
Radiation necrosis, 2599–2602, *2600, 2601, 2602, 2603,* 2604
treatment of, 52, 2602
Radiation optic neuropathy, 590–591, 2619–2622, *2620, 2621*

Radiation protectors, 2596
Radiation retinopathy, 2615
Radiation sensitizers, 2596
Radiation somnolence syndrome, 2598–2599
Radiation-induced atherosclerosis, 2611, *2611*
Radiculomyelitis, sacral, 4983
Radiculoplexopathy, 5089
Radioimmunoassays for adrenocorticotropic hormone, 2197–2198
Radioimmunofluorescence assay (RIPA), 5379
Radiosurgery, stereotactic, 2595
Raeder's paratrigeminal neuralgia, 970, 1698–1701, 3040
Raeder's syndrome, 1698–1701, 3047
Ragged-red fibers, 1378–1379, *1379, 1380*
Ramsay Hunt syndrome, 1562, *1742,* 1743–1745, *1745, 5033,* 5033–5035, *5034, 5035, 5036,* 5037–5038
Rapid enzyme immunoassay (EIA) test, 4100
Rapid eye movement sleep, 1107–1108
Rapid fluorescent focus inhibition test (RFFIT), 5274
Rapid-rise OKN, 1149
Rash
  butterfly, 3813, *3813*
  heliotrope, 2528, 3839
Rathke's cleft cysts, 2098, *2107,* 2107–2108, *2108,* 3102
Rathke's pouch, 2098
Raymond-Cestan syndrome, 1250
Raynaud's disease, 1696
Raynaud's phenomenon, 2574, 3422, 3834
  in CREST syndrome, 3014
Reactivation, 4950
Reactive arsenical encephalopathy (RAE), 4719
Reactive non-Langerhans cell histiocytoses, 2413–2414
Rebound nystagmus, *1481,* 1481–1482
Reciprocal innervation, 907
Recognition deficit in prosopagnosia, 417, *417*
Recovery nystagmus, 1470
Rectocolitis, acute, 4619
Recurrent artery of Heubner, 2891, 2897
Recurrent extragenital mucocutaneous herpes simplex virus infections, *4988,* 4988–4990, *4989*
Recurrent genital herpes infections, 4989
Recurrent hemorrhage, 3144–3145
Recurrent optic neuritis, 616, 619
Recurrent perforating arteries, 2917
Recurrent proptosis, 2252
Reduced amplitudes of accommodation, 4373
Reducing body myopathy, 1358
Reed-Sternberg cells, 2352, 2356
  number and appearance of, 2351
  origin of, 2351
Reflex blepharospasm, 1569
Reflex blinks, 1523, 1526
  auditory evoked, 1530–1531, *1532*
  from stimulation of cornea, 1529, *1530*
Reflex dilation, 893–894
Reflex eye movements, 1329–1330
Reflex tears, 926
  secretion of
    anatomy of, 917–918, *918*
    neural control of, 918–919, *919, 920,* 921, *921, 922, 923,* 923–926, *924*
Reflexes
  associated with lacrimation, 930
  cervico-ocular, 1138
  after eyelid closure, 893
  otolith-ocular, 1140–1142, *1141*
  vestibulo-collic, 1138
  vestibulo-ocular, 1139–1149, *1140, 1141, 1143, 1144, 1148,* 1156–1157
Reflexive saccade, *1106*
Refraction and visual acuity, 154–155, *155*
Refsum disease, 2840–2841
Regan Low Contrast Letter Chart, 613
Regional lymphadenopathy, 4200
Reiter's syndrome, 631, *3854,* 3854–3857, *3855, 3856*
  epidemic, 3854
Relapsing fever, 4832
  clinical manifestations, 4833–4834
  diagnosing, *4834,* 4834–4835
  epidemiology, *4832,* 4832–4833, *4833*
  pathogenesis, 4833
  prevention, 4836
  treatment and prognosis, 4835, *4835, 4836*
Relapsing polychondritis, 3842–3845, *3844, 3845*
Relative accommodation, 948
Relative afferent pupil defect, 158, 719, 720, 2359, 4142
  in retinal disease, 240, *240, 241*
  testing for, 938–941, *939, 940, 941, 942, 943t,* 943–944
Relative convergence, 948
Relaxation theory of accommodation, 909–910
Release hallucinations, 457–461, *458, 459, 460, 461*
Reliability indices, 178–180
Remyelination, 628, 5644
  after central demyelination, 3981, *3981*
Renal cell carcinoma, 2690
Renal cysts, 2705
Renal failure, 529
Renal tubular acidosis as side effect of amphotericin B therapy, 4283
Renal tumors, 2705
Rendu-Osler-Weber disease, 2230, 3012
Reoviridae, 5258
  orbiviruses, *5259,* 5259–5261, *5260*
  orthoreoviruses, 5261
  rotaviruses, *5161,* 5261, 5263
Repetitive nerve stimulation, 1422–1423, *1423*
Reserpine, 1005
Residual vision. (*See* Blindsight.)
Resolution acuity, 160
Respiratory syncytial virus, *5232,* 5232–5233, *5233*
Respiratory tract candidiasis, 4346–4347
Reticuloendothelial system. (*See* Histiocytoses.)
Retina, 3–4, *4, 5*
  abnormalities in, *1367,* 1367–1369, 2656, *2657,* 2658
  angiomas in, *2245,* 2245–2246, 2696–2697, *2697,* 2698
  basic anatomy and physiology, 25–26, *26, 26t*
    amacrine cells, *38,* 40–42, *42, 43*
    bipolar cells, *38,* 39–40, *40, 41*
    blood vessels, 51–54, *52, 53*
    glial cells, 43–44
    horizontal cells, 36, *38,* 39
    inner plexiform layer, 44–45
    interplexiform cells, 42–43
    nerve fiber layer, *50,* 50–51, *51*
    outer plexiform layer, 35–36, *38*
    photoreceptors, 30–35, *32, 34*
    pigment epithelium, 26, *29, 30, 31, 32*
    retinal ganglion cell layer, *45,* 45–50, *46, 47t, 48, 49*
    superficial plexiform layer, 50
  blood vessels in, 51–54, *52, 53*
  cellular structure of, 25
  degeneration of, 30
  detachment of, 988, 3283, 5040
  disorders in, 1464–1465
  disorders of, 3670–3671
  effect of radiation therapy on, 2615, *2616*
  hamartomas in, 2676, *2677,* 2678, *2678, 2679, 2680*
  hemorrhages in, 2976
  leukemic involvement of, *2344,* 2344–2348, *2345, 2346, 2347, 2348*
  microangiopathy of, *3732,* 3732–3734, *3733*
  photocoagulation of, 1725
  pupillomotor sensitivity of, 890, *891*
  visual loss from replacement of, 1996–1997
Retinal arteries, aneurysms arising from, 3067, 3069, *3071, 3072,* 3072–3074, *3073, 3074*
Retinal arteriovenous malformations (AVMs), *2266,* 2266–2268, *2267*
Retinal asthenopia, 1731
Retinal blur, 1134
Retinal disease
  appearance of optic disc in, 252–253, *253, 254*
  color vision in, 238, 240
  relative afferent pupillary defect in, 240, *240, 241*
  visual acuity in, 237–238, *238, 239*
  visual field defects in, 240, *242,* 243, *243, 244, 245, 246,* 247, *247, 248,* 249, *249, 250, 251,* 252, *252*
Retinal disparity, 1134
Retinal ganglion cell contribution to pupillary light reflex, 868–869, *869, 870*
Retinal ganglion cell layer, *45,* 45–50, *46, 47t, 48, 49*
Retinal ganglion cells, 107–108
  anatomy and physiology of, *45,* 45–48, *46, 47t, 48, 49*
  structure and function of, 48–50
Retinal ischemia, 3759–3761, *3761, 3762,* 3763, *3763, 3764, 3765*
  permanent visual defects from, 3694
Retinal lesions of multiple sclerosis, 5577–5579, *5578, 5579, 5580,* 5581
Retinal macroaneurysms, 3067, 3069, *3071, 3072,* 3072–3074, *3073, 3074*
Retinal microaneurysms, 3067, *3069, 3071*
Retinal microangiopathy, 5424–5426, *5426*
Retinal migraine, 3687–3691, *3688, 3689, 3690*
Retinal neovascularization, 2347–2348
Retinal nerve fiber layer, blurring of peripapillary, 487–488
Retinal neurotransmitters, 54, 54*t*
Retinal periphlebitis, 5491, *5491, 5492*
Retinal pigment epithelial (RPE) lesions, 2556, 2678, *2683*
Retinal pigment epithelium, 26, *29, 30, 31, 32*
Retinal rest, 1768–1769
Retinal scarring with atresia of blood vessels and optic atrophy, 4906–4907
Retinal slip, 1123
Retinal stroke, 3444
  management of patients with, 3577
Retinal vascular changes, associated with optic atrophy, 290

Retinal vascular manifestations, 3822–3823
Retinal vascular occlusions, 813
Retinal vascular occlusive disease, 2658
Retinal vasospasm, 3688
Retinal veins, dilation of, 489, 3282–3283, *3283, 3284*
Retinitis, *5105,* 5105–5107
  and chorioretinitis, *5426,* 5426–5429, *5427, 5428, 5429*
  necrotizing, 4671, 5023
  toxic, 755
Retinitis pigmentosa, *816,* 816–817, 4907
Retinoblastoma, 1990–1999, *1992, 1993, 1994, 1995, 1996*
  chromosomal-deletion, 1992
  diffuse infiltrating, 1994, *1995*
  endophytic, 1993–1994, *1994*
  exophytic, 1994, *1995*
  mixed endophytic-exophytic, 1994
  trilateral, 1996
Retinoblastoma syndrome, 2623
Retinocephalic vascular malformation, 2725
Retinochoroiditis, *Toxoplasma gondii* in, 5428–5429
Retinochoroidopathy, birdshot, 631
Retinocochleocerebral arteriolopathy, 3733
Retino-cortical transit time (RCT), 228
Retinohypothalamic afferents, function of, 833
Retinohypothalamic pathway, support for existence of, 833
Retinoids, 2593
  neurologic toxicity, 2593
  neuro-ophthalmologic toxicity, 2593
  ocular toxicity, 2593
Retinomesencephalic excitation, 868–875, *869, 870, 871, 872, 873, 874, 875, 876*
Retinomesencephalic inhibition associated with dark reaction, 878
Retinopathy
  cancer-associated, 2533, *2534, 2535,* 2535–2537, *2536, 2537*
  hypotensive, 3453–3454, *3454, 3455, 3456,* 3457, *3457*
  leukemic, *2344,* 2344–2348, *2345, 2346, 2347, 2348*
  melanoma-associated, 39, 219, 2473, 2537–2538, *2539*
  paraneoplastic. (*See* Paraneoplastic retinopathies.)
  pigmentary, 1383, 5292
  radiation, 2615
  stasis, 3282
  vaso-occlusive, 2590–2591, *2591*
Retinoscopy, dynamic, 951
Retinotopic principle of organization, 99
Retinotopic pursuit defects, 1126
Retraction balls, 724
Retroauricular pain, 1702
Retrobulbar compressive lesions, sudden visual loss with, 656–657
Retrobulbar compressive optic neuropathies, *653, 654, 656,* 657
  progressive visual dysfunction in, *8,* 653–656, *654*
Retrobulbar hemorrhage, 716
Retrobulbar neuritis, 599, 633, 2559–2560, 2576–2577, 4769
Retrobulbar optic neuritis, 599, 2393, 4874, 4876, *4877,* 4886
Retrobulbar optic neuropathy, 4301–4302
Retrobulbar pain, 1726–1727
Retrochiasmal visual field defects, 323–324
Retrograde amnesia, 1833
Retrograde flow, 3414
Retrograde transport, 49
Retropharyngeal abscess, 4085
Retroviridae, 5263
Retroviruses. (*See also* Lentiviruses; Oncoviruses.)
  and acquired immune deficiency syndrome, 5361–5362, *5362, 5363*
Rett's syndrome, 1317
Reverse bobbing, 1328, 3511–3512
Reverse dipping, 1328, 1493
  ocular, 4375
Reverse transcriptase, 5363, 5365
Reversible ischemic neurologic disability (RIND), 3324
Rex, 5434
Reye's syndrome, 529–530, 5019–5020, 5077, 5194–5195, 5210, 5240, 5261
Rey-Osterreith Complex Figure Test (CFT), 470
Rhabdomyomas, 2690–2692, *2691, 2692, 2693*
Rhabdomyosarcoma, 2073–2074
Rhabdoviridae, 5263
  lyssaviruses, 5263–5271, *5264, 5265, 5266, 5267, 5268, 5269, 5270, 5271, 5272, 5273,* 5274–5276
  vesiculoviruses, 5263
Rheumatic diseases, 3339. (*See also* Vasculitis.)
Rheumatic fever, acute, 4085
Rheumatic mitral stenosis, 3569
Rheumatoid arthritis, 1735, 5145
Rheumatoid factor, 3845
Rhinitis, 4287
Rhinocladiella aquaspersa, 4353
Rhinorrhea, CSF, 510
Rhinoscleroma, 2413
Rhinovirus, 5258
Rhipicephalus sanguineus, 4739
Rhizomelic chondrodysplasia punctata, 2844–2845
Rhizomucor, 4318
Rhizopus, 4318
Rhodopsin, 31–32
Ribavirin, 5165
Riboflavin deficiency as cause of optic neuropathy, 670
Richardson-Olszewski syndrome, 2748
Richner-Hanhart syndrome, 2812–2813
Rickettsia burnetii, 4766
Rickettsia rickettsii, 4739
Rickettsiae
  as cause of meningoencephalitis, 3986–3987
  description, 4737–4738, *4738,* 4738*t*
  diseases caused by, 4739
    acute febrile cerebrovasculitis, *4770, 4771,* 4771–4772, *4772*
    African Tick Bite Fever, 4751–4752
    Boutonneuse Fever, *4748,* 4748–4751, *4749, 4750, 4751*
    Brill-Zinsser disease, 4755
      endemic typhus, *4755,* 4755–4758, *4756, 4757, 4758, 4759*
    ehrlichiosis, *4762,* 4762–4765, *4765*
    epidemic typhus, *4752,* 4752–4755, *4753, 4754*
    North Asian Tick Typhus, 4751
    Oriental Spotted Fever, 4751
    Q fever, 4766
      clinical manifestations, *4767,* 4767–4770, *4768, 4769*
      diagnosis, 4770–4771
      epidemiology, 4766–4767
      pathogen, 4766, *4766*
      pathology, 4770
      prevention, 4771
      treatment and prognosis, 4771
    Queensland Tick Typhus, 4751
    rickettsialpox, 4752
    Rocky mountain spotted fever, 4739
      clinical manifestations, 4740, *4740, 4741, 4742,* 4742–4744, *4743, 4744*
      diagnosis, 4745
      epidemiology, 4739–4740, *4740*
      pathogenesis, 4740
      pathology, *4744, 4745,* 4745–4746, *4746, 4747*
      prevention, 4748
      prognosis, 4747–4748
      treatment, 4746–4747
    scrub typhus, 4758–4762, *4759, 4760, 4761*
  pathology and pathogenesis, 4738–4739
Rickettsial infections, 4031
Rickettsialpox, 4752
Riddoch phenomenon of static-kinetic dissociation, 373–374
Rifampin for tuberculosis, 4142
Rift Valley fever, *5163,* 5163–5165, *5164*
Right common carotid artery, 2869
Right internal and external carotid arteries, 2869
Riley-Day syndrome, 764, 1026–1027
Ring forms, 4651
Ringing, 1124
Rippling muscle disease, 1782
River blindness, 4509–4510, *4510*
RNA viruses, 5678
  that infect central nervous system, 5154–5296
    arenaviridae, *5154,* 5154–5158, *5155, 5156, 5157, 5158*
    bunyaviridae, 5158, *5159*
      bunyaviruses, 5158–5162
        characteristics, 5159–5160, *5160*
        clinical manifestations, 5160–5161
        diagnosis, 5161
        epidemiology of, 5160, *5161*
        pathology, 5161, *5162*
        prevention, 5162
        treatment, 5161
      phlebovirus, *5163,* 5163–5165, *5164*
    coronaviridae, *5165,* 5165–5166, *5166*
    filoviridae, 5166–5167
    flaviviridae, 5167, 5179–5184, *5181, 5183*
      Central European and Russian spring-summer tick-borne encephalitis, *5186,* 5186–5188, *5188*
        clinical manifestations, 5187
        diagnosis, 5187
        epidemiology, *5186,* 5186–5187
        pathology, 5187, *5188*
        prevention, 5188
        prognosis, 5187–5188
      dengue virus, 5167–5170, *5168, 5169*
      Hepatitis C virus (HCV), 5190
      Japanese encephalitis, 5170
        clinical manifestations, *5171,* 5171–5172, 5187
        diagnosis, 5173–5174, 5187
        epidemiology, 5170–5171

RNA viruses—*continued*
pathology, *5172,* 5172–5173, *5173,* 5187, *5188*
prevention, 5174, *5175*
prognosis, 5174, 5187–5188
treatment, 5174
Kunjin virus, 5174–5175
Kyasanur Forest disease virus, 5188–5189
Louping III virus, 5189
Murray Valley encephalitis virus, 5175–5176, *5177, 5178,* 5178–5179, 5179, *5179*
clinical manifestations, 5175–5176
diagnosis, 5178–5179
epidemiology, 5175
pathology, 5176, 5178, *5178, 5179, 5180*
prevention, 5179
prognosis, 5179
treatment, 5179
Negishi virus, 5189
Powassan virus, 5189–5190
St. Louis encephalitis virus, 5179–5184, *5181, 5183*
clinical manifestations, 5182
diagnosis, 5182–5183
epidemiology, 5179, *5181,* 5181–5182
pathogenesis, 5182
pathology, 5182, *5183*
prevention, 5183–5184
prognosis, 5183
treatment, 5183
West Nile virus, 5184
yellow fever virus, 5184–5186, *5185*
clinical manifestations, 5184
diagnosis, 5185
epidemiology, 5184, *5185*
pathogenesis and pathology, 5184–5185
prevention, 5185–5186
prognosis, 5185
treatment, 5185
orthomyxoviridae
characteristics of, 5190, *5191*
influenza viruses, 5190–5198, *5191, 5194, 5195, 5197*
clinical manifestations of infections, 5192
diagnosis, 5196
epidemiology, 5190–5192
nonpulmonary complications of, 5193–5196, *5195*
prevention, 5196–5198
prognosis, 5196
pulmonary complications of, 5192–5193
treatment, 5196
uncomplicated, 5192
paramyxoviridae, 5198, *5199,* 5200
measles, 5200
clinical manifestations, 5201, *5201*
complications, 5201, *5202,* 5203–5208, *5204, 5205, 5206, 5208, 5209, 5210*
diagnosis, 5209–5210
epidemiology, 5200
pathogenesis, 5208–5209
prevention and complications of vaccination, 5210–5213, *5211, 5212, 5213*
treatment, 5210
morbilliviruses, 5200–5201, *5201, 5202,* 5203–5217, *5204, 5205, 5206, 5208, 5209, 5210, 5211, 5212, 5213, 5214, 5215, 5216, 5217, 5218, 5219,* 5220, *5220*
characteristics of, 5200
measles, 5200
parainfluenza viruses, 5231
characteristics of, 5231, *5231*
clinical manifestations, 5232
paramyxoviruses, 5220
mumps virus, 5223
characteristics of, 5223, *5225*
clinical manifestations of, 5225, *5226*
complications of, 5225–5229, *5227*
diagnosis of, 5229–5230
epidemiology of, 5223, 5225
pathogenesis of, 5225
prevention, 5231
prognosis of, 5230–5231
treatment of, 5230
pneumoviruses, *5232,* 5232–5233, *5233*
subacute sclerosing panencephalitis, 5213
clinical manifestations, *5214,* 5214–5216, *5215, 5216, 5217*
diagnosis, 5217, 5220, *5223, 5224*
epidemiology, 5213–5214
pathogenesis, 5217
pathology, 5216–5217, *5218, 5219*
treatment and prognosis, 5220, *5224*
picornaviridae, 5233–5234, *5234*
coxsackieviruses, 5235–5241
echoviruses, 5241–5243
enteroviruses, 5234–5235, 5243–5250, *5244, 5246*
polioviruses, 5250–5258, *5251, 5252, 5253, 5254*
clinical manifestations, 5253–5257
diagnosis, 5257
epidemiology, 5250–5251
pathogenesis, 5251–5252, *5252*
pathology, 5252–5253, *5253, 5254*
prevention, 5258
rhinovirus, 5258
prognosis, 5257–5258
treatment, 5257
rabdoviridae
rabies virus
pathology, *5269,* 5269–5271, *5270, 5271,* 5273
prevention, 5274–5276
prognosis, 5274
treatment, 5274
vesiculoviruses, 5263
reoviridae, 5258
Colorado tick fever virus
clinical manifestations, 5259–5260
diagnosis, 5260
epidemiology, 5259
prevention, 5261
prognosis, 5261
treatment, 5260–5261
orbiviruses, *5259,* 5259–5261, *5260*
orthoreoviruses, 5261
rotaviruses, 5261, *5261,* 5263
retroviridae, 5263
rhabdoviridae, 5263
lyssaviruses, 5263–5271, *5264, 5265, 5266, 5267, 5268, 5269, 5270, 5271, 5272, 5273,* 5274–5276
rabies virus, 5263
clinical manifestations, *5266,* 5266–5268, *5267*
diagnosis, 5274
differential diagnosis, 5273–5274
epidemiology, 5264, *5264*
pathogenesis, 5264–5266, *5265, 5266*
togaviridae, 5277
alphaviruses, 5277–5281, *5278, 5279, 5280, 5281, 5282,* 5283, *5283, 5284, 5285,* 5285–5286
clinical manifestations, 5279–5281, *5280, 5281, 5282, 5283, 5284, 5285,* 5285–5286
pathology of, 5278–5279, *5279, 5280, 5281, 5282*
rubivirus (Rubella), 5286–5293, 5296
clinical manifestations, 5287–5293, *5288, 5289, 5294, 5295,* 5296, *5296*
diagnosis, 5293
epidemiology, 5286–5287
pathogenesis, 5287
prevention, 5293, 5296
treatment, 5293
Rochalimaea henselae, 5721
Rocky Mountain spotted fever, 4739, 4832
clinical manifestations, 4740, *4740, 4741, 4742,* 4742–4744, *4743, 4744*
diagnosis, 4745
epidemiology, 4739–4740, *4740*
pathogenesis, 4740
pathology, *4744, 4745,* 4745–4746, *4746, 4747*
prevention, 4748
prognosis, 4747–4748
treatment, 4746–4747
Rod and cone contribution to pupillary light reflex, 868
Rod and cone electroretinogram (ERG) components
oscillatory potentials, 217–218, *218*
separation of, 217, *217*
testing conditions and interpretation, *217, 218,* 218–219
waveform and factors affecting it, 219
Rod and cone through pathways, 54
Rod bipolar cells, 39
Rod myopathy, 1354–1355, *1355*
Roentgenographic abnormalities in patients with *Mycoplasma pneumoniae,* 4547–4548
Rof, 5434
Rolandic artery, occlusion of, 3440
Rolandic vein, 2946
occlusion of, 4033
Rosai-Dorfman disease, *2415,* 2415–2416, *2416, 2417*
Rose bengal test, 954
Rosenthal fibers, 1930
Ross syndrome, 1027–1028
Rostellum, 4441
Rostral basilar artery syndrome, 3492, 3494
Rostral interstitial nucleus of medial longitudinal fasciculus, 1081–1082, 1307–1308, *1309, 1310, 1311, 1312, 1313*
Rotaviruses, 5261, *5261,* 5263
Roth spots, 2345, *2345,* 3025
Roundworms (nematodes), 4494, *4495*

Angiostrongylus cantonensis
clinical manifestations, *4496*, 4496–4497, *4497, 4498*
diagnosis, 4500
epidemiology, 4494, 4496
life cycle, 4494, *4496*
pathogenesis and pathology, 4497–4499, *4498, 4499*
treatment and prognosis, 4500
Gnathostoma spinigerum
clinical manifestations, 4501–4503, *4504, 4505*
diagnosis, 4503
epidemiology, 4500–4501
life cycle, 4500, *4500, 4501*
pathogenesis and pathology, 4501, *4502*
treatment and prognosis, 4503
Loa loa, 4503, 4505–4507, *4506, 4507, 4508*
treatment of, 4507
miscellaneous, of neuro-ophthalmologic significance, 4528–4529, *4529, 4530*, 4531, *4531*
Onchocerca volvulus, 4507–4511, *4509, 4510*
diagnosis of, 4510–4511
treatment of, 4511
Strongyloides stercoralis, 4511, 4511–4512, *4512, 4513, 4514*, 4514–4515
Toxocara, 4515–4516, *4516, 4517*, 4518, *4518, 4519, 4520, 4521, 4522*, 4522–4523, *4523*
Trichinella spiralis, 4523–4525, *4524, 4526, 4527*, 4527–4528, *4528*
Rubella
congenital, 5289–5293, *5290, 5291*
and development of viral encephalitis, 3986
postnatally acquired, 5287–5289, *5288, 5289*
Rubeosis iridis, 1997
Rubivirus (Rubella). (*See also* Rubella.)
clinical manifestations, 5287–5293, *5288, 5289, 5294, 5295*, 5296, *5296*
congenital, 5289–5293, *5290, 5291*
diagnosis, 5293
epidemiology, 5286–5287
pathogenesis, 5287
postnatally acquired, 5287–5289, *5288, 5289*
prevention, 5293, 5296
treatment, 5293
Ruptured saccular aneurysms, natural history of, 3142–3144, *3143*
Russell's syndrome, 1814–1815, *1815*

S

S-100, 1919
Sabin-Feldman dye test in diagnosing toxoplasmosis, 4692
Saccades, 1102, 1154, *1155*
amplitude, 1105, *1105*
clinical examination of, 1183–1184
feedback control of, 1113–1114, *1114*
localization using, *392*, 393, *393, 394, 395*
in Parkinson's disease, 1316–1317
slow, from pontine lesions, 1303, 1303*t*
Saccadic accuracy, 1105–1107
Saccadic contrapulsion, 1293
Saccadic dysmetria, 1184, 1326, 1848
Saccadic eye movement, 1103, 1286
basal ganglia, 1120
central midbrain reticular formation, 1120
cerebellar control of, 1120, *1121*, 1122–1123
cerebral control of, 1114
basal ganglia, 1120
central midbrain reticular formation, 1120
frontal eye fields, 1114–1115, *1115, 1116, 1117*
parietal cortex, 1118–1120
prefrontal cortex, 1118, *1119*
superior colliculus, 1115–1118
supplementary eye field, 1118
thalamus, 1120
characteristics of, 1103–1107
neurophysiology of, 1109
parietal cortex, 1118–1120
prefrontal cortex, 1118, *1119*
processing of visual information for, 1108–1109, *1109*
quick phases of nystagmus, 1107, *1108*
during sleep, 1107–1108
studies of, 2754
superior colliculus, 1115–1118
supplementary field, 1118
testing, 1776
thalamus, 1120
vision during, 1109
Saccadic hypometria, 2722
Saccadic intrusions, 1462, 1487, 1869, 5599
common features of, 1486, *1487, 1488*
macrosaccadic oscillations, 1487
macrosquare-wave jerks, 1487
pathogenesis of, 1490–1491
square-wave jerks, 1486–1487, 1496–1497
treatments for, 1494–1499, 1495*t*
Saccadic latency, 1105, *1106*
Saccadic omission, 1109
Saccadic oscillations
cerebellum and, 1491
from pontine lesions, 1303
Saccadic premotor neurons, neurotransmitters for, 1114
Saccadic pulses, 1103, 1487
neural integration of, 1113
Saccadic velocities, 1105
Saccadomania, 1487
Saccular aneurysms, 2977, 2978, *2979*, 3014
as cause of spontaneous subarachnoid and intracranial hemorrhage, 3020
clinical manifestations according to site, 3037
arising from anterior cerebral artery, 3091–3093, *3094, 3095, 3096, 3097*
arising from anterior choroidal artery, 3084–3085, *3086*
arising from anterior communicating artery, 3100–3104, *3101, 3102, 3103*
arising from anterior inferior cerebellar artery, 3122, *3122*
arising from basilar artery, 3111, 3113, *3114, 3115, 3116*, 3116–3122, *3117, 3118, 3119, 3120, 3121*
arising from bifurcation of internal carotid artery, 3085, *3087*, 3087–3091, *3088, 3089, 3090, 3091, 3092, 3093*
arising from cavernous portion of internal carotid artery, *3040*, 3040–3041, *3041, 3042, 3043, 3044, 3045, 3046*, 3046–3047, *3047, 3048, 3049*, 3050, *3050, 3051, 3052, 3053*, 3054, *3054*
arising from clinoid segment of internal carotid artery, *3055, 3056*, 3056–3059, *3057, 3058*
arising from conjunctival arteries, 3074–3075
arising from extracranial portion of internal carotid artery, 3037–3038, *3038, 3039*
arising from intradural portion of internal carotid artery and its branches, 3054, 3056
arising from junction of internal carotid and anterior choroidal arteries, 3084, *3085, 3086*
arising from junction of internal carotid and ophthalmic arteries, *3059*, 3059–3060, *3060, 3061, 3062*, 3062–3063, *3063, 3064, 3065*, 3065–3066, *3066, 3067*
arising from junction of internal carotid and posterior communicating arteries, *3075*, 3075–3083, *3076, 3077, 3078, 3079, 3081, 3082, 3083*
arising from junction of internal carotid and superior hypophyseal arteries, 3059
arising from ophthalmic artery, 3066–3067, *3067, 3068, 3069, 3070*
arising from petrous portion of internal carotid artery, 3038, *3039*, 3040
arising from posterior cerebral artery, 3123, *3125*, 3125–3127, *3126*
arising from posterior communicating artery, 3083, *3084*
arising from posterior inferior cerebellar artery, 3108–3109, *3112, 3113*
arising from proximal supraclinoid portion of internal carotid artery, 3075
arising from retinal arteries, 3067, 3069, *3071, 3072*, 3072–3074, *3073, 3074*
arising from superior cerebellar artery, *3122*, 3122–3123
arising from vertebral artery, 3104, *3106*, 3106–3108, *3107, 3108, 3109, 3110, 3111*
arising from vertebrobasilar arterial system, 3104, *3104, 3105*
clinical manifestations according to site, arising from middle cerebral artery, 3095, 3097, *3097, 3098, 3099*, 3099–3100, *3100*
diagnosis
of aneurysm, 3130–3133, *3132, 3133, 3134, 3136*, 3136–3139, *3137, 3140, 3141, 3142*
of subarachnoid hemorrhage, 3130
location and laterality, 3015, *3016, 3017*
manifestations of ruptured
general considerations, 3019–3020, *3020*
hydrocephalus after rupture of intracranial, *3035*, 3035–3036
intracerebral hemorrhage associated with, 3033–3034, 3034*t*
intraventricular hemorrhage associated with, 3034
neurologic and neuro-ophthalmologic intracranial, 3021–3024, *3022, 3023*
orbital and intraocular effects of subarachnoid and intracranial hemorrhage, *3024*, 3024–3026, *3025, 3026, 3027, 3028*, 3028–3029, *3029, 3030, 3031, 3032*, 3032–3033, *3033*
subdural hematoma from intracranial, *3036*, 3036–3037
warning signs and symptoms before major rupture of intracranial, 3021
medical therapy for, 3175–3176
multiple, 3016–3018, *3019*

Saccular aneurysms—*continued*
general clinical manifestations, 3018–3019
natural history, 3139
delayed cerebral ischemia and vasospasm, 3145–3147, *3146, 3147*
medical complications, 3144
recurrent hemorrhage, 3144–3145
ruptured, 3142–3144, *3143*
unruptured, 3139–3142
natural history of ruptured, 3142–3144, *3143*
prevalence, 3014–3015
sex and age distribution, 3015
size, 3015–3016, *3018*
surgery for
direct approach, 3147
endovascular, 3178–3180, *3179*
for unruptured, 3154–3155, *3156, 3157,* 3157–3159, *3158, 3159, 3160, 3161, 3162,* 3162–3165, *3164, 3165, 3166, 3167*
ruptured, 3176–3178
timing of, and its relationship to neurologic status, 3172–3175
unruptured, 3165–3166, *3168,* 3168–3169, *3169*
treatment and results, 3147
of delayed cerebral ischemia, 3170–3172
of ruptured intracranial, 3169–3170
Sacral radiculomyelitis, 4983
Sagittal sinus
inferior, 2956, 2959
thrombosis of, 4079
SAH from rupture of intracranial aneurysm, 3021–3022
Sahlgren Saturation Test, 407
St. Louis encephalitis, 5179–5184, *5181, 5183*
clinical manifestations, 5182
diagnosis, 5182–5183
epidemiology, 5179, *5181,* 5181–5182
pathogenesis, 5182
pathology, 5182, *5183*
prevention, 5183–5184
prognosis, 5183
treatment, 5183
St. Louis encephalitis type A, 5722
St. Louis encephalitis type B, 5722
Saksenaeaceae, 4318
Salmonella, 4221–4224, *4222, 4223,* 5421
in bacteremia, 4221, *4222*
carrier state, 4223
clinical manifestations, 4221–4223, *4222, 4223*
in empyema, 3983
in intracranial abscess, 3950
prevention, 4223–4224
Salmonella enterocolitis, 4221
carrier state, 4223
prevention, 4223–4224
Salmonella meningitis, 4222–4223, *4223*
Salmonella typhi, 5679
in bacterial meningitis, 3994
Salt-and-pepper fundus, 4906
Sandfly fever virus, 5163
Sandhoff disease, 2826–2827
Sanfilippo syndrome (MPS III), 2820, *2820, 2821*
Sarcoid meningitis, 5495–5496, *5496*
Sarcoidosis, 530, *705,* 705–706, *706, 707, 708,* 709, 3346
central nervous system, 5471–5472
clinical manifestations, 5476, 5478–5479
cardiac, 5483–5484
cutaneous and subcutaneous, 5479–5480, *5480, 5481, 5482*
endocrine, 5482
hepatic, 5480–5481
joint, 5482
lymphadenopathy, 5480, *5483*
muscle, 5484, 5486
neurologic, 5491–5493, 5495, *5495, 5496, 5497,* 5498
neuro-ophthalmologic, 5498
ocular, *5475,* 5487–5488, *5488, 5489, 5490,* 5490–5491, *5491, 5492, 5493, 5494*
ocular motor dysfunction, 5508–5509, *5509*
orbital, *5486,* 5486–5487, *5487*
pupillary dysfunction, 5509–5510, *5510*
renal, 5481–5482
respiratory, 5479, *5480*
salivary gland, 5483, 5485
skeletal, 5482, *5484*
splenic, 5481
visual sensory dysfunction, *5498, 5499,* 5499–5501, *5500, 5501, 5502, 5503, 5504,* 5505–5508, *5506, 5507, 5508*
diagnosis, *5509, 5516, 5517,* 5518, *5518, 5519, 5520, 5521, 5522,* 5522–5523, *5524, 5525, 5526, 5527*
epidemiology, 5465–5466
etiology, 5466–5467
historical background, 5465
laboratory findings, 5514, 5516, 5518
optic neuritis in, 629
orbital, 5470, 5486–5487
pathogenesis, 5472, 5475–5476, *5479*
pathology, *5466,* 5467, *5467,* 5467–5468
prognosis, 5528–5529
radiographic and other imaging findings, 5510–5511, *5511, 5512,* 5514, *5514*
treatment, 5526, 5528, *5529*
Sarcomas
granulocytic, 2338–2339, 2341
of meninges and brain
chondrosarcoma, 2068–2069
osteogenic, 2069–2070
rhabdomyosarcoma, 2072–2073
osteogenic, 2069–2070
polymorphic cell, 2071
primary intracranial, 2071–2072
Sarcotubular myopathy, 1359
Sardonicus, 4112
Satiety center, 1814
Scalloped pupils, 1008
Scalp tenderness in giant cell arteritis, 3756
Scedosporium apiospermum in fungal aneurysms, 3004, 3971
Schaumann bodies, 5467
Scheie syndrome (MPS IS), 2818–2819, *2819*
Schilder's disease, 617, 622, 626–628, 5539
Schirmer test, 954–955
Schistosoma, 4485, *4485*
clinical manifestations, 4487–4489, *4488, 4489*
diagnosis, 4491–4492, *4493*
epidemiology, 4486
life cycle, 4485–4486, *4486*
pathogenesis and pathology, 4489–4491, *4490, 4491, 4492*
treatment, 4492
Schistosoma haematobium, 4485, 4486, 4487, 4490
Schistosoma intercalatum, 4486, 4487–4488
Schistosoma japonicum, 4485, 4486, 4487, 4488, 4490
in intracranial brain abscess, 3952
Schistosoma mansoni, 4485, 4486, 4487, 4488, 4490
Schistosoma mekongi, 4486, 4487
Schistosomal myelopathy, 4488
Schistosomiasis, 4485, *4485*
acute, 4487, 4489
chronic, 4487–4488, 4489
clinical manifestations, 4487–4489, *4488, 4489*
diagnosis, 4491–4492, *4493*
epidemiology, 4486
intestinal, 4488
intracranial, 4488–4489
life cycle, 4485–4486, *4486*
pathogenesis and pathology, 4489–4491, *4490, 4491, 4492*
pulmonary, 4488
treatment, 4492
vesical, 4488, *4488*
Schizogony, 4651
Schizonts, 4650, 4651
Schwann cells
structure and function of, 2297–2298, *2298, 2299*
tumors containing
neurofibromas, 2319, *2320,* 2321
schwannomas, 4–6, *5, 6, 7,* 8–13, *9, 10, 11, 13, 14,* 15–23, *16, 19, 21, 22*
Schwannoma, 2300
acoustic, 1294
bilateral vestibular, 2667
of facial nerve, 2306–2308, *2307*
intracranial, 2300–2302, *2301, 2302,* 2660
intraocular, 2656
of lower cranial nerves, 2316
of ocular motor nerves, 2302, *2303*
within orbit, 2655–2656
and peripheral nerves, 2316
of spinal nerve roots, 2316
of trigeminal nerve, 1672, 2302, 2304–2306, *2305, 2306*
vestibular, 2308
of vestibulocochlear nerve, 2308–2309, *2309, 2310,* 2311–2316, *2312, 2315*
Schwannomataosis
cutaneous, 2668
spinal, 2668
Schwartz-Jampel syndrome, 1377
Scintillating scotomas, 3672
differential diagnosis of, 3670–3672, *3672*
Scintillography, lacrimal, 956
Sclera, 4901
leukemic involvement of, 2349–2350
sensory nerve endings in, 1601
Sclera angiomas, 2712, *2714, 2715*
Scleritis, 3796, 3822, 5037–5038, 5488, *5489,* 5490, *5490*
anterior, 1724
posterior, 1724
Sclerodactyly in CREST syndrome, 3014
Scleroderma, *3832, 3833,* 3833–3838, *3834, 3835, 3836, 3837, 3838*
Sclerosis
Baló's concentric, 5539
multiple, 2664
myelinoclastic diffuse, 622, 5539

clinical manifestations, 5639
neurologic, 5639
neuro-ophthalmologic, 5639–5641
diagnosis, 5642
laboratory and neuroimaging findings, 5641–5642, *5643, 5644, 5645*
pathogenesis, 5639
pathology, 5639, *5640, 5641, 5642*
treatment and prognosis, 5642
primary lateral, 2799
tuberous. (*See* Tuberous sclerosis.)
Sclerotic bodies, 4353
Scoliosis, 2661–2662
Scopolamine, 1001
Scotomas
cecocentral, 602
central, 602, 674
paracentral, 602
positive, 154
quadrantic, 3691–3692
that originate from visual cortex, *3666,* 3666–3668, *3667, 3668*
Scrapie, 4567
Scrub typhus, 4758–4762, *4759, 4760, 4761*
Sea snake venom, 1406
Season of onset and relationship between optic neuritis and multiple sclerosis, 618
Secondary bacterial pneumonia, 5193
Secondary cortical visual areas, anatomy and physiology of, 139
area 19 (peristriate cortex), 140
area V2 (parastriate cortex: area 18 of Brodmann), 139–140
area V3 and area V3A, *127,* 140–141, *141*
area V4 and color discrimination, 142–143
area V5 (MT, MST) and motion processing, 143
area V6 and relative position in space, 145, *145*
interactions among areas V1, V2, V3, V3A, and 19, 141–142
other areas of visual sensory system, 145
Secondary deviation, 1176
Secondary erythrocytosis, 2332
Secondary glaucoma, 1997
Secondary neurologic complications, 5385
Secondary oculomotor nerve synkinesis, 1224–1225, 3047, *3049*
Secondary optic nerve sheath meningiomas, 2051
Secondary syphilis, 4857–4861, 4858*t*
Secondary systemic amyloidosis, 4173
Secretomotor nerves to salivary glands, anatomy of, 1022–1024
See-saw anisocoria, 1782–1783
Seesaw nystagmus, 1477, 1496, 2180, 3501
Segmental motor weakness, 5031–5032
Segmental neurofibromatosis, 2664
Segmental optic nerve hypoplasia, *783,* 783–784, *784*
Seizures, 5165. (*See also* Epilepsy.)
arteriovenous malformations (AVMs) presenting with, 2277
disturbances during, 994–995
focal, 1570
headaches following, 1720
and multiple sclerosis, 5574
in patients with neurofibromatosis, 2660
in patients with Sturge-Weber syndrome, 2712, 2716–2717
in patients with temporal lobe tumors, 1833–1834
relationship between migraine and, 3701
as sign of tumors, 1791–1792
in systemic lupus erythematosus, 3819
in tuberous sclerosis, 2679, 2684
visual, 461–463, *462, 463, 464*
Selective intra-arterial angiography, 3544–3545, *3548*
Sella turcica, 87, 2141–2142, *2143,* 2144, *2144*
metastases to, 2206
Semilunar ganglion, 1618–1620, *1619, 1620*
Sensory ataxic neuropathy with dysarthria and ophthalmoplegia (SANDO), 1390
Sensory cortex, involvement of, 1685
Sensory disturbances, 1860
Sensory extinction, 1841
Sensory inattention, 1841
Sensory suppression, 1841
Sensory-motor stroke, 3517
Sentinal headaches, 1710
Septic cavernous sinus thrombosis
causes, 3894–3895, *3896, 3897*
clinical manifestations, 3895–3897, *3896, 3897*
prognosis, 3898
treatment, 3897–3898
Septic emboli, 3379, *3382*
Septic embolization, 3943
Septic foci on scalp or face, 3946
Septic occlusion
of deep cerebral veins, 4034
of superficial cerebral veins, 4032–4034
Septic thrombophlebitis, 4032
diagnosis of, 4042–4043, *4043*
treatment, 4043
Septic thrombosis, 4088
of cavernous sinus, 4034–4039, *4035, 4036, 4037, 4038*
of cerebral and dural venous sinuses, 4070, *4072*
of cerebral venous sinuses, 4073
of cortical veins and venous sinuses, 4236
of jugular vein, 3926–3927
of lateral sinus, *3899,* 3899–3901, *3900, 3901, 4039,* 4039–4041, *4040*
of superior sagittal sinus, 3905–3907, *3906,* 4042
Septic venous occlusion, 3887
Septicemia, *Neisseria meningitidis,* 4104
Septicemic plague, 4227
Septo-optic dysplasia, 779, 780, 783
Septum pellucidum, 1855, *1855, 1856*
astrocytomas of, 1937
cysts of, 2124–2126, *2128*
Seroconversion, 5369
Seroconversion illness, 5372
Seronegative HLA-B27-associated spondyloarthropathies, 3852
Seronegative Lyme disease, 4828–4829
Serotonin, role of, in migraine, 3705
Serotying, 4101–4102
Serratia, 4224
Serratia marcescens, 4224
Serum antitoxoplasma antibodies, 5410
Serum lipoprotein disorders, abetalipoproteinemia, 2851–2852
Servomechanism, pupillary light response as, 891–892
Setting-sun sign, 1304
Sex in incidence of saccular aneurysms, 3015
Sex-linked recessive optic atrophy, ataxia, deafness, tetraplegia, and areflexia, 760
Sexual activity, headache associated with, 1704–1705
Sexual dysfunction and multiple sclerosis, 5573
Sézary cells, 2386
Shadow plaques, 5555, 5558, *5559*
Shagreen patches, 2671, *2674,* 2675, *2675*
Shearing injury, 725
Sheridan-Gardiner test, 161
Sherrington's law of reciprocal innervation, 1173
Shiga toxin, 4224
Shigella, 4224–4225
Shigella dysenteriae in vasogenic cervical edema, 3981
Shigellosis, 4224–4225
Short posterior ciliary arteries, 2881
Short stature, 2662
Short Wavelength Automated Perimetry (SWAP), *204,* 204–205, *205, 206*
Short-term immunotherapies, 1429–1430
Shy-Drager syndrome, 1028
Sialidoses, 2822
Sick sinus syndrome, 3389
Sickle cell anemia, 3012
Sickle cell disease, 3349–3350, 3889
Sickle hemoglobin C disease, 3349
Sigmoid sinus, 2959, 2961
thrombosis of, 3912
Simple cells, 130
Simultagnosia, 3491
Simultanagnosia, 428, 445
Simultaneous recording of visual-evoked potential and PERG, *228,* 228–229
Single cover test, 1180–1181
Single deletions of mtDNA in sporadic ophthalmoplegia, 1389–1390
Single-fiber electromyography, 1423
Single-photon emission computed tomographic (SPECT) scanning, 3532–3533
in diagnosing aneurysms, 3152
Sinus disease and optic neuritis, 630–631
Sinus headache, 1732–1733
Sinus histiocytosis with massive lymphadenopathy, 2415
Sinus rectus, 2959
Sinuses
basilar, 2964
cavernous, 2962–2964, *2963, 2964*
dural, 2954, *2955,* 2956, *2956, 2957, 2958,* 2959, *2959, 2960, 2961,* 2961–2964, *2962, 2963, 2964, 2965*
intercavernous, 2964
lateral, 2959, *2962*
occipital, 2961
paranasal, 5470
petrosal, 2964, *2965*
sagittal, 2953, *2955,* 2956, *2956, 2957*
superior, 2953, *2955,* 2956, *2956, 2957*
sigmoid, 2959, 2961
sphenoparietal, 2964
tentorial, 2961
Sinusitis, 4025–4026, 4035, 4071
allergic, 4287–4288
as cause of septic cavernous sinus thrombosis, 3894, *3897*
Sinusoidal oscillations, 1142
Sipple's syndrome, 2459
Sjögren-Larsson syndrome, 2795
Sjögren's syndrome, 3822, 3841–3842, *3842, 3843*
and multiple sclerosis, 5544

Skeletal abnormalities in patients with neurofibromatosis, 2661
Skeletal blastomycosis, 4334–4335
Skew deviation, 1286, 1296, *1296*, 1854, 1869, 3767, 4375, 5433, 5602
Skiametry, dynamic, 951
Skin
basal and squamous cell carcinomas of, *2457*, 2457–2458
thermal sensation in, 1604
touch and pressure sensation in, 1603–1604, *1604*
Skin lesions in cryptococcosis, 4381, *4382*
Skull, tuberculosis of bones of, 4163
Sleep, saccadic eye movements during, 1107–1108
Sleep test, 1418, *1418*
Sleeping sickness, 4710, *4710*, 4711
Slime, 4072
Slit lamp biomicroscopy in diagnosing traumatic optic neuropathy, 720
Slit lamp examination, 158
Slow channel syndrome, 1434, *1435*
Slowly progressive ION, 3450
Slow-rise OKN, 1149
Sluggish pupillary responses, 1367
Sly syndrome (MPS VII), 2821–2822
Smallpox, 5148–5149, *5150*
vaccinia virus, 5149–5154, *5151, 5152, 5153*
Smith-Lemli-Opitz syndrome, 766
Smoking
and incidence of atherosclerosis, 3329–3330
as risk factor for stroke, 3567
as risk factor in aneurysms, 3012
Smooth pursuit movements, 1102, 1154–1155, 1317
brainstem generation of, 1132–1134, *1133*
cerebellum and, 1131–1132
cerebral initiation and maintenance of, 1125–1126, *1126, 1127*
recovery of, 1131
Smooth pursuit system
characteristics of, 1123–1125, *1124*
neurophysiology of, 1125–1134, *1126, 1127, 1133*
Sneddon's syndrome, 3363
Snellen chart, 160
Snellen notation, 160
Snout reflex, 1659
Snowshoe hare virus, 5159
Soft fibromas, 2675, *2676*
Somatic muscles, weakness of, 1387, *1387*
Somatic mutation, 1990
Somatic sensation, 1649–1650
Somatization disorder, 1766
Somatosensory evoked potentials (SEPs), 5626–5627, 5690
Somnambulism, 3698
South American blastomycosis, 4407
Space, relative position in, and area V6, 145, *145*
Space centroid, 1171
Sparganum erinacei, 4453
Sparganum mansoni, 4453
Sparganum mansonoides, 4453
Sparganum proliferum, 4453
Sparganum ranarum, 4453
Sparganums, 4443
Spasm of near reflex, 1780–1782, *1781*
Spasmus mobilis, 1782
Spasmus nutans, 1484–1485, *1485*
Spastic miosis, 936
Specific antitreponemal antibody tests, 4927
Specific toxic optic neuropathies, *671*, 671–675
Spectral sensitivity of pupillary light reaction, 889–890, *890*
Speech, disturbances of, 1860, 5568
Spelling alexia, 424
Sphenocavernous syndrome, 1212, 1668, 1805
Sphenoid bone, fractures of, in patients with traumatic optic neuropathy, 722–723
Sphenoid ridge meningiomas, *2056*, 2056–2062, *2057, 2058, 2059, 2061*
Sphenoid sinus mucoceles, 4019–4023, *4022*
Sphenopalatine artery, 2946
Sphenopalatine ganglion, 923–924
lesions affecting, 1019–1021, *1022*
Sphenoparietal sinuses, 2964
Spherules, 35, 4355
Sphincter muscle, *851, 854*, 855, *855*
Sphingolipidoses
Fabry disease, 2831–2832, *2832, 2833*
Farber disease, 2830–2831, *2831*
gangliosidoses, 2824–2828, *2825, 2826, 2828*
Gaucher disease, 2828–2830, *2829, 2830*
Niemann-Pick disease, 2832–2837, *2834, 2835, 2836, 2837*
Spinal cord
complications of radiation therapy, 2604–2609, *2606, 2607, 2608*
hemorrhage of, 2607, *2608*
papilledema and lesions of, 518
tumors of, 1893
Spinal cysticercosis, 4472
Spinal epidural empyema, 4069
Spinal nerve roots, schwannomas of, 2316
Spinal neurocysticercosis, 4467, 4476
Spinal paralytic poliomyelitis, 5255
Spinal schwannomatosis, 2668
Spinal tract, nucleus of, 1630–1631
Spinocerebellar ataxia, 762
type 1, 763
type 2, 763
type 3, 763
type 4, 763
type 5, 763
Spinocerebellar disorders. (*See* cerebellar and spinocerebellar disorders.)
Spiral computed tomography angiography, 3544, *3545, 3546*
in diagnosing aneurysms, 3015, 3109–3110
Spiral of Tillaux, 1043, *1044*
Spirochetal aneurysms, 3004–3005, 3973
Spirochetes and spirochetoses, 4779, *4780*, 4780*t*, *4781*
Borrelia species, 4779, *4780, 4782*
Lyme disease, 4779–4780, 4783
arthritis, 4809, *4810*
cardiac manifestations, 4789, *4789*
chronic disseminated, 4808–4818, *4810, 4811, 4812, 4813, 4814, 4815, 4816, 4817, 4818*
clinical course, 4787
clinical manifestations, 4786–4787
cutaneous manifestations, 4787, *4788*, 4788–4789, *4789*, 4809–4810, *4810*
diagnosis, 4820, 4822, *4822, 4823, 4824*, 4824–4825, *4825, 4826, 4827*, 4827–4828
early disseminated, 4787–4791, *4789, 4790, 4792, 4793*, 4793–4797, *4794, 4796, 4797, 4798, 4799*, 4799–4803, *4800, 4801, 4802, 4803, 4804*, 4805, *4805, 4806, 4807*, 4807–4808, *4808, 4809*
early localized, 4787
epidemiology, 4783–4786, *4784, 4785*
neurologic manifestations, 4787, 4789–4791, *4790, 4792, 4793*, 4793–4795, *4794, 4796*, 4810–4816, *4811, 4812, 4813, 4814, 4815, 4816*
neuro-ophthalmologic manifestations, 4800–4803, *4802, 4803, 4804*, 4805, *4805, 4806*, 4807–4808, *4808, 4809*, 4816–4818, *4817, 4818*
ocular manifestations, 4787, 4795–4797, *4796, 4798, 4799*, 4799–4800, *4800, 4801, 4816*, 4816–4818, *4817, 4818*
pathogen, 4786
pathogenesis, 4818–4820
pathology, 4820, *4820, 4821*
prevention, *4831*, 4831–4832
seronegative, 4828–4829
systemic manifestations, 4787
treatment, 4829–4831
relapsing fever, 4832
clinical manifestations, 4833–4834
diagnosing, *4834*, 4834–4835
epidemiology, *4832*, 4832–4833, *4833*
pathogenesis, 4833
prevention, 4836
treatment and prognosis, 4835, *4835, 4836*
Leptospira species
clinical manifestations, 4837–4842, *4840, 4841, 4842, 4843*
diagnosis, 4842–4843
epidemiology, 4836–4837
pathology and pathogenesis, 4837, *4838, 4839, 4840*
treatment, 4843
Treponema species, *4780, 4781*, 4844, *4844*
bejel, 4850, *4852*, 4853, *4853, 4854*
pinta, 4844, *4845, 4846*
syphilis, 4853
cardiovascular, *4881*, 4881–4884
clinical manifestations, 4855–4857
congenital, 4902–4903
cutaneous manifestations, 4858–4860, *4859, 4860, 4861, 4862*
epidemiology, 4854–4855, *4856*
gummatous, *4892*, 4892–4895, *4893, 4894, 4896, 4897, 4898*, 4898–4900, *4899*, 4900
human immunodeficiency virus infection and AIDS, 4916–4918, *4919, 4920, 4921, 4922*, 4922*t*, *4923, 4924, 4925*, 4925–4929, *4926*, 4928*t*
incubation stage of, 4856–4857
latent stage of, 4856–4857, 4880–4881
natural history, 4929–4930
neurologic manifestations, 4861, *4863*, 4863–4864, *4864*
neuro-ophthalmologic manifestations, *4872*, 4872–4874, *4873, 4874, 4875*, 4876, *4876*, 4878–4880, *4879*, 4907–4908, *4908*
neurosyphilis, 4882*t*, 4882–4884, 4883*t*

ocular involvement in tertiary, 4900–4902
ocular manifestations, 4864–4868, *4865, 4866, 4867, 4868, 4869, 4870,* 4871–4872, 4903–4907, *4904, 4905, 4906, 4907*
pathogenesis, 4855
pathology, 4908–4909, *4909, 4910, 4911, 4912,* 4912–4913, *4913, 4914, 4915,* 4916, *4917, 4918, 4919, 4920, 4921, 4922, 4923, 4924*
primary stage of, 4856–4857, 4857, *4857, 4858*
prognosis with treatment, 4931
secondary stage of, 4856–4857, 4857–4861, 4858*t*
systemic manifestations, 4860–4861, *4902,* 4902–4903, *4903*
tertiary stage of, 4856–4857, 4881
treatment, 4930–4931
yaws, 4845, *4847,* 4847–4848, *4848, 4849,* 4850, *4850, 4851, 4852*
Spirochetoses in neuroretinitis, 636
Spirometra species and *Sparganum proliferum* (Sparganosis), 4453–4455, *4455, 4456, 4457, 4458, 4459,* 4460, *4460*
Spiromustine, 2568
Splenectomy, 5084
Splenic rupture, 5084
Splenium, 1859
Spondylitis, tuberculous, 4163–4164, *4166*
Spondylosis, cervical, 1722
Spongioblastomas, 2355
polar, 1934, *1935*
Spontaneous abortion, 5226
Spontaneous blinks, 1523, 1532–1533
Spontaneous blood loss as causes of decreased cerebral perfusion, 3409–3411, *3411,* 3412
Spontaneous eye movements in unconscious patients, 1492–1494, *1493,* 1493*t*
Spontaneous eyelid retraction, 1411
Spontaneous intracranial hypotension, 1252–1253, 1715–1716
Spontaneous thrombosis of unruptured aneurysm, 3142
Sporadic Creutzfeld-Jakob disease, 4571–4574, *4572, 4574, 4575,* 4576, *4576*
Spores, 4282
tuberculated, 4389
Sporogony, 4651
Sporothrix schenckii, 4282, 4415, *4416,* 4417, *4417, 4418*
Sporozoites, 4644, 4650
Spotted fever, 4737
Spumaviruses, 5362
Squamous cell carcinomas of skin, *2457,* 2457–2458
Square pupils, 1006
Square-wave jerks, 1486–1487
Stagnant hypoxia, 3324
Staphylococci, 4068
Staphylococcus, in intracranial abscess, 3950
Staphylococcus agalactiae, 4086–4089
Staphylococcus albus, 4071
Staphylococcus aureus, 4068–4071, *4069, 4070, 4071, 4072*
in bacterial aneurysms, 2999, 3967, 3968
in bacterial meningitis, 3994
in empyema, 3983
in intracranial abscess, 3950
Staphylococcus epidermidis
in bacterial meningitis, 3993, 3995
in intracranial brain abscess, 3955
and other coagulase-negative, 4071–4073, *4073, 4074*
Staphylococcus salivarius, 4092–4093
Staphylococcus warneri, 4072
Starburst amacrine cell, 42
Startle myoclonus, 4568
Stasis retinopathy, 3282
Static counter-roll, 1141
Static countertorsion, 1172
Static perimetry, 177, *177*
suprathreshold, 177–178, *179*
Stavudine (D4T), 5365
Steal phenomenon, 3425
Steele-Richardson-Olszewski syndrome, 2771
epidemiology, 2772
etiology, 2773
eyelid manifestations, 2775
laboratory and neuroimaging findings, 2775–2776
neurologic manifestations, 2773
neuro-ophthalmologic manifestations, 2773–2775, *2775*
pathology, *27,* 2772–2773, *2774*
prognosis, 2776
treatment, 2776
Stellate ganglion, 838
Stellate maculopathy, 634
Stem cells
lymphoid, 2329
myeloid, 2329
pluripotential, 2329
Stenosis, aqueductal, 2660
Step of neural activity, 1103, *1104*
Stereoacuity, 155–156
Stereopsis
in optic neuritis, 613
testing of, 1773
Stereotactic instrumentation in aneurysm clipping, 3149–3150
Stereotactic radiosurgery, 1902, 2595, 2598
for arteriovenous malformations (AVMs), 2282, 2284
Steroids, anabolic, 3362
Stevens-Johnson syndrome, 4547
Stiff-man syndrome, 2531–2532
Stilling-Turk-Duane syndrome, *1240,* 1240–1242, *1241, 1242, 1243,* 1244, *1244, 1245*
Stimulus intensity, effect of, on pupillary light reaction, 889, *889*
Stomatitis, aphthous, 3803
Stomatococcus mucilaginosus, 4092–4093
Storage diseases and cerebral degenerations of childhood, 764–767
Stormorken syndrome, 1009
Strabismus, 1997, 2656
congenital, 1170
comitant, 1176
in meningococcal meningitis, 4096
Strachan's syndrome, 671
Straight sinus, 2959
thrombosis of, 3910, 3912
Stratum moleculare layer of Brodmann, 128
Streptococcus, 4073–4075, *4074,* 5421
in bacterial aneurysms, 3968
in intracranial abscess, 3950
nonhemolytic, 4074, 4075
Streptococcus agalactiae in bacterial meningitis, 3993, 3994
Streptococcus anginosus, 4081, 4083, 4089
in sinusitis, 4025
Streptococcus avium, 4090
Streptococcus bovis, 4088
in intracranial brain abscess, 3952
Streptococcus casseliflavus, 4090
Streptococcus constellatus, 4083, 4089
in sinusitis, 4025
Streptococcus durans, 4090
Streptococcus dysgalactiae, 4088
Streptococcus equinus, 4088
Streptococcus equisimilis, 4088
Streptococcus faecalis, 4075, 4089
Streptococcus faecium, 4075, 4089
Streptococcus gallinarum, 4090
Streptococcus intermedius, 4081, 4083, 4084–4085, 4089
in sinusitis, 4025
Streptococcus malodoratus, 4090
Streptococcus milleri, 4081, 4082–4085, 4089
in bacterial aneurysms, 2999
in meningitis, 3111, 3113
Streptococcus morbillorum subacute bacterial endocarditis, 3111, 3113
Streptococcus pneumoniae, 3943, *4075,* 4075–4080, *4076, 4077, 4078, 4079, 4080*
in acute bacterial meningitis, 4004
in bacterial meningitis, 3993, 3994, 3995
in sinusitis, 4025
in vasogenic cervical edema, 3981
Streptococcus pyogenes in bacterial aneurysms, 2999
Streptococcus salivarius in bacterial aneurysms, 3001, 3967
Streptococcus viridans, 4080, *4081,* 4081–4085, *4082, 4083, 4084, 4085, 4086*
Streptococcus zooepidemicus, 4088
Streptokinase, 3562
Streptomyces nodosus, 4283
Streptomycin for tuberculosis, 4143–4144
Stress in development of multiple sclerosis, 5543
Stretch reflex blepharospasm, 1569
Striate cortex, 126
color vision mechanisms in, *138,* 138–139, *139*
lesions of, without defects in visual field, 371
permanent homonymous visual field defects from ischemia of, 3691–3692
representation of brightness in, 138
representation of visual field in, 135–137, *137*
visual disturbances originating in, *3665,* 3665–3670, *3666, 3667, 3668, 3669*
Strict aerobes, 4066
Strobilization, 4461
Stroke
completed, 3324
ischemic, 3142
in Lyme disease, 4795, *4796,* 4814–4816
management of patients with acute, 3577–3581
partial nonprogressing, 3324
Stroke-in-evolution, 3324
Stroke-like syndromes and transient, 5413–5415, *5414*
Strongyloides stercoralis, 4511, 4511–4512, *4512, 4513, 4514,* 4514–4515, 5423
Stupor, eye movements in, 1327–1330

Sturge-Weber syndrome, 324, 2707
  seizures in patients with, 2712, 2716–2717
Subacute ascending polyradiculomyelopathy, 5111–5112
Subacute bacterial endocarditis, 4028
Subacute cerebellar degeneration, 2505
  clinical features, 2505–2507
  diagnostic evaluations, 2507, *2509*
  differential diagnosis, 2507
  pathogenesis, 2507–2509, *2510*
  pathology, 2507, *2508*
  prognosis, 2509–2510
  treatment, 2509
Subacute cerebellar syndrome, 2559
Subacute cutaneous skin lesions, 3814–3815, *3815*
Subacute disseminated histoplasmosis, 4393, 4397
Subacute encephalitis, 3988
Subacute encephalopathy, 2554–2555
Subacute measles encephalitis (SME), 5213, 5418–5419
Subacute meningitis, *4015,* 4015–4017, *4016*
Subacute motor neuropathy, 2522
Subacute myelitis, 2501
Subacute sclerosing leukoencephalitis, 5213
  clinical manifestations, *5214,* 5214–5216, *5215, 5216, 5217*
  diagnosis, 5217, 5220, *5223, 5224*
  epidemiology, 5213–5214
  pathogenesis, 5217
  pathology, 5216–5217, *5218, 5219*
  treatment and prognosis, 5220, *5224*
Subacute sclerosing panencephalitis, 3979, 5213
  clinical manifestations, *5214,* 5214–5216, *5215, 5216, 5217*
  diagnosis, 5217, 5220, *5223, 5224*
  epidemiology, 5213–5214
  pathogenesis, 5217
  pathology, 5216–5217, *5218, 5219*
  treatment and prognosis, 5220, *5224*
Subacute sensorimotor neuropathy, 2523–2524
Subacute sensory neuropathy, 2521–2522
Subarachnoid cisterns, 2020, *2021*
Subarachnoid hemorrhage, 2975, 3020, 3268, 4304–4305, *4306, 4307*
  diagnosis of, 3130
  headaches associated with, 1710
  papilledema from, 516–517
Subarachnoid neurocysticercosis, *4464, 4465,* 4465–4466, *4466,* 4476
Subarachnoid oculomotor nerve palsy
  from involvement at or near its entrance to cavernous sinus, 1209, *1211,* 1211–1212, *1212, 1213*
  isolated fixed, dilated pupil as sole manifestation of, 1203–1204
  with pupillary involvement, 1204–1208, *1205, 1206, 1207, 1208, 1209*
  with pupillary sparing, 1208–1209, *1210*
Subarachnoid space, 2018
Subarcuate artery, 2917
Subclavian artery, collateral occlusion of, 3417
Subclavian steal syndrome, 3417, 3519–3521, *3520*
Subconjunctival hemorrhage, 3029
Subconjunctival loiasis, 4505, *4506*
Subcortical angiomas, 2236
Subcortical dementia, 2748
Subcortical hematomas, 3611
Subcortical hemorrhage, *3596,* 3596–3597, 5061, 5068
Subcutaneous nodules, 4334
Subdural abscess, 3943–3944
  Aspergillus in, 4308
Subdural effusions, 4004–4005, 4016
Subdural empyema, 4016, 4179, 4224
  cause of, 4214
  Pseudomonas aeruginosa, 4242
Subdural hematoma
  headaches associated with, 1709
  papilledema from acute and chronic, 516
  from ruptured intracranial aneurysm, *3036,* 3036–3037
Subdural tuberculomas, 4163
Subependymal giant-cell astrocytomas, 1935, 2687–2688, *2689, 2690*
Subependymal nodules, 2686–2687, *2688*
Subependymal veins, *2950,* 2950–2951, *2951*
Subependymomas, 1966–1967, *1967*
Subjective relative, afferent defect testing for, 944–945
Subjective visual complaints in optic neuritis, 614
Subjunctival gnathostomiasis, 4501
Subpial spaces, local infiltration of, 1928
Substance abuse, headaches associated with, 1717–1720
Substance P, 1005
Substantia nigra, 1863
Substantia nigra pars reticulata, 1519
Subthalamic nucleus, 1863
Subungual fibromas, 2675, *2675*
Sucking reflex, 1821
Suction ophthalmodynamometry (ODM), 3537–3538, *3538*
Sudden Infant Death Syndrome (SIDS), 4121
Sudden visual loss with retrobulbar compressive lesions, 656–657
Sulcus chiasmatis, 85
Sulfadiazine, 4699, *4699*
Sulfhemoglobinemia and headaches, 1718
Sulfinpyrazone, 3560–3561
Sulfonamides and headaches, 1718
SUNCT syndrome, 1752
Superficial cerebral veins
  septic occlusion of, 4032–4034
  thrombosis of, *3891,* 3891–3893, *3892, 3893*
Superficial corneal disease, 1723–1724
Superficial plexiform layer, 50
Superficial temporal artery, 2942, *2944*
Superior cerebellar artery, 2917, *2918, 2919,* 2920–2921, *2921*
  aneurysms arising from, *3122,* 3122–3123
Superior cervical ganglion, 838, *880, 881,* 881–882
Superior colliculus, 1519
  ocular motor syndromes caused by lesions of, 1315
  in saccadic eye movements, 1115–1118
Superior hypophysial artery, aneurysms arising from junction of internal carotid artery and, *3059,* 3059–3060, *3060, 3061, 3062,* 3062–3063, *3063, 3064, 3065,* 3065–3066, *3066, 3067*
Superior laryngeal neuralgia, 1747
Superior medullary velum, 1884
Superior oblique microtremor, 1259–1261, 1491–1492
Superior oblique myokymia, 1259–1261, 1491–1492, 1497
Superior orbital fissure, syndrome of, 1667–1668
Superior orbital fissure, tumors in, 1804–1805, *1805, 1806,* 1807, *1807, 1808, 1809*
Superior orbital fissure syndrome, 1727
Superior parietal arteries, 2897
Superior sagittal sinus, thrombosis of, 3905–3910, *3906, 3907, 3908, 3909, 3910, 3911, 3912,* 4042
Superior thyroid artery, 2940
Superior vena cava, occlusion of, 3929
Superoxide dismutase, 4067, 4548
Supplementary eye field in saccadic eye movements, 1118
Supraclinoid aneurysms, 3054
Supranuclear and premotor inputs to orbicularis oculi motoneurons, *1518, 1519,* 1519–1520
Supranuclear bilateral eyelid retraction, 1549, *1551*
Supranuclear disorders, insufficiency of eyelid closure caused by, 1560–1565, *1561, 1562, 1565*
Supranuclear gaze disturbances, 4078
  in patients with tetanus, 4113–4114
Supranuclear gaze palsy, 5509
Supranuclear gaze pareses, 5729
Supranuclear influences on iris sphincter muscle, 868
Supranuclear lesions, 1018, 5603, *5604*
  eyelid retraction from, 1548–1550, *1551, 1552*
Supranuclear ophthalmoparesis, 4184
Supranuclear pathways for tear secretion, 925–926
Supranuclear trigeminal connections and projections
  corticofugal fibers to nuclei, 1633
  pathways between nuclei and other brainstem areas, 1632
  pathways from nuclei to thalamus, *1632,* 1632–1633, *1634*
  thalamus and thalamocortical, 1633–1634, *1635, 1636,* 1636–1637
Supranuclear vertical gaze paresis, 4375
Supraoptic commissural fibers, 99
Supraoptic nucleus, 830
Suprasellar arachnoid cysts, 2123–2125
Suprasellar epidermoid cysts, 2098, 2108–2110, *2109*
Suprasellar germinomas, 2085
Suprasellar region, tumors involving, 1807, *1811,* 1811–1815, *1812, 1813, 1814*
Supratentorial arachnoid cysts, 2118–2120, *2119, 2120*
Supratentorial arteriovenous malformations, 2257–2261, *2258, 2259, 2260, 2261*
Supratentorial hemangioblastomas, 2223–2224, 2225
Suprathreshold static perimetry, 177–178, *179*
Suramin, 2580–2581
Surface dyslexia, 435
Surgery. (*See also* Stereotactic radiosurgery.)
  for arteriovenous malformations (AVMs), 2279–2280
  for bacterial meningitis, 4011
  cataract, 556
  decompression, 562
  endovascular, for ruptured saccular aneurysms, 3154–3155, *3156, 3157,* 3157–3159, *3158, 3159, 3160, 3161, 3162,* 3162–3165, *3164, 3165, 3166, 3167*
  for pituitary adenomas, 2188–2191

for septic thrombosis, 4038–4039
transsphenoidal, 2195–2196
for pituitary adenomas, 2199
Susac's syndrome, 3727, *3732,* 3732–3734, *3733,* 3734
Sustained opsoclonus, 1489
Swim-goggle headache, 1702
Swinging flashlight test, 939–941, *941,* 944
Swiss cheese visual field, 614
Sydenham's chorea, 1319
Sylvian aqueduct syndrome, 1868
Sympathectomy, cervicothoracic, 1696
Sympathetic hyperactivity, *973,* 973–974
Sympathetic hyperfunction, eyelid retraction from, 1555
Sympathetic nervous system and cerebral blood flow, 2970
Sympathetic outflow pathway, 879–883, *880, 881, 882*
Sympathetic pathway, to lacrimal gland, 924–925
Sympatholytic drugs, 1005
Sympathomimetic drugs, 1003–1004, *1004*
Symptomatic neurosyphilis, 4883
Symptomatic treatment of migraine, 3710
Synapse, 841
Synaptophysin, 1919
Syncephalastraceae, 4318
Synchronous adenomas, 2152
Syncytia, 5366
Syncytial meningiomas, *2026,* 2026–2027
Syndrome of anterior inferior cerebellar artery (AICA), 1287, *1288*
skew deviation and ocular tilt reaction, 1287–1289
Syndrome of diabetes insipidus, 1812
Syndrome of distal optic nerve, 1807, 1811, *1811,* 2171
Syndrome of floor of orbit, 1804
Syndrome of optic chiasm, 1811, *1812*
Syndrome of optic neuropathy, 674
Syndrome of optic tract, 1811–1812, *1813, 1814*
Syndrome of orbital apex, 1668
Syndrome of superior orbital fissure, 1667–1668
Syndrome of uncal herniation, 997–998
Syndrome of unilateral optic nerve dysfunction, 292, 294
anterior optic chiasm syndrome, 294, *297, 298*
distal optic neuropathy, 294, *297, 298*
distal syndrome, 294, *297, 298*
Foster Kennedy syndrome, 296, 298
optociliary shunts and syndrome of chronic optic nerve compression, 294
prechiasmal compression syndrome, 294
Synkinesis
involving ocular motor and other cranial nerves, 1261
levator palpebrae, 1553
lid-triggered, 1570–1571
oculomotor nerve, 3128, *3129*
primary oculomotor nerve, 3047, *3050*
secondary oculomotor nerve, 3047, *3049*
Synovitis, 3805
Syphilis, 3339, 3973, 4030, *4030,* 4853
cardiovascular, *4881,* 4881–4884
clinical manifestations, 4855–4857
congenital, 4902–4903
cutaneous manifestations, 4858–4860, *4859, 4860, 4861, 4862*
direct diagnosis of, 4918, 4925, *4925, 4926*
epidemiology, 4854–4855, *4856*
gummatous, *4892,* 4892–4895, *4893, 4894, 4896, 4897, 4898,* 4898–4900, *4899,* 4900, *4900*
human immunodeficiency virus infection and AIDS, 4916–4918, *4919, 4920, 4921, 4922,* 4922*t, 4923, 4924, 4925,* 4925–4929, *4926,* 4928*t*
incubation stage of, 4856–4857
indirect diagnosis of, 4925–4927
latent stage, 4856–4857, 4880–4881
natural history, 4929–4930
neurologic manifestations, 4861, *4863,* 4863–4864, *4864*
neuro-ophthalmologic manifestations, *4872,* 4872–4874, *4873, 4874, 4875,* 4876, *4876,* 4878–4880, *4879,* 4907–4908, *4908*
neurosyphilis, 4882*t,* 4882–4884, 4883*t*
ocular involvement in tertiary, 4900–4902
ocular manifestations, 4864–4868, *4865, 4866, 4867, 4868, 4869, 4870,* 4871–4872, 4903–4907, *4904, 4905, 4906, 4907*
optic neuritis from, 629–630
pathogenesis, 4855
pathology, 4908–4909, *4909, 4910, 4911, 4912,* 4912–4913, *4913, 4914, 4915,* 4916, *4917, 4918, 4919, 4920, 4921, 4922, 4923, 4924*
primary stage, 4856–4857, 4857, *4857, 4858*
prognosis with treatment, 4931
secondary stage, 4856–4857, 4857–4861, 4858*t*
systemic manifestations, 4860–4861, *4902,* 4902–4903, *4903*
tertiary stage, 4856–4857, 4881
treatment, 4930–4931
Syphilitic meningitis, 636, 4879, 5423–5424
Syphilitic neurosyphilis, 5423–5424
Syphilitic periostitis, 1722
Syringobulbia, 1680
Syrinxes, 2702–2703
Systemic angiomatosis, 2275
Systemic corticosteroids, 4699, 5692
Systemic diffuse large-cell lymphoma, 2361–2364, *2362, 2363, 2365*
Systemic disease and marantic endocarditis, 3391
Systemic fever, headaches associated with, 1716
Systemic hypertension, headaches associated with, 1713
Systemic hypotension
causes of, 3407, *3408,* 3409–3413
general considerations, 3407
headaches associated with, 1713
Systemic infections
with bone marrow transplantation, 2627
headaches associated with, 1716
Systemic lupus erythematosus (SLE), 530, 3005, 3888
optic neuritis in, 630
Systemic necrotizing vasculitides, *3743, 3744,* 3744–3751, *3745, 3746, 3747, 3748, 3750, 3751*
Systemic sclerosis, *3832, 3833,* 3833–3838, *3834, 3835, 3836, 3837, 3838*
Systemic toxicity
of chemotherapeutic medications, 2554, 2558, 2560, 2562, 2563, 2565–2567, 2568, 2573, 2578, 2579, 2580, 2581, 2583, 2584, 2587, 2589, 2593
from radiation therapy, 2596–2598

T

Tabes dorsalis, 4886–4887
Taboparesis, 4886, 4891, *4892*
Tachyzoites, 4667
Tactile agnosia, 1839
Tactile anomia, 1839
Tactile aphasia, 1839
Tadpole pupils, *973,* 973–974
Taenia multiceps, 4440
Taenia solium, 4460
Taeniasis, 4460
Tahyna virus, 5159–5160
Takayasu's arteritis, 3012, 3342, *3344,* 3523, 3727, *3788,* 3788–3792, *3789, 3791,* 3792, *3793*
demographics, 3788
diagnosis, 3791–3792
history, 3788, *3788, 3789*
neurologic manifestations, 3789, *3791*
ocular manifestations, 3789–3790, *3791, 3792*
pathogenesis, 3790–3791
pathology, 3790, *3793*
systemic manifestations, 3789, *3790*
treatment and prognosis, 3792, *3793*
Takayasu's disease, 3523
Talwin, 3586
Tamoxifen
neuro-ophthalmologic toxicity, 2585–2586, *2587, 2588*
neurotoxicity, 2584
ocular toxicity, 2584–2585, *2585, 2586*
systemic toxicity, 2584
Tangent screen, *175,* 175–176, *176*
testing, 156–157
Tapeworms. (*See* Cestodes (tapeworms).)
Tapia's syndrome, 4410
Tardive dyskinesia, blepharospasm associated with drug-induced, 1569–1570
Tarsitis, polypoid or vegetative, 4901
Tau, 2749, 5723
Tax, 5434
Taxoids
neuro-ophthalmologic toxicity, 2583
neurotoxicity, 2583
systemic toxicity, 2583
Tay-Sachs disease, 1326, 2824–2826, *2825, 2826*
Tear secretion
basal, 955
neurophysiology of, 926, *927*
regulation of, 926–927, *928, 929*
supranuclear pathways for, 925–926
Tears
continuous, 926
induced, 926
psychogenic, 926
reflex, 926
Technetium-99m hexamethylpropylenamine oxime (99mTc-HMPAO) in diagnosing aneurysms, 3152
Tectum, 16
Teeth, pain related to, 1733
Tegmentum, 16
Teichopsia, 3666
Tela choroidea, 17, 1884, 2021

Telangiectasia, 2721. (*See also* Ataxia telangiectasia.)
capillary, 2230–2231, *2231, 2232,* 2233, *2233*
hereditary hemorrhagic, 2230, 2275
Telangiectatic lesions in CREST syndrome, 3014
Telencephalon, 17–18
Teleopsia, 1842
Temperature regulation, disturbances of, 1813–1814
Temporal arteritis. (*See* Giant cell arteritis.)
Temporal lobe
abscesses of, 3957, 3958, 4076, *4076*
anatomy and functions of, 1827, *1829, 1830*
hematomas, 3597
lesions of, 339–340, *340, 341, 342,* 344, 347, 1323–1324
tumors involving, *1823,* 1827, *1829, 1830,* 1830–1835, *1836,* 1837
general symptoms and signs, 1830
ocular symptoms and signs, 1834–1835, *1836,* 1837
symptoms and sign produced by, 1827, 1830, *1830*
Temporal raphe, 50
Temporomandibular joint (TMJ) disease, 1733–1735, *1734*
Tensilon test, 1420–1421, *1421*
Tension-type headache, 1697–1698, 1790
Tentorial artery, 2873
Tentorial meningiomas, 2055–2056
Tentorial sinus, 2959, 2961
Tentorium, tumors situated below, 1791
Tentorium cerebelli, 2018
dural arteriovenous malformations (AVMs) of, 2273–2274
meningiomas of, 2055–2056
Teratomas, 2089–2091, *2090, 2091*
atypical, 2085
Terson's syndrome, 2348, 3025–3026, *3027,* 3028
Tertiary syphilis, 4881
Tetanospasmin, 4110, 4116
Tetanus, 1013, 1440, 4109, *4109,* 4109–4117
cephalic, 4111, 4113, *4113*
diagnosis, 4115
epidemiology, 4111
general manifestations, 4111–4113, *4112, 4113*
generalized, 4110, 4112–4113
localized, 4111, 4113
in neuritis, 4026
neurologic manifestations, 4114–4115
neurological manifestations, 4114–4115
ocular and neuro-ophthalmologic manifestations, 4113–4114, *4114*
pathogenesis, 4109–4111, *4110, 4111*
prevention, 4116–4117
prognosis, 4116
treatment, 4115–4116
in vasogenic cervical edema, 3981
Tetanus toxoid, 4116
Tetrahydrozoline hydrochloride, 1004
Thalamic dementia, 3483
Thalamic hemorrhage, 3594–3596, *3595*
Thalamic pain, 1750
Thalamic syndrome of Déjerine and Roussy, 1683
Thalamic-subthalamic hemorrhage, *3022,* 3022–3023
Thalamocortical connections, 1637
Thalamocortical projections, 1683, *1684, 1685*
Thalamus, 1634, *1635, 1637, 1638,* 1683, *1684, 1685*
abscesses of, 3957
infarction of, 3483
ocular motor syndromes caused by lesions of, *1315,* 1315–1316
in saccadic eye movements, 1120
tumors involving, 1859–1861
Thalidomide, 1263–1264
Thallium, 1264
Thamnidiaceae, 4318
Thiamine deficiency, 669–670
Thiotepa, 2578–2579
neurotoxicity, 2578–2579
ocular toxicity, 2579
systemic toxicity, 2578
Third disease, 5286
3rd ventricle, astrocytomas of, 1936–1937, *1937*
Thorazine and headaches, 1718
3-D Block Construction Test, 470
Thrombocythemia, essential, 2335, 3357
Thrombocytopenia, 2337, 3817, 5103, 5288
neonatal isoimmune, 783
Thrombocytopenic purpura, 530
Thrombocytosis, 3772
Thrombogenic metallic wires or coils, 3158, *3158*
Thrombolytic therapy, *3561,* 3561–3562
Thrombophlebitis, septic, 4032
diagnosis of, 4042–4043, *4043*
treatment, 4043
Thrombosis
amyloid angiopathy, 3351, *3353*
arterial wall constriction and compression, 3353–3355, *3354, 3355, 3356, 3357*
arteritis, 3339–3340, *3340, 3341,* 3342, *3343,* 3344, *3345, 3346,* 3346–3348, *3347*
atherosclerosis, 3329–3330, *3331,* 3332–3335, *3333, 3334*
causes, 3328–3329
of cavernous sinus, 3894–3898, *3896, 3897*
of deep cerebral veins, 3893, *3894*
drug abuse, 3363–3364
dural sinus, 2518–2520, *2520*
of dural sinuses, 3893
fibromuscular dysplasia, 3348, *3349*
general considerations, 3328
hypercoagulability, 3357–3359, *3358, 3359, 3360, 3361,* 3361–3362, *3362*
hypertension, *3335,* 3335–3336, *3336, 3337, 3338*
of internal carotid artery, 4303
of jugular vein, 3926–3927
causes, 3926–3927
clinical manifestations, 3927, *3928,* 3929
diagnosis, 3929
treatment, 3929
of lateral (transverse) sinus, *3899,* 3899–3903, *3900, 3901, 3902, 3903, 3904, 3905*
migraine and vasospasm, 3336–3339, *3338*
miscellaneous systemic disorders affecting arterial wall, 3351–3353
miscellaneous vasculopathies, 3362–3363
Moyamoya, 3348–3349, *3350*
neoplastic angiopathy, 3351
of ophthalmic vein, 3915–3918, *3916, 3917*
radiation angiopathy, 3350–3351, *3352*
sagittal sinus, 4079
septic, 4088
of cavernous sinus, 4034–4039, *4035, 4036, 4037, 4038*
of cerebral and dural venous sinuses, 4070, *4072*
of cerebral venous sinuses, 4073
of dural sinuses, 4034
of lateral sinus, *4039,* 4039–4041, *4040*
of superior sagittal sinus, 4042
sickle cell disease, 3349–3350
of sigmoid sinus, 3912
spontaneous and traumatic dissection, 3348
of straight sinus, 3910, 3912
of superficial cerebral veins, *3891,* 3891–3893, *3892, 3893*
of superior sagittal sinus, 3905–3910, *3906, 3907, 3908, 3909, 3910, 3911, 3912*
venous sinus, 2518–2520, *2520*
Thrombotic disorders, 3817
Thrombotic therapy, 3579–3581, *3580*
Thromboxane A_2, 3557
Thrombus, mural, 3207
Thunderclap headaches, 1710–1711, *1711*
before rupture of intracranial aneurysm, 3021
Thymectomy for myasthenia gravis, 1425
Thymoxamine hydrochloride, 1005
Thymus, role of, in myasthenia gravis, 1409–1410
Thyroid dysfunction, role of radiation therapy in, 2598
Thyroid orbitopathy, 1556–1557
Thyroid-stimulating hormone (TSH), 2146–2147
Thyrotropin, 2146–2147
Tic douloureux. (*See* Trigeminal neuralgia.)
Tick-borne encephalitis, *5186,* 5186–5188, *5188*
clinical manifestations, 5187
diagnosis, 5187
epidemiology, *5186,* 5186–5187
pathology, 5187, *5188*
prevention, 5188
prognosis, 5187–5188
treatment, 5187
Ticlopidine, 3561
Tics and Gilles de la Tourette syndrome, 1570
Tilted optic disc, 274, *278, 279*
Tilts, 1170
Tirilazad mesylate for delayed cerebral ischemia, 3172
Tissue hypersensitivity, 4137
Tissue hypoxia, 4653
Tissue plasminogen activator (TPA), 3562
for delayed cerebral ischemia, 3170
and incidence of atherosclerosis, 3330
Titmus Stereo Tester, 156
Titmus test, 437
T-lymphocytes, 2329, 2330
in myasthenia gravis, 1409–1410
Tobacco, 674–675
Tobacco amblyopia, 674–675
Tobacco-alcohol amblyopia, 674
Tof, 5434
Togaviridae, 5277
alphaviruses, 5277–5281, *5278, 5279, 5280, 5281, 5282,* 5283, *5283, 5284, 5285,* 5285–5286
characteristics of, 5277, *5278*
rubivirus (Rubella), 5286–5293, 5296
clinical manifestations of, 5279–5281, *5280, 5281, 5282, 5283, 5284, 5285,* 5285–5286

pathogenesis of, 5277–5278
pathology of, 5278–5279, *5279, 5280, 5281, 5282*
Tolosa-Hunt syndrome, 1213, 1724, 1727–1729, 3972
Tonic convergence, 948
Tonic downward deviation, 1328
Tonic pupil syndromes, 1014
Tonic pupils, 2543–2544, *2544,* 3767, 5052–5053, 5433, 5509–5510, *5510*
areflexia, and progressive segmental hypohidrosis, 1027–1028
from ischemia of ciliary ganglion or short posterior ciliary nerves, 3694–3695
Tonic upward deviation, 1328
Tonsillectomy, 969
Tonsillitis, 3947
Tonus ptosis, 1540
Tooth-bud growth arrest, role of radiation therapy in, 2597
Topographical ERG, 223, *223*
Torsional angular vestibulo-ocular reflex (VOR), 1143–1145, *1144*
Torsional nystagmus, 1473, 1473*t*
Torsional saccades, brainstem generation of, 1111–1113, *1112*
Torsipulsion, 1286
Torticollis, benign paroxysmal, 3698
Torula histolytica, 4367
Total Deviation Plot, 182
Touch and pressure sensation, 1603–1604, *1604*
Tourette syndrome, 1319, 2855–2856
Tournay's phenomenon, 984–986, 4127
Touton giant cell, 2421, *2421,* 3989
Toxic and deficiency optic neuropathies, 663
clinical characteristics of, 664–666
differential diagnosis, 666–667
etiologic criteria, 663–664
evaluation, 667
specific nutritional amblyopias, 667–671
Toxic and drug-induced ocular myopathies, 1406
Toxic and metabolic optic neuropathies, 264–265
Toxic encephalopathy in Lyme disease, 4814–4816
Toxic megacolon, 4619
Toxic optic neuropathy, 664, 2560, 4142
Toxic reactions and facial dysesthesias, 1751
Toxic retinitis, 755
Toxic shock syndrome, 5193
Toxocara canis, 4515, 4516, 4522, 4531
Toxocara canis infections, 1997
Toxocara catis, 4522
Toxocara encephalitis, 4522
Toxocariasis, 4515–4516, *4516, 4517,* 4518, *4518, 4519, 4520, 4521, 4522,* 4522–4523, *4523*
association with neuroretinitis, 636
intraocular, 4516, 4522–4523
ocular, 4516
Toxoplasma chorioretinitis, 4681–4682
Toxoplasma gondii, 4667
acute, in immunocompetent patient, *4671,* 4671–4672, *4672*
clinical manifestations, 4670–4671
acute acquired toxoplasmosis in immunocompetent patient, *4671,* 4671–4672, *4672*
acute toxoplasmosis in immunodeficient patient, 4672–4673, *4674,* 4675, *4675, 4676,* 4677–4678, *4678, 4679*
congenital toxoplasmosis, 4678, *4680,* 4681
ocular toxoplasmosis, *4681,* 4681–4683, *4682, 4683*
diagnosis, 4691–4694, *4694, 4695, 4696,* 4696–4699
epidemiology, 4668–4670
in intracranial brain abscess, 3952
life cycle, *4666,* 4667–4668, *4668, 4669, 4670*
pathogenesis, 4670, *4671*
pathology, 4683, 4685
of acquired central nervous system toxoplasmosis, *4686,* 4686–4687, *4687, 4688*
of central nervous system toxoplasmosis, 4685
neuro, of congenital toxoplasmosis, 4687, *4690*
of ocular toxoplasmosis, 4687, *4690,* 4691, *4691, 4692*
of toxoplasmic lymphadenitis, 4685
prevention, 4701
retinochoroiditis caused by, 5428–5429
treatment and prognosis, *4699,* 4699–4701
Toxoplasma seronegative, 5411
Toxoplasma seropositive, 5411
Toxoplasmic lymphadenitis, pathology of, 4685
Toxoplasmosis, 5409
acute
in immunocompetent patient, *4671,* 4671–4672, *4672*
in immunodeficient patient, 4672–4673, *4674,* 4675, *4675, 4676,* 4677–4678, *4678, 4679*
diagnosis of, 4693–4694, *4694, 4695, 4696*
acute acquired
diagnosis of, in immunocompetent patient, 4693
treatment of
in immunocompetent patient, 4699–4700
in immunodeficient patient, 4700
in pregnant women, 4700
association with neuroretinitis, 636
cerebral, 5409–5411, *5410*
in immunocompetent patient, *4671,* 4671–4672, *4672*
in immunodeficient patient, 4672–4673, *4674,* 4675, *4675, 4676,* 4677–4678, *4678, 4679*
diagnosis of, 4693–4694, *4694, 4695, 4696*
ocular, *4681,* 4681–4683, *4682, 4683*
diagnosis of, 4698–4699
pathology of, 4687, *4690,* 4691, *4691, 4692*
treatment of, 4700–4701
Tranexamic acid for aneurysms, 3175
Transcortical motor aphasia, 3434
Transcortical sensory aphasia, 3484
Transcranial Doppler sonography, 3548–3549
Transcranial Doppler velocimetry, *3543,* 3543–3544, *3544*
Transesophageal echocardiography, 3548, *3549*
Transfer ratio, 109–110
Transformed migraine, 1752, 3699
Transforming growth factor beta (TGF-β), 3334
Transfrontal operation for pituitary adenomas, 2189–2190
Transient aphasia, 3676
Transient bilateral abducens nerve paresis, 5151–5152
Transient hemiparesis, 3676–3677
Transient ischemic attacks (TIAs), 3324
and headaches, 1706–1707
management of, 3570–3576
prognosis of patients with, 3552–3553
Transient miosis, 2567
Transient monocular loss of vision, 3420, 3423–3424, 3444
management of patients with, 3576–3577
prognosis of patients with, 3553–3555
Transient neurologic deficits, 5414–5415
Transient visual disturbances, *3665,* 3665–3670, *3666, 3667, 3668, 3669*
Transient visual loss, 813–814
Transient visual obscurations, 510, 512
Transitional meningiomas, 2027
Translational otolith-ocular responses, 1140
Transmissible amyloidoses, 4561
Transmissible spongiform encephalopathies, 4561
Transmission, 841
Transplants. (*See also* Bone marrow transplantation.)
corneal, 5264
Transport phase of reaching, 450
Transsphenoidal encephalocele, 786
Transsphenoidal procedure for removal of pituitary adenomas, 2190–2191
Transsphenoidal surgery, 2195–2196
for pituitary adenomas, 2199
Transthoracic echocardiography, 3548
Transverse myelitis, 3821–3822, 4113, 5088, 5104, 5195, 5239–5240, 5243
Transverse myelopathy, 2555
Trapping of aneurysm, 3152
Trauma, *3588, 3589,* 3589–3590, *3590*
as cause of aneurysms, 2989–2990
and facial dysesthesias, 1751
headache associated with, 1705–1706, 1725–1726
in intracranial abscess in, 3947
papilledema after, 517
Traumatic aneurysms, 2989–2990, *2991,* 2991*t*, 2992, *2992, 2993, 2994,* 2994–2998, *2995, 2996, 2997, 2998*
cervical, 2990
Traumatic dissections of cervical segment of internal carotid artery, 3210–3215, 3211*t*, *3212, 3213*
Traumatic hydrocephalus, 3908
Traumatic intracranial aneurysm, treatment of, 2997
Traumatic myopathies, 1391–1392, *1392, 1393*
Traumatic optic neuropathy, 715–735
classification of, 717, *717*
clinical assessment, 717–718
examination, 718–720
history, 718
imaging studies, 720–722, *721*
visual-evoked potentials, 720
epidemiology, 716*t*, 716–717
management, 731–735, 733*t*
pathogenesis
general concepts, 724–725
primary mechanisms of nerve injury, 725
secondary mechanisms of nerve injury, 725–729, *726, 727*
pathology, *722,* 722–724, *723, 724*
pharmacology
clinical applications, 730–731
experimental, 729–730
types of injury, 715

Trematodes (flukes), 4479, *4480*
miscellaneous, of neuro-ophthalmologic significance, 4492, *4493,* 4494
Paragonium species, 4479, *4481,* 4481–4483, *4482, 4483, 4484,* 4485
Schistosoma species, 4485, *4485*
clinical manifestations, 4487–4489, *4488, 4489*
diagnosis, 4491–4492, *4493*
epidemiology, 4486
life cycle, 4485–4486, *4486*
pathogenesis and pathology, 4489–4491, *4490, 4491, 4492*
treatment, 4492
Tremor, 2627
intention, 5568
Treponema, 4780, 4781, 4844, *4844*
bejel, 4850, *4852,* 4853, *4853, 4854*
pinta, 4844, *4845, 4846*
syphilis, 4853
cardiovascular, *4881,* 4881–4884
clinical manifestations, 4855–4857
congenital, 4902–4903
cutaneous manifestations, 4858–4860, *4859, 4860, 4861, 4862*
epidemiology, 4854–4855, *4856*
gummatous, *4892,* 4892–4895, *4893, 4894, 4896, 4897, 4898,* 4898–4900, *4899,* 4900
human immunodeficiency virus infection and AIDS, 4916–4918, *4919, 4920, 4921, 4922,* 4922*t*, *4923, 4924, 4925,* 4925–4929, *4926,* 4928*t*
incubation stage of, 4856–4857
latent, 4856–4857, 4880–4881
natural history, 4929–4930
neurologic manifestations, 4861, *4863,* 4863–4864, *4864*
neuro-ophthalmologic manifestations, *4872,* 4872–4874, *4873, 4874, 4875,* 4876, *4876,* 4878–4880, *4879,* 4907–4908, *4908*
neurosyphilis, 4882*t*, 4882–4884, 4883*t*
ocular involvement in tertiary, 4900–4902
ocular manifestations, 4864–4868, *4865, 4866, 4867, 4868, 4869, 4870,* 4871–4872, 4903–4907, *4904, 4905, 4906, 4907*
pathogenesis, 4855
pathology, 4908–4909, *4909, 4910, 4911, 4912,* 4912–4913, *4913, 4914, 4915,* 4916, *4917, 4918, 4919, 4920, 4921, 4922, 4923, 4924*
primary, 4856–4857, 4857, *4857, 4858*
prognosis with treatment, 4931
secondary, 4856–4857, 4857–4861, 4858*t*
systemic manifestations, 4860–4861, *4902,* 4902–4903, *4903*
tertiary, 4856–4857, 4881
treatment, 4930–4931
yaws, 4845, *4847,* 4847–4848, *4848, 4849,* 4850, *4850, 4851, 4852*
Treponema pallidum
in intracranial brain abscess, 3952
in spirochetal aneurysms, 3004–3005
Treponema pallidum hemagglutination (TPHA) test, 5614
Triazoles for fungal infections, 4284
Trichinella spiralis (Trichinosis), 4523–4525, *4524, 4526, 4527,* 4527–4528, *4528*
Trichinosis, 524, 4523–4525, *4524, 4526, 4527,* 4527–4528, *4528*
central nervous system, 4525, *4526,* 4527–4528
Trichloroethylene, 1264
Trichomegaly of eyelashes, 5374
Trichosporon beigelit, 4282, 4417–4418
Trigeminal arteries, 2917
Trigeminal axons, sensory nerve endings of afferent
conjunctiva, 1601, *1602*
cornea, 1595–1596, *1596, 1597,* 1598, *1598, 1599, 1600,* 1600–1601
eyelids, 1601–1602
limbus, 1601
orbit, 1602
sclera, 1601
uvea, 1601
Trigeminal fibers, afferent, 1624, *1627,* 1627–1628
Trigeminal ganglion, 1618–1620, *1619, 1620*
Trigeminal nerve, 1628, *1628, 1629, 1630*
dysfunction, 3047, 3283–3284
involvement of Gasserian ganglion or sensory root of, 1672–1675
neuroparalytic (neurotrophic) keratitis, *1676,* 1676–1677
involvement of Gasserian or sensory root of, 1672–1675
involvement of mandibular division of, *9,* 1669–1671, *1671*
involvement of maxillary division of, 1668–1669
involvement of opthalmic division of, 1667, 1667*t*
frontal branch lesions, 1667
lacrimal branch lesions, 1667
nasociliary branch lesions, 1667, *1668*
syndromes of orbital apex, superior orbital fissure, and anterior cavernous sinus, 1667–1668
lesions of, 1655
major divisions of, 1606, *1607*
mandibular, 1616, *1617,* 1618, *1618*
maxillary, 1616, *1616*
ophthalmic, 1606–1607, *1607, 1608, 1609,* 1610, *1610, 1611, 1612, 1613, 1614,* 1615, *1615*
mesencephalic nucleus, 1628–1629
motor nucleus, 1628
in pathogenesis of migraine, 3704–3705, *3705*
reflex blinks from stimulation of supraorbital branch of, *1526,* 1526–1529, *1527,* 1527*t*, *1528*
sensory nuclear complex, 1629–1632
tests for cutaneous sensation
clinical tests, 1649–1650
evoked potentials, 1650
tests of corneal sensation, *1651,* 1651–1652
tests of motor function
clinical tests, 1652
neurophysiologic, 1652–1653
in transmission of painful impulses, 1695–1696
Trigeminal nerves
dysfunction of, 1796, 2236
schwannomas of, 2302, 2304–2306, *2305, 2306*
Trigeminal neuralgia, 1796, 5569–5571, *5570*
central causes of head and facial pain other than, 1749–1750
differential diagnosis of, 1737
etiology and pathology of, 1736–1737
occurrence of, 1735
symptoms of, 1736
treatment of, 1737–1741
Trigeminal neuropathy, 2619, 4373
Trigeminal nuclei
location of corneal afferents in, 1631
location of dural and blood vessel afferents in, 1631–1632
Trigeminal pain, during and after herpes zoster ophthalmicus, 1729
Trigeminal pathways, involvement of, in brainstem, 1677–1678
lesions of medulla, *1678,* 1678–1680, *1679*
Trigeminal receptors, physiology of, in skin and cornea
general considerations, 1602–1603
ocular sensitivity, 1606
pain, 1605–1606
thermal sensation, 1604–1605
touch and pressure sensation, 1603–1604, *1604*
Trigeminal reflex blinks, *1526,* 1526–1529, *1527,* 1527*t*, *1528*
excitability of, and spasms of lid closure, 1529–1530, *1531, 1532*
Trigeminal reflexes
blink, 1653–1656, *1656*
corneomandibular, 1657–1658
masseter, 1658–1659
palpebromandibular reflex, 1658
snout, 1659
trigeminovagal, 1656–1657
Trigeminal root, 1620, *1621,* 1622
motor, 1622, 1624, *1624, 1625, 1626*
sensory, 1622, *1623, 1624*
Trigeminal schwannoma, 1252
Trigeminal sensory neuropathy, 1675
Trigeminal sensory nuclear complex, 1629–1632
Trigeminal spinal nuclei and subnuclei, interconnections among, 1631
Trigeminal system, role in afferent control of extraocular movements and other visual functions, 1640–1644, *1642, 1643*
Trigeminal-evoke potentials, 1650
Trigeminal-lacrimal reflexes, 930
Trigeminovagal reflexes, 1656–1657
Trigeminovascular system, 1696
Trilaminar muscle fiber disease, 1359
Trilateral retinoblastoma, 1996
Trimethaphan, impact of, on postsynaptic neuromuscular transmission, 1441
Trismus, 4112
Trisomy 18, 783
Trochlear nerve, 1066, *1066, 1067*
dysfunction, 1795
fascicular portion of, 1064, *1065*
lesions of
within cavernous sinus and superior orbital fissure, 1235
within orbit, 1235–1236
in subarachnoid space, 1234–1235, *1235*
paresis in, 3043, 3046, 3128, 4113, 5087
Trochlear nerve fascicle, lesions of, 1229, 1231–1232, *1232, 1233,* 1234
Trochlear nerve function and basilar aneurysms, 3119–3120
Trochlear nerve nucleus, lesions of, 1227, 1229, *1230, 1231, 1232*
Trochlear nerve palsies, 1227, *1228, 1229, 1230*
acquired, 1227, 1229, *1230, 1231,* 1231–1232, *1232, 1233,* 1234–1236, *1235*

congenital, 1227	miliary, 4144, 4145	ependymoblastoma, 1979
differential diagnosis of acquired, 1236	nonreactive, 4138	medulloblastoma, 1979-1984, 1981, 1982,
evaluation and management of, 1236-1237	ocular, 4144-4145	1983
Trochlear nucleus, 1064, 1064	orbital, 4144-4145	medulloepithelioma, 1984-1985, 1985,
Γrolard, vein, 2947	pulmonary, 4138	1986
Tropheryma whippelii, 4180–4189, 4182,	clinical manifestations, 4138-4139, 4164,	neuroblastoma, 1985-1990, 1987, 1988,
4183, 4184, 4185, 4186, 4187, 4188,	4165, 4166, 4166–4167	1989, 1991
5721	Tuberculous abscesses of brain, 4161–4162,	primitive neuroectodermal, 1999,
diagnosis, 4184, 4187-4188, 4188	4165	1999–2000, 2000
general clinical manifestations, 4181–4182	Tuberculous encephalitis, 4149, 4151	retinoblastoma, 1990–1999, 1992, 1993,
general manifestations, 4181–4182	Tuberculous meningitis, 4145, 4148,	1994, 1995, 1996
nature of bacterium, 4181	4148–4149, <i>4149</i> , <i>4150</i> , 4151, <i>4151</i> ,	endodermal sinus, 2092, 2093, 2094, 2094
neurologic manifestations, 4182, 4183, 4184	4152, 4153, 4153–4154, 4154,	endolymphatic sac, 2703–2704
neuro-ophthalmologic manifestations, 4184–4186, 4186	4154–4157, 4155, 4156 Tuberculous otitis media, 4162	ependymal, 1963, 1963–1966, 1964, 1965
ocular manifestations, 4182–4184, 4185,	Tuberculous spondylitis, 4163–4164, 4166	ependymomas, 1963, 1963–1966, 1964, 1965
4186	Tuberculum sellae meningiomas, 2062,	subependymomas, 1966–1967, 1967
pathology, 4186, 4187, 4188	2062–2065, 2064, 2992	extra-axial, at base of brain, 1887–1890,
treatment and prognosis, 4189, 4189,	Tuberin, 2669	1888, 1889, 1890, 1891, 1892, 1893
4189–4192, <i>4190</i> , <i>4191</i>	Tuberohypophyseal system, 2145, 2146, 2147t	false localizing symptoms and signs of
Trophozoites, 4614, 4644	Tuberothalamic infarction, 3483	cerebellar dysfunction, 1797
Γropical optic neuropathy, 670–671	Tuberous sclerosis, 2669, 3012	cranial neuropathies, 1794-1797
Tropical spastic paraparesis, 5436	associations, 2693	dementia, 1794
Γropicamide, 1001–1002	cutaneous findings, 2670, 2671, 2672, 2673,	extrapyramidal signs, 1797
Γropism, 4952	2674, 2675, 2675–2676, 2676	generalized limitation of eye movements,
Γrousseau's syndrome, 2515	diagnosis, 2693–2694, 2695t	1797–1798
Γrue pursuit cells, 1129	genetics, 2669	hydrocephalus, 1792–1794, 1793
Trypanosoma, 4701 Trypanosoma brucei, 4710, 4710	management, 2694–2696 neuroimaging, 2692	nystagmus, 1797 protosis, <i>1797</i> , 1798
clinical manifestations, 4714, 4714–4715	neurologic findings, 2679, 2684	pyramidal signs, 1797
diagnosis, 4717–4719	occurrence, 2669	visual field defects, 1794
epidemiology, 4711, 4713-4714	ocular findings, 2676, 2677, 2678,	visual hallucinations, 1794
life cycle, 4710, 4710–4711, 4711, 4712	2678–2679, 2679, 2680, 2681, 2682,	of 4th ventricle, 1884, 1884-1887, 1885,
pathology and pathogenesis, 4715–4717	2683	1887
prognosis, 4719	visceral findings, 2690, 2690–2692, 2691,	frontal lobe, 1818–1825, 1819, 1820, 1821,
treatment, 4719	2692, 2693, 2694 Tubular aggregate myonethy, 1350	1823, 3425
Trypanosoma cruzi, 4701–4702, 4702 clinical manifestations, 4705–4706	Tubular aggregate myopathy, 1359 Tularemia, 4228, 4228–4229	ocular symptoms and signs produced by, 1824–1825
diagnosis, 4708–4709	glandular, 4229	ganglioglioma, 689–690
epidemiology, 4703–4705	oculoglandular, 4229	generalized limitation of eye movements as
life cycle, 4702, 4702–4703, 4703	oropharyngeal, 4229	sign of, 1797-1798
pathogenesis, 4708	typhoidal, 4229	germ cell, 2083-2085, 2084
pathology, 4706-4708, 4709	Tullio's phenomenon, 1289, 4829	giant cell, 2443-2444
prevention, 4710	Tumbling E Cube, 161, 163	glomus jugulare, 2468, 2469, 2470–2471
treatment, 4709–4710	Tumor emboli, 3376–3377, 3378, 3379, 3380	and headaches, 1725, 1726
Γrypanosomes in neuritis, 4026	Tumor markers, 2084	hydrocephalus as sign of, 1792–1794, 1793
Frypanosomiasis African, 4710, <i>4710</i>	Tumor necrosis factor alpha (TNF- α , cachectin), 3996	intracranial, 1898–1902, 1899, 1900, 1901
American, 4701–4702, 4702	Tumors, 681, 1010, 2987, 2989, 2989, 2990	intrinsic, of brainstem, 1871–1875, <i>1872</i> , <i>1874</i> , <i>1876</i> , <i>1877</i> , 1877–1878
East African, 4713–4714, 4715	astrocytic hamartoma, 690, 691	involving basal ganglia, 1861, 1861–1865,
West African, 4713, 4714, 4714, 4715	of blood vessels	1862, 1864
Γrypomastigotes, 4702, 4711	hemangioblastomas, 2223-2226, 2224,	involving cerebellum, 1878, 1878-1884,
Tryptophan, conversion to melatonin, 1866	2225, 2226, 2227, 2228	1879, 1881
ГSH, 2146–2147	hemangiopericytomas, 2228, 2228-2230,	involving corpus callosum, 1855, 1857,
TSH toxicosis, 2163–2164	2229	1857–1859, <i>1858</i>
Γsutsugamushi disease, 4758–4762, 4759,	of bone cartilage, 2437	involving frontal lobe, 1818–1825, 1819,
4760, 4761 Tubercle, 4137	benign, 2442–2444, 2443, 2444, 2445 chordomas, 2437–2442, 2438, 2439,	1820, 1821, 1823 involving lateral geniculate body, 1815,
Tuberculated spores, 4389	2440, 2441, 2442	1818, <i>1818</i>
Tuberculin skin test, 4140	capillary and cavernous hemangiomas,	involving lateral ventricles, 1848–1849,
treatment, 4140-4144	691–694, 692, 693, 694	1849, 1850
Tuberculoid leprosy, 4169	cardiac, 3396, 3398, 3400, 3401	involving occipital lobe, 1844-1848, 1845,
Tuberculoma, 709, 4154, 4157–4161, 4158,	containing Schwann cells	1846, 1847
4159, 4160, 4161	neurofibromas, 2319, 2320, 2321	involving parietal lobe, 1837–1844, 1838,
intracranial, 4167	schwannomas, 4–6, 5, 6, 7, 8–13, 9, 10,	1839, 1843
subdural, 4163	11, 13, 14, 15–23, 16, 19, 21, 22	involving pineal gland, 1851, 1865,
Tuberculomas en plaque, 4163 Tuberculosis, 4136, 5419	diagnostic techniques, 1893–1894, 1894, 1895, 1896, 1896–1902, 1897, 1898,	1865–1871, <i>1866</i> , <i>1868</i> , <i>1869</i> involving suprasellar region, 1807, <i>1811</i> ,
of bones of skull, 4163	1899, 1900, 1901	1811–1815, 1812, 1813, 1814
central nervous system (CNS), 4145, 4167	dysembryoplastic neuroepithelial,	involving temporal lobe, 1823, 1827, 1829,
extrapulmonary, 4144	1978–1979, <i>1979</i>	1830, 1830–1835, 1836, 1837
intraocular, 4145, 4146, 4147	embryonal, 1979	involving thalamus, 1859-1861

Tumors—*continued*
involving 3rd ventricle, 1849, *1851, 1852,* 1852–1855, *1853*
Koenen's, 2675, *2675*
lymphoma, 701–702, 701–703, *702*
lymphoreticular malignancies, 701
malignant teratoid medulloepithelioma, 691
of medulla, 1878
melanocytomas, *696,* 696–697, *697, 698*
meningeal carcinomatosis, 700–701
of mesencephalon, 1873–1874, *1874*
metastatic, 2477
bone, 2477, *2480*
meningeal carcinomatosis, 2485–2488, *2486, 2487*
parenchymal, 2477, 2479, *2479, 2480, 2481, 2482, 2483,* 2483–2484, *2484, 2485, 2486*
metastatic and locally invasive, 698–700, *699, 700*
nerve glioma, 681–689, *682, 683, 684, 685, 686, 687, 688, 689*
neuroectodermal, 1999
of neuroglia, 1920
astrocytic, 1920, *1921*
astrocytomas, 1921–1922
histologic classification, 4–17, *5, 6, 7, 8, 9, 10, 11, 12, 13, 14, 15, 16, 17*
topographic classification, 17–39, *19, 20, 22, 23, 24, 25, 26, 27, 28, 30, 31, 34, 39, 40, 41*
ependymal
ependymomas, *1963,* 1963–1966, *1964, 1965*
subependymomas, 1966–1967, *1967*
oligodendroglia, 1958, *1960,* 1960–1963, *1961*
of neurons, 1975
ganglion cell
central neurocytoma, 1977–1978, *1978*
disembryoplastic infantile gangliogliomas, 1977
dysembryoplastic neuroepithelial, 1978–1979, *1979*
dysplastic cerebellar gangliocytoma, 1977, *1978*
gangliocytomas, 1975–1977, *1976*
gangliogliomas, 1975–1977, *1976*
nonlocalizing symptoms and signs of
abducens nerve pareses, 1792
headache, 1790–1791
papilledema, 1791
seizures, 1791–1792
of occipital lobes, 1844–1848, *1847*
of olfactory groove, *1825,* 1825–1827
oligodendroglia, 1958, *1960,* 1960–1963, *1961*
optic nerve hemangioblastoma, 694, *695,* 696, *696*
in orbit, *1798,* 1798–1804, *1800, 1801, 1802, 1803, 1804*
orbital, 1897–1898, *1898*
of paranasal sinuses, 2450–2453, *2451, 2452, 2453*
parenchymal metastatic, 2477, 2479, *2479, 2480, 2481, 2482, 2483,* 2483–2484, *2484, 2485, 2486*
parietal lobe, 1838–1844, *1839, 1843*
pearly, 2108–2110, *2109*
peripheral nerve sheath, 2316–2318, *2317, 2318*
of pineal gland, *1851, 1865,* 1865–1871, *1866, 1868, 1869*
of pineal parenchymal cells, pinealomas, 1972–1973, *1974,* 1975
of pons, 1874–1875, *1876, 1877,* 1877–1878
pyramidal signs as sign of, 1797
renal, 2705
of septum pellucidum, 1855, *1855, 1856*
of spinal cord, 1893
in superior orbital fissure, 1804–1805, *1805, 1806,* 1807, *1807, 1808, 1809*
in superior orbital fissure and cavernous sinus, 1804–1805, *1805, 1806,* 1807, *1807, 1808, 1809*
treatment of, 1902–1903
Turner's syndrome, 2165
Type A tissue of Antoni, 2300
Type B tissue of Antoni, 2300
Typhoid fever, 4221–4222
Typhoidal tularemia, 4229
Typhus, 4737
louse-borne, 4752
Typhus nodules, 4753
Tyramine hydrochloride, 1003
Tyrosinemia, 2812–2813, *2813*
hepatorenal, 2812
Tyrosinosis, 2812
Tzanck smear in diagnosing varicella-zoster virus infections, 5075–5076

U

Uhthoff's symptom, 154, 745, 5628
inverse, 5577
of multiple sclerosis, 5575–5577, *5576*
in optic neuritis, 614–615
Ulcerative colitis, 3857
Ulceroglandular tularemia, 4229
Ulcers, genital, 3803, *3804*
Ultrasonography, 3533
Ultrasound in diagnosis of patients with arterial dissections, 3207
uMRD, 1538
Uncal herniation, syndrome of, 997–998
Uncinate fit, 1834
Unclassified botulism, 4122–4123
Uncoating, 4948
Unconscious patients, spontaneous eye movements in, 1492–1494, *1493,* 1493*t*
Unilateral apraxia, 1859
Unilateral cortical ptosis, *1538,* 1538–1539
Unilateral dyschromatopsia, 653
Unilateral facial nerve paresis, 5248
Unilateral internal ophthalmoplegia, 5022–5023
Unilateral internuclear ophthalmoplegia, 3509
Unilateral nasal hemianopia, 302–304, *303, 304, 305, 306, 307*
Unilateral optic nerve dysfunction, syndrome of, 292, 294
anterior optic chiasm syndrome, 294, *297, 298*
distal optic neuropathy, 294, *297, 298*
distal syndrome, 294, *297, 298*
Foster Kennedy syndrome, 296, 298
optociliary shunts and syndrome of chronic optic nerve compression, 294
prechiasmal compression syndrome, 294
Unilateral optic neuropathy, 4487
Unilateral papilledema, *498,* 498–499, *499, 500*
Unilateral proptosis, 2260–2261
Unilateral ptosis, 2260, *2263*
Universal angiomatosis, 2275
Unmyelinated fibers, 5705
Unpigmented ciliary epithelium, 900
Unruptured saccular aneurysms, natural history of, 3139–3142
Upbeat nystagmus, 1326, 1472–1473, 1473*t,* 1495–1496
Upper eyelid crease, 1510
Upper visual field, 115
Ureaplasma urealyticum, 4555–4556
Urethral candidiasis, 4347
Urinary calculi, 5257
Urinary tract candidiasis, 4347–4348
Urokinase, 3562
Usher's syndrome, 5544
Utilization behavior, 1822
Uvea, sensory nerve endings in, 1601
Uveal tract
abnormalities of, 2658
damage to, 5041
leukemic involvement of, 2348–2349, *2349, 2350*
Uveitis, 1724, 2357, 4850, 5488, *5489,* 5490, *5490*
anterior, 5581
of multiple sclerosis, 5581, *5581, 5582*
posterior, 5581
Uveomeningitis syndromes, 2541
Uveoparotid fever, 5483

V

Vaccines
for acellular pertussis, 4210–4211
antirabies, 1261
antituberculosis, 4167
Bacille Calmette-Guérin (BCG), 4167, *4168*
for bacterial meningitis, 4012
formalin-inactivated, 5196–5197
influenza
complications following, 5197
and multiple sclerosis, 5544
for Lyme disease, 4832
for measles, 5210–5213, *5211, 5212, 5213*
optic neuritis after, 629
passive, for bacterial meningitis, 4012
polyvalent pneumococcal polysaccharide, 4079–4080
in preventing HIV infection, 5385
against rabies, 5275–5276
Vaccinia necrosum, 5152
Vaccinia virus, 5149–5154, *5151, 5152, 5153*
Vagal reflex activity, 1657
Vaginal epithelium, cornification of, 4102
Vagoglossopharyngeal neuralgia, 1746
Varicella, 5013
clinical manifestations, 5014, *5015, 5016,* 5016–5025, *5018, 5020, 5021, 5022,* 5024
epidemiology, 5013
pathogenesis, 5013
pathology, 5013, *5014*
Varicella meningoencephalitis, 5017–5018
Varicella pneumonitis, 5016
Varicella-zoster virus, 5012–5013, *5013,* 5417
Varices, *2250,* 2250–2252, *2251, 2252*
Variola, 5148–5149, *5150*
vaccinia virus, 5149–5154, *5151, 5152, 5153*
Vascular candidiasis, 4348
Vascular cutaneous lesions, 3815

Vascular disorders, headache associated with, 1706–1714, *1711*
Vascular malformations, *3587*, 3588–3589
Vascular optic disc swelling without visual loss, 580–581, 583
Vasculature, appearance atrophic optic disc with special reference to, 286
Vasculitides, 3725, 3727, *3729*
primary central nervous system
acute posterior multifocal placoid pigment epitheliopathy, 3739–3741, *3740, 3741, 3742,* 3743–3744
Cogan's syndrome, *3734,* 3734–3736, *3735*
Eales' disease, 3736–3737, *3737, 3738,* 3739, *3739*
granulomatous angiitis of, 3727–3729, *3728, 3729, 3730,* 3731–3732
microangiopathy of brain, retina, and inner ear, *3732,* 3732–3734, *3733*
systemic necrotizing
allergic angiitis and granulomatosis, *3752,* 3752–3754, *3753, 3754*
associated with drug abuse and hepatitis B virus, 3754–3755, *3755*
giant cell arteritis, 3755–3761, *3756, 3757, 3758, 3759, 3760*
Henoch-Schönlein purpura, 3783
hypersensitivity, *3782,* 3782–3783, *3783*
lethal midline granuloma, 3802, *3803*
lymphomatoid granulomatosis, *3786,* 3786–3788, *3787*
mixed cryoglobulinemia, 3783–3786, *3785*
polyarteritis nodosa, *3743, 3744,* 3744–3751, *3745, 3746, 3747, 3748, 3750, 3751*
Takayasu's arteritis, *3788,* 3788–3792, *3789, 3791,* 3792, *3793*
Wegener's granulomatosis, 3792, *3794*
Vasculitides other than giant cell arteritis, 578, *579,* 580, *580, 581, 582*
Vasculitis, 4028, 4148–4149, *4150,* 4686, 4738, 5206
arthritides, 3845
juvenile rheumatoid arthritis, 3850–3852, *3852*
rheumatoid arthritis, 3845, *3846, 3847,* 3847–3850, *3848, 3849, 3850, 3851*
seronegative (HLA-B27-associated spondyloarthropathies), 3852
ankylosing spondylitis, 3852–3854, *3853*
arthritis with inflammatory bowel disease, 3857–3859, *3859, 3860, 3861, 3862, 3863*
Reiter's syndrome, *3854,* 3854–3857, *3855, 3856*
associated with drug abuse and hepatitis B virus, 3754–3755, *3755*
Behçet's disease, 3802–3803
clinical manifestations, 3803–3808, *3804, 3805, 3806, 3807*
demographics, 3803
diagnosis, 3809, 3811
pathogenesis, 3808–3809
pathology, 3808, *3810*
treatment and prognosis, 3811
central nervous system (CNS) in, 4361, *4361, 4363,* 4341
connective tissue diseases
associations, 3829–3830
cardiovascular manifestations, 3815–3816, *3816*
constitutional symptoms, 3812
demographics, 3812
diagnosis, 3830–3831, 3831*t*
drug-induced lupus, 3830
gastrointestinal manifestations, 3817–3818
hematologic manifestations, 3816–3817
mucocutaneous lesions, *3813,* 3813–3815, *3814, 3815*
musculoskeletal symptoms and signs, *3812,* 3812–3813
neurologic and psychiatric manifestations, 3819–3822, *3820, 3821, 3822*
neuro-ophthalmologic manifestations, 3826–3829, *3827, 3828, 3829*
ocular manifestations, 3822–3823, *3823, 3824, 3825, 3826*
orbital manifestations, 3825–3826, *3826*
pathogenesis, *3818,* 3830, *3830*
prognosis, 3831
pulmonary manifestations, 3815, *3816*
renal manifestations, *3817,* 3817–3818, *3818, 3819*
systemic lupus erythematosus, 3811
history, 3811–3812
treatment, 3831–3833, *3832*
delayed cerebral, *5020,* 5020–5022, *5021*
dermatomyositis, 3838–3841, *3839, 3840, 3841, 3842*
idiopathic retinal, *3864,* 3864–3865
malignant atrophic papulosis, 3859, 3861, 3863–3864
pathophysiology, 3725–3727
polymyositis, 3838–3841, *3839, 3840, 3841, 3842*
poststreptococcal, 4086
relapsing polychondritis, 3842–3845, *3844, 3845*
scleroderma, *3832, 3833,* 3833–3838, *3834, 3835, 3836, 3837, 3838*
Sjögren's syndrome, 3841–3842, *3842, 3843*
vasculitides, 3727, *3729*
primary central nervous system
acute posterior multifocal placoid pigment epitheliopathy, 3739–3741, *3740, 3741, 3742,* 3743–3744
Cogan's syndrome, *3734,* 3734–3736, *3735*
Eales' disease, 3736–3737, *3737, 3738,* 3739, *3739*
granulomatous angiitis of, 3727–3729, *3728, 3729, 3730,* 3731–3732
microangiopathy of brain, retina, and inner ear, *3732,* 3732–3734, *3733*
systemic necrotizing
allergic angiitis and granulomatosis, *3752,* 3752–3754, *3753, 3754*
associated with drug abuse and hepatitis B virus, 3754–3755, *3755*
giant cell arteritis, 3755–3761, *3756, 3757, 3758, 3759, 3760*
Henoch-Schönlein purpura, 3783
hypersensitivity, *3782,* 3782–3783, *3783*
lethal midline granuloma, 3802, *3803*
lymphomatoid granulomatosis, *3786,* 3786–3788, *3787*
mixed cryoglobulinemia, 3783–3786, *3785*
polyarteritis nodosa, *3743, 3744,* 3744–3751, *3745, 3746, 3747, 3748, 3750, 3751*
Takayasu's arteritis, *3788,* 3788–3792, *3789, 3791,* 3792, *3793*
Wegener's granulomatosis, 3792, *3794*
Vasculopathy, 5067
Vasogenic cerebral edema, 3981–3982
Vasogenic edema, 3942, *3942*
Vasogenic theory of migraine, 3701–3703
Vaso-occlusive retinopathy, 2590–2591, *2591*
Vasopressin, 835, 1867, 2146
Vegetative tarsitis, 4901
Veiled cells, 2404
Veillonella, 4104
Veillonella parvula, 4104
Vein of Galen
aneurysms of, 2263–2266, *2264, 2265*
natural history of arteriovenous malformations (AVMs) of, 2278
Vein of Labbé, 2947
Vein of Trolard, 2947
Velocity storage, 1476
for vestibulo-ocular reflex (VOR), 1145–1146
Velocity-to-position integration and vestibulo-ocular reflex (VOR), 1145
Venezuelan equine encephalitis, *5282,* 5285–5286
Venous angiomas, 2246, *2247, 2248, 2249, 2250,* 2250–2252, *2251, 2252*
Venous compression, cranial neuropathies caused by, 3930, *3930*
Venous emboli, *3405,* 3405–3407, *3406*
Venous occlusive disease, 3887
branch retinal vein occlusion (BRVO), 3925–3926, *3926*
central retinal vein occlusion (CRVO), 3918–3925, *3920, 3921, 3922, 3923, 3924*
cerebral, and dural sinus thrombosis
causes, 3887–3890
of cavernous sinus, 3894–3898, *3896, 3897*
of deep cerebral veins, 3893, *3894*
diagnosis, *3905,* 3912–3914, *3913*
of dural sinuses, 3893
evaluation, 3914–3915
of lateral (transverse) sinus, *3899,* 3899–3903, *3900, 3901, 3902, 3903, 3904, 3905*
pathophysiology, 3890–3891
of sigmoid sinus, 3912
of straight sinus, 3910, 3912
of superior sagittal sinus, 3905–3910, *3906, 3907, 3908, 3909, 3910, 3911, 3912*
thrombosis of superficial veins, *3891,* 3891–3893, *3892, 3893*
treatment, 3915
cerebral embolism via vertebral system, 3929–3930
cranial neuropathies caused by compression, 3930, *3930*
occlusion of superior vena cava, 3929
pulmonary veno-occlusive, 3929
thrombosis of jugular vein
causes, 3926–3927
clinical manifestations, 3927, *3928,* 3929
diagnosis, 3929
treatment, 3929
thrombosis of ophthalmic vein, 3915–3918, *3916, 3917*

Venous pulsations, lack of spontaneous, 489
Venous sinus thrombosis, 1708–1709, 2518–2520, *2520*
Venous stasis retinopathy, 3453–3454, *3454, 3455, 3456,* 3457, *3457*
Venous system of brain, 2946
 cerebral veins, 2946–2947, *2948, 2949,* 2949–2952, *2950, 2951, 2952*
  posterior fossa, 2952–2953
 diploic veins, 2954, *2955*
 dural sinuses, 2954, *2955,* 2956, *2956, 2957, 2958,* 2959, *2959, 2960, 2961,* 2961–2964, *2962, 2963, 2964, 2965*
 extracranial cerebral veins, *2957, 2962,* 2966–2967, *2968*
 meningeal veins, 2954
 orbital veins, *2964, 2965,* 2965–2966, *2966*
Ventral medial mesencephalic syndrome, 3506
Ventral nucleus, 105
Ventral pontine infarction, 3512
Ventral syndrome, 1678–1679
Ventricles
 colloid cysts of 3rd, 1970–1972, *1971*
 cysts and tumors involving, 1849, *1851, 1852,* 1852–1855, *1853*
 meningiomas in 4th, 2055
 meningiomas in lateral, *2065,* 2065–2066, *2066*
 meningiomas in 3rd, 2065, 2067, *2067*
 tumors involving lateral, 1848–1849, *1849, 1850*
 tumors of 4th, *1884,* 1884–1887, *1885, 1887*
Ventriculitis, 5056
Ventriculoencephalitis, 5108–5110
Vergence, 1155
Vergence eye movements, 1102
 cerebellar control of, 1136
 cerebral control of, 1135–1136
 characteristics of, 1134
 neurophysiology of, 1134–1136, *1135*
Vergence pendular oscillations, 1469
Vernet's syndrome, 2448
Versions, 1173
Vertebral arteries, 2869
 aneurysms arising from, 3104, *3106,* 3106–3108, *3107, 3108, 3109, 3110, 3111*
 dissecting aneurysms of, 3216–3218, *3217, 3218, 3219, 3220,* 3220*t*, *3221,* 3221–3223
 fusiform aneurysms of, 3195–3198, *3197*
 and its branches, 2904–2905, *2905, 2906, 2907,* 2907–2911, *2908, 2909, 2910, 2911*
 occlusion, 3494–3496
 reversal of blood flow in, 3475
Vertebral artery to common carotid artery transposition, 3576
Vertebral vein, 2967
Vertebral venous system, cerebral embolism via, 3929–3930
Vertebrobasilar arterial disease, hemiparesis from, 3477
Vertebrobasilar arterial system
 aneurysms arising from, 3104, *3104, 3105*
 brainstem signs of occlusive disease of, *3496,* 3496–3497, *3497, 3498, 3499,* 3499–3502, *3500, 3501, 3502, 3503, 3504, 3505,* 3506, *3506, 3507, 3508, 3509,* 3509–3516, *3510, 3511, 3513, 3514, 3515*
 cerebellar signs of occlusive disease of, 3516
 neurologic and ocular signs of occlusive disease of, *3475,* 3475–3477, *3476, 3477, 3478, 3479,* 3479–3480, *3480, 3481, 3482,* 3482–3487, *3486, 3487, 3488, 3489, 3490*
 transient ischemic attacks from intermittent insufficiency of, 3471–3475
Vertebrobasilar arterial system transient ischemic attacks
 pathophysiology of, 3474–3475
 symptoms of, 3472–3474
Vertebrobasilar arteries, generalized disease of, 3518–3519
Vertebrobasilar artery system ischemia, symptoms and signs of, 3471, *3471*
Vertebrobasilar system, head movement and cervical arthritis in, 3474–3475
Vertical eye, lid movements that accompany, 1533–1536, *1534, 1535*
Vertical gaze paresis, 3510, 5433, 5727
Vertical hemifield slide phenomenon, 300, 302, *302*
Vertical heterotropia, 1183
Vertical myoclonus, 1328
Vertical ocular deviation, 1181
Vertical one-and-a-half syndrome, 3499
Vertical retraction syndrome, 1192, *1194, 1195, 1196*
Vertical saccades, brainstem generation of, 1111–1113, *1112*
Vertical vestibulo-ocular reflex (VOR), 1143–1145, *1144*
Vertigo, 1170, 3472, 5165
 in patients with basilar artery migraine, 3677
Very low-density lipoprotein (VLDL), 3335
Vesical schistosomiasis, 4488, *4488*
Vesiculoviruses, 5263
Vessel fenestration, aneurysm formation in association with, 2982
Vestibular imbalance
 nystagmus caused by central, 1472*t*, 1472–1475, 1473*t*
 nystagmus caused by peripheral, 1470–1472
 nystagmus from, 1495–1496
Vestibular nystagmus, 1462
Vestibular responses, 1317
Vestibular schwannoma, 2308
Vestibular symptoms, 1170
Vestibular system, 1087–1092, *1088, 1089, 1090, 1091*
 clinical examination of, 1185
Vestibulocochlear nerve
 dysfunction of, 1797
 schwannomas of, 2308–2309, *2309, 2310,* 2311–2316, *2312, 2315*
Vestibulocochlear neuropathy, role of radiation therapy in, 2612–2613
Vestibulo-collic reflex, 1138
Vestibulo-ocular reflex, 1139–1149, *1140, 1141, 1143, 1144, 1148,* 1156–1157, 1184–1185
 angular, 1139
 horizontal angular, 1142–1143, *1144*
 indirect, 1143
 linear, 1139
 measurement of, 1142
Vestibulo-ocular system and eye-head coordination, 1138
 cervico-ocular reflex, 1138
 combined head and eye pursuit, 1139
 reflex, 1138, 1139–1149, *1140, 1141, 1143, 1144, 1148*
Vibrio cholerae, 4244, *4244*
 central nervous system (CNS) infection, 4145
 cholera, 4244–4245
Vidian artery, 2871
Vidian nerve and nasopharyngeal carcinoma, 2448
Viliuisk encephalomyelitis, 5741–5744, *5742*
 cause, 5744
 clinical manifestations, 5743
 epidemiology, 5741
 laboratory findings, 5743
 pathology, 5742–5743
 treatment and prognosis, 5743
Vimentin, 1919–1920, 2392
Vinca alkaloids, 2581
 neuro-ophthalmologic toxicity, 2581–2583
 neurotoxicity, 2581
 ocular toxicity, 2581
 systemic toxicity, 2581
 taxoids, 2583
Viral disease, 5416–5419, *5418*
 optic neuritis from, 628–629
Viral encephalitis, 3985–3986, *3986*
Viral hemorrhagic fever, 5166
Viral meningitis, 5424
Virchow-Robin spaces, granulomas in, 5492
Virion attachment proteins (VAPs), 4947
Virus-cell interactions, 4947–4950, *4952*
Virus-environment interactions, 4953–4954
Viruses, 4945, 4946*t*, 4947*t*, *4948.* (*See also* DNA viruses; RNA viruses.)
 and central nervous system, 4954
 and central nervous system (CNS) infection, 3943
 structure and classification, 4945–4947, *4949, 4950, 4951*
Virus-host interactions, 4950–4952, *4953*
Virus-induced demyelination, 3978
Visceral larval migrans, 4515
Visceral neurofibromas, 2661
Visceral oculomotor nuclei, 860–861, *862*
Vision
 blurred, 1170
 dyslexia related to abnormal, 432–434, *434, 435*
 loss of, with traumatic intracavernous aneurysms, 2995–2996
 during saccadic eye movements, 1109
Vistech chart, *167,* 167–168
Visual acuity, 160*t*, 160–164, *161, 162, 163, 164*
 in assessing traumatic optic neuropathy, 719
 in optic neuritis, 602, 612
 and refraction, 154–155, *155*
 in retinal disease, 237–238, *238, 239*
Visual agnosia, 413, 1848
 and cyclosporine, 2634
Visual allesthesia, 3473, 3673, 5596
Visual areas, cortical connections between, *146,* 147
Visual association areas, 139
Visual attention and parietal lobes, 1129–1130
Visual cancellation of vestibulo-ocular reflex (VOR), 1146–1147
Visual claudication, 3523
Visual complications of multiple myeloma, 2392–2393
Visual confusion, 1170
Visual discrimination, 145

Visual distortions, 467–469
Visual enhancement of vestibulo-ocular reflex (VOR), 1146
Visual evoked blinks, 1531–1532
Visual field
in assessing traumatic optic neuropathy, 719
lesions of extrastriate cortex with defects in, *371*, 371–372
lesions of striate cortex without defects in, 371
loss of, in optic neuritis, 601
in optic neuritis, 602, *603*, 612
representation of, in striate cortex, 135–137, *137*
Visual field defects, 307, *308*, *309*, 309–311, *310*, *312–313*, 313, *314–315*, *316*, *317*, *318*, *1775*, 1775–1777, *1776*, *1778*, 1835, *1836*, 1843, *1843*, 1846
as complication in peripheral visual field defects, 810–812, *812*
and cyclosporine, 2634
homonymous, 3444
in papilledema, 512, *512*, *513*, 514
in patients with carotid-ophthalmic aneurysm, 3063, *3065*, *3066*
in retinal disease, 240, *242*, 243, *243*, *244*, *245*, *246*, 247, *247*, *248*, 249, *249*, *250*, *251*, 252, *252*
as sign of tumors, 1794
Visual field examination, 156–157, *157*
Visual field indices, 180, 182
Visual field information
graphic representation of, 178, *180*
interpretation of, 178
Visual field interpretation, five-step approach to, 185–186, *186*, *187*, *188*, *189*, *190*, *191*, *192*, *193*, 194, 194*t*, *195*, *196*, *197*, *198*, *199*, *200*, *201*, *202*, *203*
Visual field loss, progression of, 182, *184*, 184–185, *185*
Visual function, tests of higher, *470*, 470–471, *471*, *472*
Visual hallucinations, 457–464, *458*, *459*, *460*, *461*, *464*, *465*, *466*, 466–467, 1842, 1846–1848, 3765, 4878
and cyclosporine, 2634
as sign of tumors, 1794
in systemic lupus erythematosus, 3829
Visual information, processing of, for saccadic eye movements, 1108–1109, *1109*
Visual inputs, segregation of, 388–391, *390*, *391*
Visual involvement in non-Hodgkin's lymphomas, *2381*, 2381–2385, *2382*, *2383*
Visual loss, 3128, 3130
in aging and dementia, 469–470
associated with direct carotid-cavernous sinus fistula, 3281–3282
bilateral simultaneous, 3426
in neuromyelitis optica, 623–624
from replacement of retina, 1996–1997
transient, 813–814
vascular optic disc swelling without, 580–581, 583
Visual manifestations in papilledema, 510, *511*, 512, *512*, *513*, 514
Visual masking, 1109
Visual Naming Test from the Multilingual Aphasia Examination, 470
Visual pathways
acquired pendular nystagmus and its relationship to disease of, 1466–1468, *1467*, 1467*t*
clinical features of nystagmus with lesions affecting visual pathways, 1464–1466
origin and nature of nystagmus associated with disease of, 1464
Visual perceptions, dissociation of, 372–374
Visual perseveration, 454–457, 1842
Visual phenomena, positive, 601
Visual psychophysics, 159
Visual recovery, following decompression, 657–658
Visual seizures, 461–463, *462*, *463*, *464*
Visual sensory dysfunction, *2166*, *2167*, 2168, *2169*, *2170*, 2170–2171, *2172*, *2173*, 2174, *2174*, *2175*, 2176, *2177*, *2178*, *2393*, 2393–2394, *2394*
Visual sensory function, miscellaneous abnormalities in, 514
Visual sensory manifestations of multiple sclerosis, 5575
asymptomatic involvement of visual sensory system, 5596
inverse Uhthoff's symptom, 5577
ocular motor system, 5596, 5599
optic chiasmal neuritis, 5590, *5591*, *5592*, *5593*, *5594*, 5595, *5595*
optic neuritis, 5581–5582, *5583*, *5584*, 5584–5590, *5585*, *5586*, *5588*, *5589*, *5590*
postchiasmal demyelinating neuritis, *5595*, 5595–5596, *5597*, *5598*
retinal lesions, 5577–5579, *5578*, *5579*, *5580*, 5581
Uhthoff symptom, 5575–5577, *5576*
uveitis, 5581, *5581*, *5582*
visual perceptual disorders, 5596
Visual sensory pathway, embryology of, 3
lateral geniculate body and postgeniculate, 16–17, *17*, *18*, *19*, 29
myelination, *20*, 21–22, *22*
optic chiasm, *14*, 14–15
optic nerve, 4, *6*, 6–8, *7*, *8*, *9*, *10*, *11*
optic tract, 15, *16*
retina, 3–4, *4*, *5*
Visual sensory system
clinical examination, 154, 155*t*
color vision and brightness comparison, 156, 156*t*
cranial nerves, exophthalmometry, external examination, and anterior segment, 158
fundus, 158–159
other procedures, 159
photo stress test, 157–158
Pulfrich phenomenon, 158
pupillary, 158
refraction and acuity, 154–155, *155*
stereoacuity, 155–156
visual field, 156–157, *157*
electrophysiologic test, 215, 216*t*
electro-oculogram (EOG), 223–225, *224*
electroretinogram (ERG), 215–223, *216*, *217*, *218*, *219*, *220*, *221*, *222*, *223*
other retinal potentials, 225
visual-evoked potential (VEP), 225–229, *226*, *227*, *228*, 228*t*
history, 154
psychophysical tests, 159–160
acuity, 160*t*, 160–164, *161*, *162*, *163*, *164*
color vision, 209–212, *210*, *211*, *212*, *213*, 213*t*, 214, 214*t*
contrast sensitivity, 164–169, *165*, *166*, *167*, *168*, *269*
dark adaptation, 214–215, *215*
perimetry and visual field
Amsler grid, *157*, 174–175
ancillary information, 178, *181*
confrontation, 172–174, *173*, *174*
five-step approach to interpretation, 185–186, *186*, *187*, *188*, *189*, *190*, *191*, *192*, *193*, 194, 194*t*, *195*, *196*, *197*, *198*, *199*, *200*, *201*, *202*, *203*
general principles, 169–171
Goldmann manual projection perimeter, 176–177, *177*
graphic representation of data, 178, *180*
indices, 180, 182
interpretation of information, 178
new, *204*, 204–209, *205*, *206*, *207*, *208*, *209*
probability plots, 182, *182*, *183*
progression of loss, 182, *184*, 184–185, *185*
psychophysical basis for, *171*, 171–172, *172*
reliability indices, 178–180
static, 177, *177*
suprathreshold static, 177–178, *179*
tangent (Bjerrum) screen, *175*, 175–176, *176*
techniques for, 172
Visual stimulus for saccade, 1104
Visual-evoked potential, 159, 161, 225–229, *226*, *227*, *228*, 228*t*, *5625*, 5625–5626
abnormal, 1369
in assessment of optic nerve function, 720
clinical ophthalmology and nerve-ophthalmology, 227–228, 228*t*
in patients with migraines, 3709
Visual-evoked responses in cortical and cerebral blindness, 369–370
Visually guided reaching and grasping, *450*, 450–451
anatomic correlates, 451, *452*, *453*, 453–454
disorders of, *450*, 450–451
optic ataxia, 451, *451*, *452*
Visuospatial disorders. (*See* Bálint's syndrome.)
Vitamin A deficiency, retinopathy of, 32
Vitamin A in phototransduction, 32
Vitamin A-induced headache, 1718–1719
Vitamin B_1 deficiency, 669
Vitamin B_{12} deficiency, 668–669
association between multiple sclerosis and, 5544
Vitamin B_{12}-intrinsic factor complex, 4443
Vitamin E deficiency, 1331, 2785
encephalomyopathy with ophthalmoplegia from, 1391
Vitreous, disorders of, 3670–3671
Vitreous fluorophotometry in diagnosing optic neuritis, 608
Vitreous hemorrhage, 3025–3026, *3027*, 3028
Vitreous opacities, 4182–4183, *4185*
Vitritis, 3855
Vogt-Kayanagi-Harada uveomeningitis syndrome, 5091
Volitional saccadic function, 2754–2755
Volume expansion, 3170–3171
Voluntary blinks, 1523
Voluntary convergence, 948
Voluntary enhancement and cancellation of vestibulo-ocular reflex (VOR), 1147
Voluntary eye movements, 1185
Voluntary nystagmus, 1490, 1777, 1779, *1779*

Voluntary saccadic oscillations, 1490, 1779–1780
Von Economo's encephalitis, 5722
  clinical manifestations, 5723, 5725
    acute and subacute, 5725
      amyostatic-akinetic type, 5729
      hyperkinetic type, 5729
      somnolent-ophthalmoplegic type, 5725–5729, *5727*
    chronic, 5729
      Parkinsonian syndrome, 5729–5732
    miscellaneous deficits, 5732
  diagnosis, 5732
  epidemiology, 5722
  etiology, 5733
  laboratory studies, 5732
  pathology, 5722–5723, *5723, 5724, 5725, 5726, 5727*
  prognosis, 5733
  treatment, 5733
von Hippel-Lindau (VHL) disease, 2245–2246, 2696
  associations, 2705
  clinical features, 2696
    ocular findings, 2696–2698, *2697, 2698, 2699, 2700, 2701, 2702, 2703*
  diagnosis, 2705, 2707
  genetics, 2696
  and hemangioblastomas, 2223, 2225, 2226
  management, 2707
  neurologic findings, 2698, 2700, 2702–2704, *2704, 2705*
  occurrence, 2696
  visceral findings, 2704–2705, *2706*
von Hippel-Lindau (VHL) syndrome, 2459
von Recklinghausen's neurofibromatosis, 1801
Von Sölder reflex, 1657–1658
VP-16, 2593
  neurotoxicity, 2593
  systemic toxicity, 2593
Vpr, 5365
Vpu, 5365

W

WAIS-R, Block Design subtest from, 471
Waldenström's macroglobulinemia, 2389, 2399–2400, *2400*, 2565
Walker-Warburg syndrome, 788, 1362
Wallace mutation, 751
Wallenberg lateral medullary syndrome, 1750
Wallenberg's syndrome, 968, 1170, *1285*, 1285–1287, *1286, 1287*, 1293, 3217, *3218*, 3513, 3514–3515
Wall-eyed bilateral internuclear ophthalmoplegia (WEBINO) syndrome, 5605
Wandering macrophages, 2329, 2404
Warning leak headache, before rupture of intracranial aneurysm, 3021
Waterhouse-Friderichsen syndrome, 4099, *4099*
Watershed regions, 3407
Watson syndrome, 2664
W-cells, 48
Weber-Christian disease, 3012
Weber's Law, 171
Weber's syndrome, 1200, 1873–1874, *1874*, 3599–3601
Wegener's granulomatosis, 3727, 3792, *3794*
  demographics, 3792
  diagnosis, 3802
  laboratory tests, 3800–3802
  neurologic manifestations, 3795–3796
  ocular and neuro-ophthalmologic manifestations, 3796–3797, *3797, 3798, 3799, 3800, 3801*
  pathogenesis, 3799–3800
  pathology, 3798–3799, *3801*
  systemic manifestations, 3792, 3794, *3794*
  treatment and prognosis, 3802
Wegener's granulomatosis sarcoidosis, 3888
Weil's disease, 4842, *4843*
Wernicke's disease, 670, 1284
Wernicke's encephalopathy, 670, 1331, 5415
Wernicke's pupil, 990
Wernicke's speech area, 1837
West African trypanosomiasis, 4713, 4714, *4714*, 4715
West Nile encephalitis, 5184
West Nile virus, 5184
Westergren method, 576
Western blot analysis, 5379
Western equine encephalitis, 5280, 5281, 5283, *5283, 5284, 5285*
Wheezing, 5479
Whipple's disease, 1314–1315, 1326, 1469, 2413, 4180–4189, *4182, 4183, 4184, 4185, 4186, 4187, 4188*, 5721
White matter
  degeneration of
    Krabbe disease, 2857–2859, *2858, 2859*
    Pelizaeus-Merzbacher, 2856–2857
  heterotopias, 2686
White rami communicantes, 880
Whitnall's ligament, 1511, *1512*
Whooping cough, *4209*, 4209–4210
Whorl, 2027
Wide Range Achievement Test, 436, 470
Wiesel, Torsten, 129, *130*, 131
Wilbrand's knee, *80*, 81, 97, *98*, 294, *297*, 2171–2172
Willaertia in encephalitis, 3987
Willis, circle of, 85, 3414, *3414, 3415*
  incidence of asymmetry in, 3018
Wilson's disease, 1014, 1319, 1331, 1568
  diagnosis, 2803–2804
  epidemiology, 2800–2801
  etiology and genetics, 2801
  laboratory findings, 2803
  neuroimaging, 2803, *2803*
  neurologic and psychiatric manifestations, *2801*, 2801–2802, *2802*
  ocular manifestations, 2802–2803, *2803*
  pathology, 2801
  prognosis, 2804
  treatment, 2804
Winterbottom's sign, 4714
Wiskott-Aldrich syndrome, 2364
Wolff-Parkinson-White syndrome, 746
Wolfram's syndrome, 761
Wolfring, glands of, 918
Women, effects of migraine on, 3659, *3659*
Wool sorters' disease, 4106
Word deafness, 1831
World Health Organization (WHO) and classification of nasopharyngeal carcinomas, 2445
Wound botulism, 1438, 4117, 4121–4122, *4122*
Wyburn-Mason syndrome, 2266, 2267, 2275, 2725, *2726, 2727*, 2727–2729, *2728*

X

X, Y, W pathways, *118*, 119
Xanthoastrocytomas, pleomorphic, 1934, *1934*
Xanthogranuloma, juvenile, 2416, 2418, *2418, 2419, 2420, 2421*
Xanthopsia, 33
Xenodiagnosis, 4708–4709
Xenon inhalation technique, 3530
Xenon-enhanced CT scanning, 3530
X-linked adrenoleukodystrophy, 2845–2847, *2846, 2847, 2848*
Xylohypha bantiana, 4353, 4354, *4356*

Y

Yawning as coordinated act, 1522
Yaws, 4844, 4845, *4847*, 4847–4848, *4848, 4849*, 4850, *4850, 4851, 4852*
Yeast fungi, 4282, *4282*
Yeasts
  Blastomyces dermatitidis, 4332, *4333*
    clinical manifestations, 4333
      acute pulmonary blastomycosis, 4333, *4335*
      central nervous system blastomycosis, 4336–4338, *4338*
      chronic pulmonary blastomycosis, 4333
      cutaneous blastomycosis, 4333–4334, *4336, 4337*
      extrapulmonary blastomycosis, 4333
      genitourinary tract blastomycosis, 4335–4336
      ocular and orbital blastomycosis, 4338, *4339–4340, 4341*, 4341–4342, *4342*
      paranasal sinus blastomycosis, 4338
      skeletal blastomycosis, 4334–4335
    demographics, 4332
    diagnosis, 4342, *4343*
    pathophysiology, 4333, *4334*
    treatment, 4342–4343
  Blastoschizomyces capitatus, 4343, *4344*
  Candida species, 4343, *4345*
    clinical manifestations, 4345
      deep organ involvement, 4346–4349, *4348, 4349, 4350*, 4351–4352, *4352*
      disseminated candidiasis, 4352–4353
      mucocutaneous candidiasis, 4345–4346, *4347*
    pathology, 4344, *4346*
    pathophysiology, 4343–4344
    treatment, 4353
  chromomycosis and cerebral phaeohyphomycosis, 4353–4355, *4354, 4355, 4356*
  Coccidioides immitis, 4355
    clinical manifestations, 4357–4362, *4358, 4359, 4360, 4361, 4362, 4363, 4364, 4365, 4366*
    demographics, 4355–4356
    diagnosis, 4364–4365, *4367*
    pathology, 4357, *4357*
    pathophysiology, 4356–4357, *4357*
    prognosis, 4367
    treatment, 4365, 4367
  Cryptococcus neoformans, 4367–4368, *4368*
    clinical manifestations
      central nervous system cryptococcosis, 4370–4375, *4374, 4375, 4376, 4377*, 4378

ocular and orbital cryptococcosis, 4378–4381, *4379, 4380, 4381*
other sites of cryptococcosis, 4381–4382, *4382*
pulmonary cryptococcosis, 4370, *4373*
diagnosis, 4382–4384, *4384, 4385*
pathology, *4369,* 4369–4370, *4370*
pathophysiology, 4368–4369
prognosis, 4387
treatment, 4384–4387, *4386*
Fusarium species, *4387,* 4387–4389, *4388, 4389*
Histoplasma capsulatum, 4389, *4390*
clinical manifestations, 4392
acute pulmonary histoplasmosis, 4392
chronic pulmonary histoplasmosis, 4392
disseminated histoplasmosis, 4393–4401, *4394, 4395, 4396, 4397, 4398, 4399, 4400, 4401*
isolated central nervous system histoplasmosis, 4401–4402, *4403*
demographics, 4389, *4391*
diagnosis, 4402, 4404, *4404*
pathogenesis, 4389, 4391–4392
presumed ocular histoplasmosis syndrome, 4404–4406, *4405, 4406, 4407*
prevention, 4404
treatment, 4404
Paracoccidioides brasiliensis, 4406–4407, *4408*
clinical manifestations, 4408–4410, *4409, 4410*
demographics, 4407–4408
diagnosis, 4410–4411
pathology, 4410, *4411*
pathophysiology, 4408
treatment, 4411–4412
Pseudallescheria boydii, 4412, 4412–4415, *4413, 4414*
Sporothrix schenckii, 4415, *4416,* 4417, *4417, 4418*
Trichosporon beigelit, 4417–4418
Yellow fever, 5184–5186, *5185*
clinical manifestations, 5184
diagnosis, 5185
epidemiology, 5184, *5185*
jungle, 5184
pathogenesis and pathology, 5184–5185
prevention, 5185–5186
prognosis, 5185
treatment, 5185
Yersinia, 4225, 4225–4228
Yersinia enterocolitica, 4225, 4228
Yersinia pestis, 4225, 4226, 4227
Yersinia pseudotuberculosis, 4225
Yoke pair, 1173
Yolk sac tumors, 2092, *2093,* 2094, *2094*

Z

Zalcitabine (DDC), 5365
Zebra body myopathy, 1359
Zellweger cerebrohepatorenal syndrome, *2842,* 2842–2843
Zellweger syndrome, 765–766, 2843
Zellweger-like disease, 2844
Zidovudine, 5365
Zinn-Haller, circle of, 61–62
Zona fasciculata, 2458
Zona glomerulosa, 2458
Zona reticularis, 2458
Zoonotic disease, 4642, 4643
Zoster-related encephalitis, 5053–5055
Zygomaticotemporal nerve, lesions of, 1021
Zygomycetes, 4318